Prosthodontics

Editor

LILY T. GARCIA

DENTAL CLINICS OF NORTH AMERICA

www.dental.theclinics.com

January 2014 • Volume 58 • Number 1

ELSEVIER

1600 John F. Kennedy Boulevard • Suite 1800 • Philadelphia, Pennsylvania, 19103-2899

http://www.dental.theclinics.com

DENTAL CLINICS OF NORTH AMERICA Volume 58, Number 1
January 2014 ISSN 0011-8532, ISBN: 978-0-323-26386-3

Editor: John Vassallo
Developmental Editor: Yonah Korngold

Dental Clinics of North America (ISSN 0011-8532) is published quarterly by Elsevier Inc., 360 Park Avenue South, New York, NY 10010-1710. Months of issue are January, April, July, and October. Business and Editorial Offices: 1600 John F. Kennedy Boulevard, Suite 1800, Philadelphia, PA 19103-2899. Periodicals postage paid at New York, NY and additional mailing offices. Subscription prices are $280.00 per year (domestic individuals), $485.00 per year (domestic institutions), $135.00 per year (domestic students/residents), $340.00 per year (Canadian individuals), $628.00 per year (Canadian institutions), $410.00 per year (international individuals), $628.00 per year (international institutions), and $200.00 per year (international and Canadian students/residents). International air speed delivery is included in all *Clinics* subscription prices. All prices are subject to change without notice. **POSTMASTER:** Send address changes to *Dental Clinics of North America*, Elsevier Health Sciences Division, Subscription Customer Service, 3251 Riverport Lane, Maryland Heights, MO 63043. **Customer Service (orders, claims, online, change of address): Elsevier Health Sciences Division, Subscription Customer Service, 3251 Riverport Lane, Maryland Heights, MO 63043. Tel: 1-800-654-2452 (U.S. and Canada). Fax: 314-447-8029. E-mail: journalscustomer service-usa@elsevier.com (for print support); journalsonlinesupport-usa@elsevier.com (for online support).**

Reprints. For copies of 100 or more, of articles in this publication, please contact the Commercial Reprints Department, Elsevier Inc., 360 Park Avenue South, New York, NY 10010-1710. Tel.: 212-633-3874; Fax: 212-633-3820; E-mail: reprints@elsevier.com.

The *Dental Clinics of North America* is covered in *MEDLINE/PubMed (Index Medicus), Current Contents/Clinical Medicine, ISI/BIOMED* and *Clinahl.*

Printed and bound by CPI Group (UK) Ltd, Croydon, CR0 4YY

Transferred to digital print 2012

Contributors

EDITOR

LILY T. GARCIA, DDS, MS, FACP
Professor and Associate Dean for Education, The University of Iowa College of Dentistry and Dental Clinics, Iowa City, Iowa

AUTHORS

NADIM Z. BABA, DMD, MSD
Professor of Restorative Dentistry and Director, Hugh Love Center for Research and Education in Technology, Loma Linda University, School of Dentistry, Loma Linda, California

REVA MALHOTRA BAREWAL, DDS, MS
Private Practice, Portland, Oregon

AVINASH S. BIDRA, BDS, MS, FACP
Assistant Professor and Maxillofacial Prosthodontist, Assistant Program Director, Post-Graduate Prosthodontics, Department of Reconstructive Sciences, University of Connecticut Health Center, Farmington, Connecticut

DAVID M. BOHNENKAMP, DDS, MS, FACP
Clinical Associate Professor, Department of Prosthodontics, The University of Iowa College of Dentistry and Dental Clinics, Iowa City, Iowa

MATTHEW BRYINGTON, DMD, MS
Assistant Director of Graduate Prosthodontics, Restorative Dentistry, School of Dentistry, West Virginia University, Morgantown, West Virginia

LYNDON F. COOPER, DDS, PhD
Stallings Distinguished Professor, Department of Prosthodontics, School of Dentistry, University of North Carolina, Chapel Hill, North Carolina

INGEBORG J. DE KOK, DDS, MS
Associate Professor, Department of Prosthodontics, School of Dentistry, University of North Carolina, Chapel Hill, North Carolina

CHARLES J. GOODACRE, DDS, MSD
Professor, Department of Restorative Dentistry, Loma Linda University, School of Dentistry, Loma Linda, California

CHAD CAMERON HAGEN, MD, DABPN
Co-Medical Director, Sleep Disorders Program, Oregon Health and Science University, Portland, Oregon

RAMI JEKKI, DDS
Assistant Professor, Department of Restorative Dentistry, Loma Linda University, School of Dentistry, Loma Linda, California

JOHN D. JONES, DDS
Professor, Department of Comprehensive Dentistry, The University of Texas Health Science Center at San Antonio, San Antonio, Texas

LISA A. LANG, DDS, MS, MBA
Associate Professor and Chair, Department of Comprehensive Care, Assistant Dean of Clinical Education, School of Dental Medicine, Case Western Reserve University, Cleveland, Ohio

HAMILTON H. LE, DMD, FACP
Diplomate American Board of Prosthodontics, Fellow American College of Prosthodontists, Adjunct Professor, President, California Section, Department of Post Graduate Prosthodontics, American College of Prosthodontists, Tufts University School of Dental Medicine, Boston, Massachusetts

NORMA OLVERA, DDS, MS
Assistant Professor, Department of Comprehensive Dentistry, The University of Texas Health Science Center at San Antonio, San Antonio, Texas

MARY NORMA PARTIDA, DDS, MPH
Associate Professor, Department of Comprehensive Dentistry, The University of Texas Health Science Center, San Antonio Dental School, San Antonio, Texas

JENNIFER W. PRIEBE, DDS, MS, FACP
Department of Restorative Dentistry, University of Detroit Mercy, School of Dentistry, Detroit, Michigan

GHADEER THALJI, DDS, PhD, FACP
Assistant Professor, Department of Prosthodontics, The University of Iowa College of Dentistry, Iowa City, Iowa

IBRAHIM TULUNOGLU, DDS, PhD
Associate Professor, Department of Comprehensive Care, School of Dental Medicine, Case Western Reserve University, Cleveland, Ohio

JONATHAN P. WIENS, DDS, MS, FACP
Department of Restorative Dentistry, University of Detroit Mercy, School of Dentistry, Detroit, Michigan

JOHN WON, DDS, MS
Assistant Professor, Department of Restorative Dentistry, Loma Linda University, School of Dentistry, Loma Linda, California

ROY T. YANASE, DDS, FACP
Diplomate and Past President, American Board of Prosthodontics, Fellow American College of Prosthodontists, Clinical Professor, Advanced Prosthodontic Education; Clinical Professor, Continuing Dental Education, Ostrow School of Dentistry at USC, Los Angeles, California

ROYA ZANDPARSA, DDS, MSc, DMD
Clinical Professor, Tufts University School of Dentistry, Postgraduate Prosthodontics Division, Boston, Massachusetts

Contents

Evidence-Based Prosthodontics: Fundamental Considerations, Limitations, and Guidelines   1

Avinash S. Bidra

> Evidence-based dentistry is rapidly emerging to become an integral part of patient care, dental education, and research. Prosthodontics is a unique dental specialty that encompasses art, philosophy, and science and includes reversible and irreversible treatments. It not only affords good applicability of many principles of evidence-based dentistry but also poses numerous limitations. This article describes the epidemiologic background, fundamental considerations, scrutiny of levels of evidence, limitations, guidelines, and future perspectives of evidence-based prosthodontics. Understanding these principles can aid clinicians in appropriate appraisal of the prosthodontics literature and use the best available evidence for making confident clinical decisions and optimizing patient care.

Occlusal Stability   19

Jonathan P. Wiens and Jennifer W. Priebe

> Occlusion is the foundation for clinical success in fixed, removable, and implant prosthodontic treatment. Understanding those principles is critical when restoring a patient's occlusion. Many philosophies, devices, and theories of occlusion have evolved based on anecdotal clinical observations and applied geometric perceptions. The literature has reported these classic and contemporary occlusal concepts. As evidence-based dentistry emerged, it championed scrutiny of previously held beliefs, resulting in the abandonment of many pragmatic, yet beneficial occlusal procedures. The impetus toward scientific discovery, whereby factual information might be universally applied in dental education and clinical practice, has renewed interest in occlusal studies.

Gingival Displacement for Impression Making in Fixed Prosthodontics: Contemporary Principles, Materials, and Techniques   45

Nadim Z. Baba, Charles J. Goodacre, Rami Jekki, and John Won

> The clinical success and longevity of indirect restorations depend on the careful and accurate completion of several procedures. One of the challenging procedures is management of the gingival tissues and gingival esthetics. The goal for management of gingival tissues and gingival esthetics is to maintain the normal appearance of healthy gingival. Achieving this goal requires optimal health before treatment and minimal trauma during treatment. The best way of optimizing health and minimizing trauma is to avoid contacting the gingiva with restorative materials.

> Bioceramics have been adopted in dental restorations for implants, bridges, inlays, onlays, and all-ceramic crowns. Dental bioceramics include glass ceramics, reinforced porcelains, zirconias, aluminas, fiber-reinforced ceramic composites, and multilayered ceramic structures. The process of additive manufacturing is ideally suited to dentistry. Models are designed using data from a computed tomography scan or magnetic resonance imaging. Since its development in 2001, direct ceramic machining of pre-sintered yttria tetragonal zirconia polycrystal has become increasingly popular in dentistry. There are wide variety commercially available cements for luting all-ceramic restorations. However, resin cements have lower solubility and better aesthetic characteristics.

> Dentists are becoming increasingly aware of the importance of the detection and management of obstructive sleep apnea. The anatomic and neuromuscular risk factors in the pathogenesis of obstructive sleep apnea are reviewed with particular emphasis on oral findings. Mandibular repositioning appliances hold an important role in the treatment of this condition; however, knowledge of indications and contraindications for treatment, potential areas of oropharyngeal obstruction, appliance design, and treatment steps are vital to ensure maximum treatment success. A review of the steps involved in treatment and management with particular emphasis on collaborative care with physicians is presented.

> The pivotal point in treatment planning for dental implants occurs when the location of bone is viewed radiographically in the context of the planned prosthesis. Radiographic planning for dental implant therapy should be used only after a review of the patient's systemic health, imaging history, oral health, and local oral conditions. The radiological diagnostic and planning procedure for dental implants can only be fully achieved with the use of a well-designed and -constructed radiographic guide. This article reviews several methods for construction of radiographic guides and how they may be utilized for improving implant surgery planning and performance.

> Dental implants are an indispensible tool for the restoration of missing teeth. Their use has elevated the practice of dentistry by improving both our technical ability to rehabilitate patients and general quality of life. To routinely achieve the associated high expectations, diligent attention to details must be observed and addressed from the outset. Of central concern is the attainment of osseointegration and the location of implants to ideally support the intended restoration. The pivotal point in treatment

planning for dental implants occurs when the location of bone is viewed radiographically in the context of the planned prosthesis. This most often requires diagnostic waxing or tooth arrangement using mounted diagnostic casts.

Implant-supported dental restorations can be screw-retained, cement-retained, or a combination of both, whereby a metal superstructure is screwed to the implants and crowns are individually cemented to the metal frame. Each treatment modality has advantages and disadvantages. The use of computer-aided design/computer-assisted manufacture technologies for the manufacture of implant superstructures has proved to be advantageous in the quality of materials, precision of the milled superstructures, and passive fit. Maintenance and recall evaluations are an essential component of implant therapy. The longevity of implant restorations is limited by their biological and prosthetic maintenance requirements.

The development of an oral care path focuses on the identification of the early indicators of disease. Once the risks have been identified and diagnosed, the proper therapies can be selected and prescribed. The experienced practitioner must meld clinical experience and observation with evidence-based scientific dentistry and information on the treatment and prevention of continued disease for the prosthodontic patient after restorations have been completed. The incorporation of dental implants has not allowed for complications of caries and periodontal disease on teeth and implants. Osseoseparation is necessary for justification of continued maintenance.

A critically appraised topic (CAT) review is presented about the use of computer-aided design (CAD)/computer-aided machining (CAM) removable partial denture (RPD) frameworks. A systematic search of the literature supporting CAD/CAM RPD systems revealed no randomized clinical trials, hence the CAT review was performed. A PubMed search yielded 9 articles meeting the inclusion criteria. Each article was characterized by study design and level of evidence. No clinical outcomes research has been published on the use of CAD/CAM RPDs. Low levels of evidence were found in the available literature. Clinical research studies are needed to determine the efficacy of this treatment modality.

DENTAL CLINICS OF NORTH AMERICA

Preface

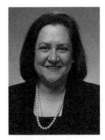

Lily T. Garcia, DDS, MS, FACP
Editor

The specialty of Prosthodontics is rich with scientific and clinically relevant information. Being invited by the publishers of *Dental Clinics of North America* has allowed me to engage friends and colleagues, primarily prosthodontists as well as other practitioners, to work together. I asked several of my "seasoned" colleagues to invite some of our best and brightest newer colleagues to join in on this endeavor. The clinical science reflects information that can be used immediately to expand our understanding and capacity in providing the highest quality of care for our patients.

The articles cover a comprehensive listing of topics that include topics that are often overlooked, ranging from fundamental information on occlusion and caries risk management to the on-going development of digital dentistry. These concepts that are innate to our general knowledge and affect patient care need to be reinforced with the most current evidence.

The challenge in dental education, as well as in private practice, remains diagnosis and treatment planning with the ultimate goal of predictable patient outcomes. This issue of *Dental Clinics of North America* represents a compilation designed to reinforce and expand on the current level of knowledge and make us better in patient care. The topics are a unique entry into sharing best concepts for all dentists to learn and implement. As with our patient care, the ability to envision the best outcome for our patients helps lead us through complex decision matrices focused on development of unique treatment plans. It is with this intent that ALL dentists should strive to build on our core competencies and provide the highest quality of care for our patients.

Dent Clin N Am 58 (2014) xi–xii
http://dx.doi.org/10.1016/j.cden.2013.11.001
0011-8532/14/$ – see front matter © 2014 Elsevier Inc. All rights reserved.

dental.theclinics.com

I offer special thanks to the authors and coauthors who devoted time and energy to create a *Dental Clinics of North America* issue of this caliber.

Thank you,

Lily

Lily T. Garcia, DDS, MS, FACP
Professor and Associate Dean for Education
The University of Iowa College of Dentistry and Dental Clinics
801 Newton Road
North Dental Sciences Building, N310 DSB
Iowa City, IA 52242, USA

E-mail address:
lily-garcia@uiowa.edu

Evidence-Based Prosthodontics
Fundamental Considerations, Limitations, and Guidelines

Avinash S. Bidra, BDS, MS

KEYWORDS

- Evidence-based dentistry • Prosthodontics • Guidelines • Systematic reviews
- Randomized controlled clinical trials • Prospective studies • Retrospective studies

KEY POINTS

- Prosthodontics is a unique specialty that offers numerous advantages and disadvantages for application of principles of evidence-based dentistry (EBD).
- An important difference between medical and dental models of care is the level of control a patient has about how, when, and whether it is necessary to treat a dental problem. This is especially true in the discipline of prosthodontics. Hence, an absolute extrapolation of evidence-based concepts from medicine to prosthodontics is not possible.
- Current lack of "strong" evidence for a particular treatment does not necessarily imply that the treatment is "inferior" or "clinically ineffective." Efforts should be targeted, however, to improve the future scientific evidence for such treatments.
- Due to the unique nature of prosthodontics, it is necessary to establish a consensus on guidelines for reporting prosthodontic outcomes. These guidelines can ensure that investigators provide standardized reporting of their studies in order for them to be clear, complete, and transparent and allow integration of their evidence into clinical practice.
- In order to teach and understand evidence-based prosthodontics, academicians and clinicians need to attain new skills pertaining to computer-based knowledge systems. These skills are necessary to use scientific evidence for the 5-step process of asking, acquiring, appraising, applying, and assessing.
- Evidence-based prosthodontics can change the future course of prosthodontics education, patient care, reimbursements, research agendas, and oral health policies that have an impact on prosthodontics.

INTRODUCTION

The traditional model of care in dentistry involves use of individual clinical expertise and patient treatment needs to provide dental care (**Fig. 1**). This model of care has been used for centuries across the world and is primarily based on observations, beliefs, and personal and expert opinions. Although this model has not led to any

Department of Reconstructive Sciences, University of Connecticut Health Center, 263 Farmington Avenue, L6078, Farmington, CT 06030, USA
E-mail address: avinashbidra@yahoo.com

Dent Clin N Am 58 (2014) 1–17
http://dx.doi.org/10.1016/j.cden.2013.09.001
0011-8532/14/$ – see front matter © 2014 Elsevier Inc. All rights reserved.

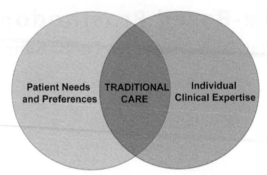

Fig. 1. Traditional model of care in dentistry involves use of individual clinical expertise and patient treatment needs to provide dental care.

devastating effects in dentistry, it precludes systematic assimilation, acceptance, and assessment of new treatment effects. Furthermore, it provides minimal confidence to clinicians for making clinical decisions for new scenarios and new treatments. The term, *evidence-based practice*, is defined as "the conscientious, explicit and judicious use of current best evidence in making decisions about the care of the individual patient. It means integrating individual clinical expertise with the best available external clinical evidence from systematic research."[1] This definition stems from the medical perspective, and dentistry is more familiar with the term, EBD.

Currently, there is no definition for evidence-based prosthodontics but it is understood that it encompasses the application of EBD with respect to prosthodontics. According to the American Dental Association (ADA), EBD is defined as "an approach to oral healthcare that requires the judicious integration of systematic assessments of clinically relevant scientific evidence, relating to the patient's oral and medical condition and history, with the dentist's clinical expertise and the patient's treatment needs and preferences."[2] Therefore, the EBD process is not a rigid methodologic evaluation of scientific evidence that dictates what practitioners should or should not do but also relies on the role of individual professional judgment and patient preference in this process (**Fig. 2**).[3]

NEED FOR EVIDENCE-BASED PROSTHODONTICS

With rapid advancements in dental materials and dental technology and improved understanding of clinical outcomes, a surfeit of research has been published in prosthodontics and dental implant–focused literature (**Box 1**). Furthermore, a surplus amount of published research exists in interdisciplinary fields that are of critical importance to prosthodontics. It is well known that not all published literature is scientifically valid and clinically useful. Therefore, a critical analysis of the quality of published research and consolidation of the excess scientific information is necessary to render them significant and useful. In an extensive analysis of scientific publications between 1966 and 2005, Harwood[4] noted that there were 44,338 published articles in prosthodontics. Of these, there were 955 randomized controlled clinical trials (RCTs) (2%). Nishimura and colleagues[5] identified 10,258 articles on prosthodontic topics between 1990 and 1999 and estimated that to stay current in the year 2002 would require reading and absorbing approximately 8 articles per week, 52 weeks per year, and across 60 different journals. These numbers do not include published articles on implant dentistry. Russo and colleagues[6] identified 4655 articles published between

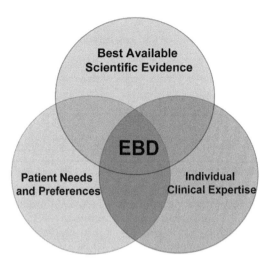

Fig. 2. EBD involves integration of best available scientific evidence along with individual clinical expertise and patient treatment needs to provide dental care.

1989 and 1999 dedicated to implant dentistry and estimated that to stay current in the year 2000 would require reading and absorbing approximately 1 to 2 articles per week, 52 weeks per year. It is not difficult to assume that these numbers are significantly higher in the year 2013 and will continue to grow due to increased growth in the number of journals and publications, underscoring the need for computer-based clinical knowledge systems and for clinicians to acquire new skills to use the best available scientific evidence (BASE) (**Box 2**).

EPIDEMIOLOGIC BACKGROUND

The epidemiologic background for evidence-based practice dates back to the nineteenth century, to the work of John Snow, who is widely regarded as the father of modern epidemiology.[7] Snow rejected the popular miasma theory as the cause of the cholera outbreaks in England. Through a systematic method of data collection and analysis, Snow established a classic case-control study and traced the cholera outbreaks to drinking water contamination from the sewage systems. His ideas were rejected, criticized, and not embraced until several years after his death. Similar to Snow's experiences, other landmark events in modern epidemiology include

---

Box 1
The need for evidence-based prosthodontics

- Enable the recognition of best available scientific evidence in prosthodontics.
- Consolidate the scientific information overload in prosthodontics and related literature.
- Scrutinize the scientific basis for existing prosthodontic treatments.
- Improve current and future treatments.
- Encourage improvement in the quality of clinical research as well as in reporting.
- Distinguish and advance the specialty of prosthodontics.

Box 2
New skills required by clinicians to adopt evidence-based prosthodontics

- Asking the appropriate research question for a clinical situation of interest.
- Acquiring information through efficient scientific literature search.
- Appraising the acquired information.
- Applying the acquired information to clinical practice, along with individual clinical expertise and patient preferences.
- Assessing the results of the applied intervention to optimize the clinical situation.

Semmelweis'[8] important discoveries on hand washing intervention to drop maternal mortality rates and childbed fever and Doll and colleagues'[9] systematic observations on cigarette smoking and its association with lung cancer. Several other similar events have all had a significant impact on worldwide public health.

Pioneering efforts in the twentieth century by Archibald Cochrane called for state-of-the-art systematic reviews (SRs) of all relevant RCTs in health care,[10] leading to the creation of the world-renowned Cochrane Collaboration in 1993 to organize all medical research information in a systematic manner in the interests of evidence-based medicine. The term, evidence-based medicine, itself was first described in the medical literature in 1992 by a working group of a similar name, who stated that this would be a new way of teaching the practice of medicine.[11] The ADA has espoused the principles of evidence-based practices since its inception and has made remarkable progress over the past 20 years to render popularity to the current known principles of EBD for use in clinical practice and dental education.

CONSIDERATIONS IN PROSTHODONTICS

An important difference between medical and dental models of care is the level of control a patient has about how, when, and whether it is even necessary to treat a dental condition. This is especially true in the discipline of prosthodontics. Prosthodontics is a unique dental specialty that encompasses art, philosophy, and science and includes reversible and irreversible treatments. Therefore, an absolute extrapolation of evidence-based concepts from medicine to prosthodontics is not possible. Treatment outcomes, which are a core element of prosthodontics, however, render themselves well for application of principles of EBD. There are 3 predominant items that are important to understanding challenges in reporting treatment outcomes in prosthodontics.

Defining the Outcomes of Clinical Interest

Key issues in defining clinical outcomes in prosthodontics are multifaceted due to the inherent nature of the treatment. Some examples of these issues include differentiating success versus survival, complications versus consequences, and prosthesis outcomes versus patient-centered outcomes. Another important characteristic is defining the appropriate endpoint of a clinical study. Hujoel and DeRouen[12] have categorized clinical endpoints (outcomes) as surrogate endpoints and true endpoints. Surrogate outcomes include measures that are not of direct practical importance but are believed to reflect outcomes that are important as part of a disease/treatment process. True outcomes, however, reflect unequivocal evidence of tangible benefit to patients. Both types of outcomes are important in prosthodontics, because surrogate outcomes are helpful for preliminary evidence and true outcomes are helpful for definitive evidence (**Table 1**).

Table 1 Understanding differences between surrogate and true outcomes in clinical trials in prosthodontics	
Surrogate Outcomes	**True/Definitive Outcomes**
Includes measures that are not of direct practical importance but are believed to reflect outcomes that are important as part of a disease/treatment process[12]	Reflects unequivocal evidence of tangible benefit to the patient
Examples • Pocket depth • Open margins • Peri-implant bone level • Prosthesis retention/support	Corresponding examples • Tooth/implant survival • Secondary caries • Implant survival • Patient satisfaction
Endpoints are "softer" and easier to measure and studies are relatively inexpensive.	Endpoints are "harder" and difficult to measure and studies can be more expensive.
Do not have a direct impact on changes in clinical practice or changes in public health policies.	Can have a direct impact on changes in clinical practice and/or changes in public health policies.

Duration Needed to Appropriately Study the Outcomes

The time period needed to study a clinical outcome of interest depends on the definition of a treatment outcome, surrogate or true endpoint desired, treatment effect desired, and adverse events related to a treatment under investigation. Currently, there is no consensus in prosthodontics on definitions for preliminary, short-term, or long-term studies. Therefore, it becomes the prerogative of the investigator, editor, and reader to decide if the result of a study reports on short-term or long-term outcomes. Often, a study with a follow-up period of up to 6 years is described as "long-term follow-up" where only a meager number of samples have actually made it to a 6-year follow-up and the rest have a follow-up of less than 2 years. It is understood that preliminary and short-term studies have high clinical impact when they report failures of a particular treatment; only long-term studies can have high clinical impact for treatment success. Treatment success reported in short-term studies, however, can lay the justification whether additional research is needed.

Minimum Sample Needed to Study the Outcome of Interest?

The sample size of a study depends on the difference in treatment effect desired. In prosthodontics, it is difficult to obtain large sample sizes from a single study center because of the elective and expensive nature of prosthodontic treatment, which has led to a large body of published research in the prosthodontic literature with small sample sizes. For a study to have a large clinical impact and provide sufficient evidence to change a particular clinical practice, sample size is critical. Currently, there is no consensus in prosthodontics on definitions for sample sizes as small, moderate, and large. The validity of defining such sample sizes is currently unknown.

LEVELS OF EVIDENCE AND PROSTHODONTICS

Evidence in medicine has been popularly categorized into 5 hierarchical levels and widely represented as a pyramid with the "weakest/lowest level of evidence" at the base and the "strongest or highest level evidence" at the apex (**Fig. 3**). This gradation

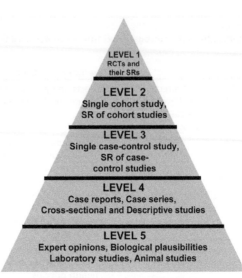

Fig. 3. Evidence in medicine has been popularly categorized into 5 hierarchical levels and widely represented as a pyramid with the "weakest/lowest level of evidence" at the base and the "strongest or highest level evidence" at the apex. This model may not be applicable to prosthodontics.

has been used by several health agencies across the world. Although the 5 hierarchical levels of evidence and the pyramidal representation may be popular in medicine, the applicability of this paradigm to prosthodontics is questionable because few articles in prosthodontics comprise RCTs and large cohort studies, implying that most current clinical practices in prosthodontics are all based on "weak evidence."

Additionally, 2 critical elements of importance to prosthodontics that are omitted from the evidence-based pyramid are sample size and duration of a study. As previously discussed, these 2 elements can significantly affect the way evidence has an impact on clinical practices. For example, results from a cohort or a case-control study with a very large sample size and/or a long-term follow-up on all-ceramic crowns can have a better impact on clinical decisions compared with results from an RCT with a small sample and a short-term follow-up. In this scenario, in spite of RCT regarded as the "strongest evidence," it would fail to be used by clinicians for confident decision making. Furthermore, major medical breakthroughs have originated from cohort and case-control studies, which are considered by many as "weaker" forms of evidence. The terms, *weak* and *strong*, are subjective and exclusive and do not lend themselves to an unbiased assessment of best available evidence in prosthodontics. Therefore, an alternative approach for prosthodontics literature is suggested. The suggested paradigm involves a horizontal spectrum encompassing 3 stages of evidence—preliminary evidence, substantive evidence, and progressive evidence (**Fig. 4**).

Preliminary Evidence

Expert/experience-based opinions, philosophies, theories, and biologic plausibilites

Expert opinion is the oldest form of evidence in health care for centuries and continues to remain one of the most popular forms of evidence in contemporary dentistry because it is easy for clinicians to acquire and apply the presented evidence. Expert/ experience-based opinions and monographs have dominated the art component of

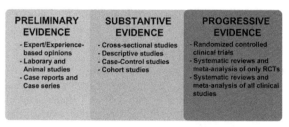

Fig. 4. The suggested new paradigm involves a horizontal spectrum encompassing 3 stages of evidence—preliminary evidence, substantive evidence, and progressive evidence.

prosthodontic literature for almost a century. Additionally, they have a strong representation in the discipline of dental occlusion, dental techniques, choice of dental materials, and dental technology. Expert opinions, philosophies, theories, and biologic plausibilities are all important, because they provide a starting point to initiate and propel new ideas, theories, and innovations and develop further research. Unfortunately, many expert opinions are biased and scientifically not validated. As a result, several popular opinions and philosophies in prosthodontics have not been clinically validated. Some examples include need for balanced occlusion in complete dentures, designs for removable partial dentures, tooth preparation designs, types of restorations in fixed prosthodontics, and many others.

Laboratory studies and animal studies

A large body of research in dentistry falls into the category of laboratory studies and animal studies. Compared to clinical research, this type of research is easier to conduct, accomplished faster and allows different types of hypotheses to be tested in a controlled setting. In prosthodontics, due to rapid emergence and advancements of new dental materials, dental technology, and improved biologic understanding, these studies are important because they provide a good foundation before proceeding with clinical studies. Pioneering work on osseointegration done by PI Branemark in his animal/laboratory studies and its subsequent development through progressive research is a testimony for this type of preliminary research. In the discipline of dental materials, independent investigators with a clinical understanding should verify research done by the industry. Studies with promising results should then be progressed to subsequent stages of research. Unfortunately, this paradigm is not often followed in prosthodontics and many dental materials and technology have been used clinically based on laboratory studies alone.

Case reports and case series

A single case report/case study describes the unique characteristics and treatment of a single patient, and a case series describes the treatment in a group of patients. With regards to sample size, currently there is no consensus on when a study can be defined as a case series versus a cohort study. It is understood, however, that case series are descriptive in nature and involve a small heterogeneous sample as opposed to a cohort study, which is observational and analytic in nature. Nevertheless, case reports and case series have high sensitivity for detecting novelty and form the basis for detecting new concepts, etiologic clues, side effects, and new treatments and have contributed to major breakthroughs in medicine.[13] In prosthodontic literature, case reports/series typically depict management of unique situations through unique techniques and/or unique materials. Such reports not only help clinicians in management of similar situations but also aid in laying the foundation for future laboratory studies and clinical trials.

Substantive Evidence

Cross-sectional studies/surveys and descriptive studies

A cross-sectional study is defined as a study measuring the distribution of some characteristic(s) in a population at a particular point in time.[14] Essentially, the exposure and outcome are measured simultaneously, at the time of the survey. This study design is helpful for preliminary analysis of the prevalence of a condition/disease at a given point of time and for investigating the potential risk factors or causes of the condition.[15] An example in prosthodontics is a cross-sectional study to analyze the prevalence of halitosis in patients with fixed complete dentures. In this example, because there is no temporal assessment, it is difficult to conclude that halitosis is related to fixed complete dentures. However, if significant numbers of samples are from a certain social or ethnic background, have a history of smoking or poor oral hygiene, then the researcher can investigate further to delineate the risk factors.

Descriptive studies are studies that describe a particular characteristic and any related changes due to an intervention. They are commonly reported in prosthodontics with respect to anatomic variations and esthetic-related characteristics. Therefore, temporal considerations, cause-effect analysis, and survival outcomes are usually not applicable to such studies, which does not mean that the evidence from these studies is "weak." Major understanding of complete denture principles and esthetic dentistry has resulted from such studies. These studies are specific to a given population, however, and describe preliminary data or trends that may or may not be extrapolated to different populations. Some descriptive studies, however, have large sample sizes encompassing different countries and races.[16]

Case-control studies

A case-control study is defined as "a study that compares people with a specific disease or outcome of interest (cases) to people from the same population without that disease or outcome (controls), and which seeks to find associations between the outcome and prior exposure to particular risk factors."[14] Case-control studies are not commonly described in the core prosthodontics literature, probably because prosthodontics typically does not deal with diseases and cure but with treatment outcomes. Compared with cohort studies, they are inexpensive and afford potential for large sample sizes. As a rule, they cannot prove causation, so cohort studies and RCTs are subsequently needed to test a causal hypothesis. Therefore, they are often associated with controversies and have a potential for propaganda by the media. A popular recent example that is relevant to prosthodontics is a case-control study linking the risk of meningiomas and dental radiographs.[17]

Case-control studies are of great value, however, when cohort studies or RCTs cannot be performed due to ethical and patient safety reasons, when controversial causal claims are made by case reports and case series. A popular recent example relevant to prosthodontics is a case series on 4 patients linking zinc-containing denture adhesives to neurologic diseases.[18] Multiple case-control studies would now be required to show converse results before obtaining ethical approval to perform prospective cohort studies and RCTs to examine cause-effect relationships between zinc-containing denture adhesives and neurologic diseases.

Cohort studies

A cohort is a well-defined group of persons who have had a common experience or exposure and are then followed-up to determine the incidence of new diseases or health events.[19] Therefore, by definition, they have the potential to establish causal relationships between exposure and disease. Historically, large cohort studies have produced powerful data that have had an impact on public health around the world. Some of these include the Framingham Heart Study examining cardiovascular disease and dietary cholesterol,[20] the Physicians' Health Study investigating aspirin and b-carotene on beta heart disease, and cancer[21] and the British doctors' cohort study examining smoking and lung cancer.[22] It is understood that to have a meaningful clinical impact, cohort studies require large sample sizes and a long follow-up period. In general, there are 4 kinds of cohort studies: prospective, retrospective, nested case-control, and case-cohort study.

Some examples of cohort studies with long-term follow-up, which have had a significant impact on prosthodontics, include Tallgren's 25-year follow-up study on reduction of the residual alveolar ridges in complete denture wearers[23] and a 20-year follow-up study by Douglass and colleagues[24] on cephalometric evaluation of vertical dimension changes in patients wearing complete dentures. Unfortunately, such studies are uncommon because they are expensive, time-consuming, and difficult to execute without a significant loss to follow-up of patients. Therefore, short-term cohort studies have become widely popular in the prosthodontics literature, but they do not have the potential to change clinical practices or provide enough data for confident clinical decision making. Furthermore, many cohort studies in prosthodontics with longer follow-up periods lack adequate sample sizes and do not report a life table (survival) analysis.

A life table (or a cohort life table) in epidemiology is defined as "a table depicting the survival data of a cohort of individuals in a clinical study or trial. This is essentially the number of items alive and under observation (not lost to follow-up) at the beginning of each year, the number surviving in each year, the number lost to follow-up each year, the conditional probability of survival for each year, and the cumulative probabilities of survival from the beginning of the study to the end of each year."[25] Life table methods subsequently allow several forms of statistical measures to be used for analysis. Some popular examples used in prosthodontics literature include Kaplan-Meier probability of survival method and the Cox proportional hazards model. Life table methods are extremely important in understanding long-term prosthodontic treatment outcomes, because they allow appreciation of attrition/loss to follow-up of samples from the beginning to the end of the study. Systematic reviews performed on observational studies that claim long-term success/survival have often exposed extremely low sample sizes remaining at the end of the study. Furthermore, different samples in a cohort study are followed-up for different time periods and, without a life table, extraction of useful data is impossible.[26] Therefore, for an observational study in prosthodontics to contribute meaningful evidence to clinicians, providing a life table is paramount.

Progressive Evidence

Randomized controlled clinical trials

RCT is defined as "an experiment in which two or more interventions, possibly including a control intervention or no intervention, are compared by being randomly allocated to participants."[14] Because they are interventional/experimental in nature, they have a high sensitivity to prove causation and also yield quantitative data. They are regarded as the best-known method to minimize/control bias, which is defined as a systematic error or deviation in results or inferences from the truth.[14] Due to these primary factors, they are often considered to provide the "highest level" of evidence in medicine. In addition to medicine, randomization is also widely popular in education, criminology, social work, food industry, and international development. Because of their interventional/experimental nature, RCTs are conducted only after observational and descriptive studies have shown no safety concerns for patients.

In contrast to medicine and even other disciplines in dentistry, RCTs are not popular in prosthodontics for various reasons. In Harwood's extensive analysis of 44,338 prosthodontic publications between 1966 and 2005, only 955 articles (2%) were RCTs.[4] In another study by Dumbrigue and colleagues in 1999,[27] only 1.7% of articles published in prosthodontic journals met the minimum criteria to be included in central register of RCTs. The same investigator in another study in 2001 noted that only 16% of RCTs published in prosthodontic journals attempted to control bias, indicating the low quality of the RCTs.[28] Similarly, Jokstad and colleagues in 2002[29] noted that methods of randomization and allocation concealment were not described in 70% of RCTs published in prosthodontic journals. A recent study by Pandis and colleagues in 2010[30] compared and ranked the quality of RCTs published in top journals across 6 different specialties of dentistry. Their results showed that RCTs published in prosthodontics ranked the lowest among all specialties. All these findings demonstrate the lack of popularity of RCTs in prosthodontics.

Due to the elective and expensive nature of prosthodontic treatment and associated heterogeneity, RCTs are expensive, time consuming, and not easily acquiescent for a large sample size and long-term follow-up. Furthermore, unlike other disciplines, controlling bias is challenging because randomization, double blinding, or even single blinding is difficult and several treatments involve patient input, making it difficult for allocation concealment. All of these are possible reasons for lack of popularity of RCTs in prosthodontics. It is important, however, to understand a few important elements of RCTs that are relevant to prosthodontics and scrutinize them in the published literature.

Methods of randomization Randomization is defined as "the process of randomly allocating participants into one of the arms of a controlled trial."[14] Broadly, they can be classified as fixed allocation randomization or adaptive randomization and both methods have inherent advantages and disadvantages.[31] Fixed allocation randomization can involve (1) a simple method, such as use of a random integer table; (2) a block method, involving blocks of integers, symbols, or alphabets (usually blocks of 4, such as ABBA); or (3) a stratified method, involving division of the members of population in homogeneous subgroups before sampling. Adaptive randomization methods include baseline adaptive randomization and response adaptive randomization. They are designed to change the allocation probabilities as the study progresses to accommodate imbalances in numbers of participants or in baseline characteristics between the two groups. They also accommodate the responses of participants to the assigned intervention.[31] Another form of allocation that is not truly random is quasirandomization. This entails allocation based on a patient's medical record number or date of birth or by simply allocating every alternate person. Such methods of allocation are easy to manipulate, leading to a selection bias.

Blinding/masking Blinding in a clinical trial is defined as "the process of preventing those involved in a trial from knowing to which comparison group a particular participant belongs. The risk of bias is minimized when, as few people as possible know, who is receiving the experimental intervention and who the control intervention. Participants, caregivers, outcome assessors, and analysts are all candidates for being blinded."[14] Due to the elective nature and the amount of control a patient has over his or her prosthodontics treatment, it is important to recognize that is difficult to perform double-blinded or triple-blinded studies.

Concealment of allocation Allocation concealment in a clinical trial is defined as "the process that is used to ensure that the person deciding to enter a participant into a RCT does not know the comparison group into which that individual will be allocated."[14] It is widely accepted that the method of allocation concealment should be used as an assessment of the quality of an RCT as it has significant potential to bias the results of a study.

Parallel-group trial or crossover trial Parallel-group trial or independent group trial is a popular form of RCT and is defined as "a trial that compares 2 groups of people concurrently, one of which receives the intervention of interest and one of which is a control group."[14] Some parallel trials have more than two comparison groups and some compare different interventions without including a nonintervention control group. In contrast, a crossover trial refers to "a type of clinical trial comparing 2 or more interventions in which the participants, upon completion of the course of one treatment, are switched to another."[14] A recent example of a well-designed crossover trial design in prosthodontics is a comparison between a 2-implant unsplinted overdenture, a 2-implant bar-supported overdenture, and a 4-implant bar-supported overdenture, where the participants were randomly allocated to receive the prosthesis in various orders of treatment.[32] After the predetermined follow-up period, the participants were then allowed to cross over and receive the subsequent prosthesis.[32] Concerns in crossover trials include the need for additional duration of the study and need for minimizing the influence of one treatment on another (called carryover effect) by allowing a pause (called a washout period).[33] An additional challenge of consideration is the first-encounter bias among patients. This form of bias may lead to a nepotism and influence treatment satisfaction among patients.

Single-mouth trial or split-mouth trial Single-mouth trials are the popular form of RCT in prosthodontics and involve allocation of 1 treatment of interest per mouth. Split-mouth trials refer to a type of clinical trial comparing 2 or more interventions in which the participants are subjected to random allocation of 1 treatment of half of the mouth and another treatment/no treatment of the second half of the mouth. Depending on the intervention, the mouth can be essentially split into maxilla versus mandible, right versus left, or anterior versus posterior areas. The primary objective of using a split-mouth design is to eliminate all components related to differences between subjects from the treatment comparisons and thereby reduce the error variance (noise) of the experiment and obtain a more powerful statistical test.[34]

Comparisons made on a within-patient basis have a disadvantage, however, in that unless a prior knowledge indicates that no carryover effects exist, reported estimates of treatment efficacy are potentially biased.[34] Therefore, an important consideration is whether treatments for each side of the mouth are performed sequentially or simultaneously. An example of a split-mouth trial in prosthodontics is a comparison between all-ceramic crowns and metal-ceramic crowns between right and left sides of the mandible. In this example, although carryover effect may be less significant, all other factors need to be homogenized between the 2 treatments, such as opposing occlusion, opposing restorations, treatment tooth number, patient's primary chewing/guiding direction, and so forth.

Intention-to-treat analysis or per protocol analysis Intention-to-treat analysis and per protocol analysis are important terms that describe strategies for analyzing data from RCTs. In an intention-to-treat analysis, all participants are incorporated in the arm to which they were assigned, whether or not they received the intervention given to that arm. Intention-to-treat analysis prevents bias caused by the loss of participants, which may interrupt the baseline equivalence established by randomization and which may reflect nonadherence to the protocol.[14] Per protocol analysis involves an analysis of the subset of participants from an RCT who complied with the protocol adequately to ensure that their data would be likely to exhibit the treatment effect. This subset may be defined after considering exposure to treatment, availability of measurements, and absence of major protocol violations. This form of analysis may be subject to bias because the reasons for noncompliance may be related to treatment.[14]

Systematic reviews and meta-analysis of RCTs only

An SR of the literature is defined as "a review of a clearly formulated question that uses systematic and explicit methods to identify, select, and critically appraise relevant research, and to collect and analyze data from the studies that are included in the review."[14] A meta-analysis is defined as "the use of statistical techniques in an SR to integrate the results of included studies."[14] They provide validity for published studies regarding the thoroughness of controlling systematic errors in research methods, sampling, data collection, and data analysis. SRs are significantly different from a traditional literature review, which does not necessarily have a focused question and does not have an accounted search or quantifiable data, and the review itself is subjected to author bias. Therefore, traditional literature reviews primarily serve to answer background questions, such as Who? When? Why? What? Where? and How?, and other descriptive information but do not necessarily answer a clinical question for a patient at hand. SRs help to answer foreground questions because they compare treatments and can answer clinical questions.[1] The focused question for an SR usually follows the PICO format, which comprises (1) patient population of interest, (2) intervention of interest, (3) control/alternative interventions, and (4) outcome of interest.

In medicine, SRs of RCTs are popularly regarded as the gold standard for evidence-based practice. This thought process may not be applicable to prosthodontics due to the well-recognized paucity of RCTs itself. The world-renowned Cochrane reviews published by the Cochrane Collaboration include SRs of only RCTs in dentistry. Cochrane reviews are distinguished from other SRs by their claim of having stringent guidelines and low risk of bias and are updated every few years. Due to stringent inclusion criteria and paucity of RCTs, a majority of Cochrane reviews in dentistry currently conclude with "lack of sufficient evidence" to recommend one treatment versus another. It is expected that with progress and better understanding of clinical research, these conclusions can be more definitive but their impact on prosthodontics is unknown at this time.

Systematic reviews and meta-analysis of observational studies or all clinical studies

SRs and meta-analyses of only observational studies or including all clinical studies (both RCTs and observational studies) are widely popular in dentistry as well as in prosthodontics because such reviews are better poised to analyze more studies/data to answer a given clinical question, in comparison to SRs of only RCTs, where data are scarce. Through an exhaustive critical analysis and data consolidation of all clinical studies, they remove the burden from a clinician to independently identify and scrutinize best studies for clinical decision making. In a study analyzing data from observational studies and RCTs, Concato and colleagues[35] concluded that the results of well-designed observational studies (with either a cohort or a case-control design) do not systematically overestimate the magnitude of the effects of treatment compared with those in RCTs on the same topic. The investigators also contended that the popular belief that only RCTs produce trustworthy results and that all observational studies are misleading does a disservice to patient care, clinical investigation, and the education of health care professionals.[35]

It is important to recognize, however, that the risk of bias is high in SRs of observational studies compared with SRs of RCTs only. The impact of this risk of bias in clinical decision making for prosthodontics is unknown at this time. Creugers and Kreulen[36] performed an SR of all SRs in prosthodontics published over a 10-year period. Two pairs of SRs were identified as dealing with comparable items (survival of fixed partial dentures and survival of single crowns). They concluded that both SRs produced similar results, but the outcomes of the evaluated SRs may be used as prognostic data and cannot be used for direct comparison of treatments.[36] With the inundation of publications related to observational studies in prosthodontics, it is expected that the popularity of SRs will continue but it is important that SRs are updated periodically to include new studies and enable prospective and accurate comparison of treatment outcomes.

GUIDELINES FOR REPORTING EVIDENCE

With the burgeoning publication growth in prosthodontics, it is necessary for investigators to comply with certain guidelines for reporting scientific evidence. Several consensus groups and task forces in medicine have suggested various guidelines. The common goal of all guidelines is to improve scientific reporting and ensure standardization so that they allow an accurate assessment of the presented evidence. Popular guidelines are described further.

CONSORT

Consolidated Standards of Reporting Trials (CONSORT) is a popular guideline for reporting RCTs.[37] A group of scientists and editors in 1996 developed this statement to improve the quality of reporting of RCTs. The objective of CONSORT is to provide guidance to investigators about how to improve the reporting of their trials and to be clear, complete, and transparent. Several medical and dental journals, including the *Journal of American Dental Association*, require investigators to report the findings of their RCTs to satisfy the CONSORT. The CONSORT checklist includes 37 items that cover the entire report of a trial, ranging from the study title to the source of funding.

TREND

Transparent Reporting of Evaluations with Nonrandomized Design (TREND) was created in 2003.[38] In contrast to CONSORT, the objective of TREND is to provide guidance to investigators to standardize and improve the reporting of studies with nonrandomized designs (cohort and case-control studies). The TREND checklist includes 22 items that cover the entire report of a study, ranging from study title to external validity.

PRISMA

The objective of Preferred Reporting Items for Systematic Reviews and Meta-Analyses (PRISMA)[39] is to provide guidance to investigators to standardize the reporting of SRs and meta-analyses. Initially, a group of scientists and editors in 1996 initiated a document called Quality of Reporting of Meta-analyses (QUOROM), and, in July 2007, QUOROM was changed to PRISMA. The PRISMA checklist includes 27 items that cover the entire report, ranging from abstract to the source of funding.

PRISMA also provides a flowchart to enable investigators to describe a standardized search process.

MOOSE

Meta-analysis of Observational Studies in Epidemiology (MOOSE) was created in 1997.[40] The objective of MOOSE is to provide guidance to investigators to standardize the reporting of meta-analyses from nonrandomized studies. The MOOSE checklist includes 35 items, ranging from background to funding source.

SORT

Strength of Recommendation Taxonomy (SORT) has emerging popularity in dentistry.[41] It was developed by a group of family physicians in 2004 to classify the level of evidence for a study and provide recommendations. The objective of SORT is to provide a patient-oriented guidance to assess the quality, quantity, and consistency of evidence and allows investigators to rate individual studies or bodies of evidence. The recommendations are rated as either A, B, or C based on consistency and quality of patient-oriented evidence.

AMSTAR

Assessment of Multiple Systematic Reviews (AMSTAR) was developed in 2007 as an instrument to assess the methodologic quality of SRs.[42] It consists of 11 questions to analyze the quality of an SR, such as "Was a comprehensive literature search performed?" and "Was a list of studies (included and excluded) provided?" Each of these questions has 4 possible answers for the investigator: "Yes," No," Can't Answer," and "Not applicable." This helps investigators critically analyze the quality of a published SR.

LIMITATIONS OF EVIDENCE-BASED PROSTHODONTICS

There are some well-known limitations to EBD, and prosthodontics is no exception. Such limitations include applicability of research to a specific patient population, publication biases, paucity of current data, cost, and ethics. Prosthodontics is a unique specialty encompassing art, philosophy, and science and an absolute extrapolation of evidence-based concepts widely described in medicine is impossible. Establishing exceptional evidence, however, for prosthodontic treatment outcomes is paramount for the present and future of the specialty. One of the most popular criticisms for applying concepts of EBD to prosthodontics is that the information gained from clinical research may not directly answer the principal clinical question of what is best for a specific patient. This is because it is acknowledged that the homogeneity and characteristics of patients participating in clinical trials may be significantly different from those seen in dental offices. It is important to recognize, however, that EBD does not advocate absolute adoption of clinical evidence but calls for an integration of the clinical evidence along with the dentists' clinical expertise and patient needs and preferences. EBD does not provide a cookbook that dentists must follow nor does it establish a standard of care.[3] According to the ADA, the EBD process must not be used to interfere in the dentist/patient relationship nor be used entirely as a cost-containment tool by third-party payers.[3]

CURRENT AND FUTURE PERSPECTIVES

Compared with the traditional model of care, EBD is relatively new and, with progress in time, multiple clinical questions for which currently there is weak evidence or minimal/insufficient evidence should be resolved. Long-term survival and success of treatment, core components of the specialty of prosthodontics, is an important arena for channeling efforts and resources to help further distinguish the specialty of prosthodontics. To facilitate this process, however, it is important to establish a consensus in prosthodontics on defining the 3 core elements previously described: defining prosthodontic outcomes, duration needed for a meaningful understanding of prosthodontic outcomes, and sample size needed to make meaningful conclusions. Because prosthodontics is a unique specialty, a consensus is necessary to establish explicit guidelines for reporting of prosthodontic outcomes (suggested acronym, GROPO). Similar to numerous guidelines described in medicine, these guidelines can be exclusive to prosthodontics and ensure that investigators provide standardized reporting of their studies in order for them to be clear, complete, and transparent and allow integration of their evidence into clinical practice.

In order to teach and understand evidence-based prosthodontics, clinicians need to attain new skills pertaining to computer-based knowledge systems. These skills are necessary for asking, acquiring, appraising, applying, and assessing scientific evidence for the pertinent clinical situation. Current popular resources include Web sites of PubMed/Medline, ADA Center for EBD, Cochrane Library, and Center for Evidence-Based Dentistry. The 2 popular journals dedicated to EBD are *Journal of Evidence-Based Dental Practice* and *Evidence-Based Dentistry*. Another important avenue for practicing prosthodontists is participation in practice-based research networks (PBRNs), which has gained national momentum in the United States. A dental PBRN is an investigative alliance of academic researchers and practicing dentists.[43] The accord provides clinicians with an opportunity to propose or participate in research studies conducted in their own offices that address everyday issues in oral health care. These clinical studies, conducted in participating dental offices with consenting patients, help expand the profession's evidence base and further refine care.[43] Perhaps a PBRN focused on prosthodontics and/or prosthodontists can be assembled in the near future that can provide answers to specific clinical questions chosen by the specialty and for the specialty of prosthodontics.

REFERENCES

1. Sackett DL, Rosenberg WM, Gray JA, et al. Evidence based medicine: what it is and what it isn't. BMJ 1996;312(7023):71–2.
2. ADA Center for Evidence-Based Dentistry. Available at: http://ebd.ada.org/about. aspx. Accessed December 1, 2012.
3. ADA Policy on Evidence-Based Dentistry. Available at: http://www.ada.org/1754. aspx. Accessed December 1, 2012.
4. Harwood CL. The evidence base for current practices in prosthodontics. Eur J Prosthodont Restor Dent 2008;16(1):24–34.
5. Nishimura K, Rasool F, Ferguson MB, et al. Benchmarking the clinical prosthetic dental literature on MEDLINE. J Prosthet Dent 2002;88(5):533–41.
6. Russo SP, Fiorellini JP, Weber HP, et al. Benchmarking the dental implant evidence on MEDLINE. Int J Oral Maxillofac Implants 2000;15(6):792–800.
7. UCLA Department of Epidemiology. John Snow. Available at: http://www.ph.ucla. edu/epi/snow.html. Accessed December 1, 2012.
8. CDC Guidelines for Hand Hygiene in Health Care Settings. Available at: http://www. cdc.gov/mmwr/preview/mmwrhtml/rr5116a1.htm. Accessed December 1, 2012.
9. Doll R, Peto R, Boreham J, et al. Mortality in relation to smoking: 50 years' observations on male British doctors. BMJ 2004;328(7455):1519.

10. The Cochrane Collaboration. History. Available at: http://www.cochrane.org/about-us/history. Accessed December 1, 2012.
11. Evidence-Based Medicine Working Group. Evidence-based medicine. A new approach to teaching the practice of medicine. JAMA 1992;268(17):2420–5.
12. Hujoel PP, DeRouen TA. A survey of endpoint characteristics in periodontal clinical trials published 1988-1992, and implications for future studies. J Clin Periodontol 1995;22(5):397–407.
13. Bidra AS, Uribe F. Successful bleaching of teeth with dentinogenesis imperfecta discoloration: a case report. J Esthet Restor Dent 2011;23(1):3–10.
14. The Cochrane Collaboration. Glossary of Terms. Available at: http://www.cochrane.org/glossary. Accessed December 1, 2012.
15. Matthews DC, Hujoel PP. A practitioner's guide to developing critical appraisal skills: observational studies. J Am Dent Assoc 2012;143(7):784–6.
16. Owens EG, Goodacre CJ, Loh PL, et al. A multicenter interracial study of facial appearance. Part 1: a comparison of extraoral parameters. Int J Prosthodont 2002;15(3):273–82.
17. Claus EB, Calvocoressi L, Bondy ML, et al. Dental x-rays and risk of meningioma. Cancer 2012;118(18):4530–7.
18. Nations SP, Boyer PJ, Love LA, et al. Denture cream: an unusual source of excess zinc, leading to hypocupremia and neurologic disease. Neurology 2008;71(9):639–43.
19. CDC Glossary of Epidemiology Terms. Available at: http://www.cdc.gov/excite/library/glossary.htm. Accessed December 1, 2012.
20. Dawber TR, Meadors GF, Moore FE Jr. Epidemiological approaches to heart disease: the Framingham Study. Am J Public Health Nations Health 1951;41(3):279–81.
21. Hennekens CH, Eberlein K. A randomized trial of aspirin and beta-carotene among U.S. physicians. Prev Med 1985;14:165–8.
22. Doll R, Hill AB. The mortality of doctors in relation to their smoking habits. BMJ 1954;1(4877):1451–5.
23. Tallgren A. The continuing reduction of the residual alveolar ridges in complete denture wearers: a mixed-longitudinal study covering 25 years. J Prosthet Dent 1972;27(2):120–32.
24. Douglass JB, Meader L, Kaplan A, et al. Cephalometric evaluation of the changes in patients wearing complete dentures: a 20-year study. J Prosthet Dent 1993;69(3):270–5.
25. Miller-Keane encyclopedia and dictionary of medicine, nursing, and allied health. 7th edition. 2003. Available at: http://medical-dictionary.thefreedictionary.com/life+table. Accessed December 1, 2012.
26. Bidra AS, Huynh-Ba G. Implants in the pterygoid region: a systematic review of the literature. Int J Oral Maxillofac Surg 2011;40(8):773–81.
27. Dumbrigue HB, Jones JS, Esquivel JF. Developing a register for randomized controlled trials in prosthodontics: results of a search from prosthodontic journals published in the United States. J Prosthet Dent 1999;82(6):699–703.
28. Dumbrigue HB, Jones JS, Esquivel JF. Control of bias in randomized controlled trials published in prosthodontic journals. J Prosthet Dent 2001;86(6):592–6.
29. Jokstad A, Esposito M, Coulthard P, et al. The reporting of randomized controlled trials in prosthodontics. Int J Prosthodont 2002;15(3):230–42.
30. Pandis N, Polychronopoulou A, Eliades T. An assessment of quality characteristics of randomised control trials published in dental journals. J Dent 2010;38(9):713–21.

31. Friedman LM, Furberg CD, DeMets DL. Fundamentals of clinical trials. 4th edition. New York: Springer; 2010. p. 97–109.
32. Burns DR, Unger JW, Coffey JP, et al. Randomized, prospective, clinical evaluation of prosthodontic modalities for mandibular implant overdenture treatment. J Prosthet Dent 2011;106(1):12–22.
33. Barnett ML, Pihlstrom BL. A practitioner's guide to developing critical appraisal skills: interventional studies. J Am Dent Assoc 2012;143(10):1114–9.
34. Hujoel PP, DeRouen TA. Validity issues in split-mouth trials. J Clin Periodontol 1992;19(9 Pt 1):625–7.
35. Concato J, Shah N, Horwitz RI. Randomized, controlled trials, observational studies, and the hierarchy of research designs. N Engl J Med 2000;342(25): 1887–92.
36. Creugers NH, Kreulen CM. Systematic review of 10 years of systematic reviews in prosthodontics. Int J Prosthodont 2003;16(2):123–7.
37. Schulz KF, Altman DG, Moher D, CONSORT Group. CONSORT 2010 statement: updated guidelines for reporting parallel group randomised trials. J Clin Epidemiol 2010;63:834–40.
38. Des Jarlais DC, Lyles C, Crepaz N, TREND Group. Improving the reporting quality of nonrandomized evaluations of behavioral and public health interventions: the TREND statement. Am J Public Health 2004;94(3):361–6.
39. Moher D, Liberati A, Tetzlaff J, PRISMA Group. Preferred reporting items for systematic reviews and meta-analyses: the PRISMA statement. J Clin Epidemiol 2009;62:1006–12.
40. Stroup DF, Berlin JA, Morton SC, et al. Meta-analysis of observational studies in epidemiology: a proposal for reporting. Meta-analysis Of Observational Studies in Epidemiology (MOOSE) group. JAMA 2000;283(15):2008–12.
41. Ebell MH, Siwek J, Weiss BD, et al. Strength of recommendation taxonomy (SORT): a patient-centered approach to grading evidence in the medical literature. Am Fam Physician 2004;69(3):548–56.
42. Shea BJ, Grimshaw JM, Wells GA, et al. Development of AMSTAR: a measurement tool to assess the methodological quality of systematic reviews. BMC Med Res Methodol 2007;7:10.
43. Dental Practice-Based Research Network. National Institute of Dental and Craniofacial Research. Available at: http://www.nidcr.nih.gov/Research/DER/Clinical Research/DentalPracticeBasedResearchNetwork. Accessed December 1, 2012.

Occlusal Stability

Jonathan P. Wiens, DDS, MS*, Jennifer W. Priebe, DDS, MS

KEYWORDS

- Occlusal • Stability • Fixed prosthodontic treatment
- Removable prosthodontic treatment • Implant prosthodontic treatment

KEY POINTS

- In dentistry, articulation is the static and dynamic contact relationship between the occlusal surfaces of the teeth during function.
- The exact maxillomandibular position at which maximum intercuspation should occur or be restored has been deliberated. Patients presenting with occlusal instability and tooth loss may require that a functional occlusion be reestablished. Understanding the accepted terminology and definitions in the *Glossary of Prosthodontic Terms* is essential before prescribing any particular occlusal scheme.
- The literature supports that bilateral mandibular manipulation, compared with gothic arch tracing or chin-point guidance is a clinical method to consistently record centric relation (CR).
- The 3 most likely temporomandibular disorders observed in clinical practice are occlusal-muscle disorders related to parafunction, internal joint derangements, and degenerative joint disease. It is important for the clinician to evaluate each patient for the range of motion during mandibular movement and observe signs and symptoms for a variety of the temporomandibular disorders.
- Selecting the occlusal scheme for dentate patients, or those requiring implant, fixed or removable prosthodontic care, should take into consideration the prevailing patient conditions and anticipated prosthetic needs to achieve occlusal stability.

INTRODUCTION

Occlusion is the foundation for clinical success in fixed, removable, and implant prosthodontic treatment.[1-5] Understanding those principles that determine its development is critical when restoring a patient's occlusion. The dynamic interface of the maxillary and mandibular occlusal surfaces has been studied for more than 3 centuries. During that time, the evolution of many philosophies, devices, and theories of occlusion has occurred, based on anecdotal clinical observations and applied

Department of Restorative Dentistry, University of Detroit Mercy, School of Dentistry, Detroit, MI 48208, USA
* Corresponding author.
E-mail address: jonatwiens@comcast.net

geometric perceptions. Peer-reviewed journals and textbooks have reported these classic and contemporary occlusal concepts.[6-28] As evidence-based dentistry emerged, it championed a closer scrutiny of previously held beliefs, resulting in the abandonment of many pragmatic, yet beneficial occlusal procedures. The impetus toward scientific discovery, whereby factual information might be universally applied in both dental education and clinical practice, has created a renewed interest in occlusal studies.[29-34]

The American College of Prosthodontists formed a Task Force on Occlusion Education, consisting of prosthodontic educators and clinicians who represented the content experts, to reexamine what should be taught about occlusion.[35] Dental educators from universities across the United States were surveyed regarding the content and methodology of their occlusion curriculum. Also, the available scientific literature regarding occlusion was explored. Many occlusal studies were noted to be at the lowest level of hierarchal evidence, lacking randomization, bias controls, examiner blinding, or satisfactory statistical power, and so forth. Other areas were identified as having equivocal evidence or lack of agreement. It was concluded that occlusal concepts should be included in dental education and clinical practice when survey consensus occurred or when supporting scientific literature was discovered, resulting in the development of an occlusion primer.[5] There remains a significant need for occlusion research to confirm educational constructs and to validate clinical procedures currently in use.

OCCLUSAL STABILITY

In dentistry, articulation is the static and dynamic contact relationship between the occlusal surfaces of the teeth during function.[36] Teeth make contact in a static manner during maximal intercuspation (MI), such as at the end of the chewing cycle or during deglutition or clenching. They may also contact in a dynamic manner during eccentric gliding tooth contacts, which occur during incising, the closing chewing cycle, or perhaps during bruxism. Condylar pathways, tooth guidance, and the overriding neuromuscular control determine mandibular movements, which affect the occlusal surfaces or interface.[37] As a result, the anatomic shapes of teeth, although genetically scripted, must morphologically and physiologically adapt to functional loading.

These tissue and organ adaptations vary by location and timing and can result in identifiable physiologic changes in the occlusal interface, which include tooth wear and pulpal and periodontal changes that affect the cementum and alveolar bone. Missing or worn teeth may alter the occlusal vertical dimension (OVD), posterior support, or anterior guidance (AG), which may be further compromised by mesial drift, malposed or tipped teeth, and aberrant eruption patterns.[38] Altered growth and development, congenital anomalies, or degenerative changes within the joints often create variant or discordant skeletal relationships and associated atypical occlusal contacts. In addition, airway obstruction, diet, erosion, and parafunctional habits generally affect tooth position, shape, and impending function.[39]

Also, muscle and joint disorders can be the result of systemic disease, trauma, arthritis, and other processes unrelated to the dentition, yet may affect the occlusal interface by creating atypical tooth contacts. In the process, the patient's physiologic adaptive capacity for repair may be breached; this may lead to signs and symptoms within the neuromusculature and the temporomandibular joints (TMJs) that may culminate in a remarkable loss of occlusal stability.[40,41]

The purpose of this article is for the clinician to recognize occlusal stability, which requires understanding normal occlusal relationships as well as appreciating the ongoing physiologic and dynamic adaptive nature in which a patient's occlusion may change before, during, and after treatment.

Features of occlusal stability (Dentate)

1. Acceptable occlusal interface
   a. Uniform bilateral and anteroposterior occlusal contacts in MI
   b. Absence of occlusal trauma, which may be indicated by:
      i. Pain
      ii. Widened periodontal membrane and increased mobility
      iii. Root resorption, cementum, and alveolar bone changes
      iv. Pulpitis
      v. Fractures
   c. Absence of tooth surface loss (other than age-appropriate wear)
   d. Absence of nonaxial loading or tooth migration
   e. Absence of anterior and posterior occlusal plane discrepancies
2. Acceptable OVD
3. Acceptable MI position (MIP) and centric occlusion CO
   a. Less than 2 mm of CO with intact proprioception
   b. Preferably MIP occurs at CO
4. Acceptable AG or group function (GF)
5. Absence of posterior balancing interferences
6. Absence of muscle disorders
7. Absence of TMJ disorders

MANDIBULAR CENTRICITY

The exact maxillomandibular position at which maximum intercuspation should occur or be restored has been deliberated. Patients presenting with occlusal instability and tooth loss may require that a functional occlusion be reestablished. Understanding the accepted terminology and definitions in the *Glossary of Prosthodontic Terms* is essential before prescribing any particular occlusal scheme.

- Centric relation (CR) is the maxillomandibular relationship in which the condyles articulate with the thinnest avascular portion of their respective disks, with the complex in the anterior-superior position against the shapes of the articular eminencies. This position is independent of tooth contact, is clinically discernible when the mandible is directed superior and anteriorly, and theoretically is restricted to a purely rotary movement about the transverse horizontal axis.
- CO is the occlusion of opposing teeth when the mandible is in CR, which may or may not coincide with the maximal intercuspal position.
- MIP is the complete intercuspation of the opposing teeth independent of condylar position, sometimes referred to as the best fit of the teeth regardless of the condylar position.

CR and MIP

CR and MIP are positions that are approached during deglutition, which occurs more than 2000 times per day.[42–44] MI occurs naturally at CO in 1 of 10 adult patients. However, in most dentate patients, MI generally occurs anterior to CO by approximately 1 mm.[45–48] This observation may develop as a result of mesial drift created by the anterior vector forces on teeth during jaw closure. Functional tooth movement and mesial drift forces can create interproximal frictional wear. Transseptal fiber shortening has been suggested as the mechanism to accommodate this wear and maintain the interproximal contacts. Other associated causes may be related to tipped teeth, a lack of posterior occlusal support, resulting in anterior posturing of the mandible, and joint laxity with anteriorly displaced disks or possibly lateral pterygoid muscle contracture.

Proprioception and mechanoreceptors function to ensure uniform and repeatable closure. They rely on the presence of a periodontal ligament and receptors found in other orofacial structures for biofeedback to achieve comfort and a best fit. Loss of the periodontal attachment or teeth reduces this valuable input. When MIP is not consistent with CO, it is usually designated as an acquired MIP. Missing or tipped teeth, mesial drift, and malocclusions creating deflective occlusal contacts greater than 2 mm may exceed the patient's adaptive capacity over time. This situation may result in nonaxial or irregular tooth loading and potentially a traumatic outcome. Before placing any restoration that alters the occlusal interface, the clinician must decide on the best maxillomandibular position to create the MI, which is typically at CO or the patient's acquired MIP.[49]

CR precepts

- The articular disk is interposed between the condyle and eminence
- The condyles are in the anterior-superior position
- There is rotary mandibular movement about a transverse horizontal axis
- CR is repeatable and can be recorded

Selecting CO as a Restorative Position

Bilateral mandibular manipulation, compared with Gothic arch tracings or chin-point guidance, is believed to be a better clinical method to consistently record CR.[1] However, factors that may alter CR mandibular closure or hinder its recording should be contemplated.[2–5] Performing an occlusal analysis as well as a careful occlusal equilibration can achieve a neuromuscular release that ensures a reprogramming of mandibular closure to CO.[50] Deprogramming can be assisted by the use of an occlusal device, along with muscle relaxants/vapocoolant spray, which may interrupt the acquired MIP propagated proprioception.[51] The restoration of MI at CO for any occlusal scheme ensures that all border movements are included and may eliminate the apparent but erroneous immediate side shift associated with an eccentric CR recording, which usually accompanies the difficult occlusal adjustment at restoration placement.[52] In addition, CO may be accurately transferred to a class III or IV articulator to facilitate the construction of restorations and prostheses.

Occlusal equilibration is performed to align the MIP with CO by eliminating prematurities or deflective occlusal contacts or to create harmonious gliding tooth contacts, which reduces off-axis loading or atypical wear patterns. Occlusal equilibration is also indicated before restoring quadrants of teeth, which alters the occlusal interface, such as when restoring the AG, OVD, or occlusal plane correction or the elimination of occlusal trauma. In addition, adequate interocclusal distance may be reestablished for patients with advanced wear or mandibular posturing. However, prophylactic occlusal equilibration is not routinely indicated for asymptomatic patients who present with occlusal stability and minimal occlusal discrepancies.[53–56] Occlusal equilibration follows a specific sequence to achieve MI at CO and to achieve harmonious gliding tooth contacts, which requires appropriate training on the exact methodology to achieve the desire result (**Box 1**).[57]

Selecting Acquired MIP as a Restorative Position

The use of the patient's existing MIP and OVD as a restorative position, without reference to CO, may be possible for the placement of a singular restoration. However, a prerequisite is the presence of occlusal stability. The placement of restorations using the acquired MIP carries the risk of introducing inaccuracies into the occlusal interface but with an added unreliable or unrepeatable jaw position, thus impeding occlusal verification and its correction. Facebow full arch casts mounted on a class III or IV articulator better represent the mandibular arc of closure in CR as well as the dynamics of the occlusal interface during eccentric jaw movements.[58–62] Arbitrarily mounted segmental casts on a class II articulator have the potential to introduce significant occlusal errors.[63] Full arch casts capture the greatest number of intercuspal contacts for cast articulation; they also may provide the contralateral laterotrusive tooth guidance, which along with the condylar guidance (CG), influences the mediotrusive pathway on the ipsilateral-restoration side. Segmental casts or triple-tray methods are lacking these aspects and may introduce occlusal errors.

Selecting the OVD

The OVD is a function of maxillary and mandibular growth, which is usually limited by the repetitive contraction length of the elevator muscles. In the dentate patient, craniofacial growth and alveolar bone formation occur as the dentition erupts, which adds to the vertical growth until the teeth occlude.[64,65] The lack of a stable occlusal contact usually results in continued tooth eruption beyond the occlusal plane. This observation may be further influenced by deflective occlusal contacts or orofacial musculature. Generally, as teeth wear, there is continued eruption and associated alveolar bone

---

Box 1
Stepwise sequencing for occlusal equilibration

1. Deprogramming

2. Mounted casts

3. Mock adjustment of casts

4. CR (MI to occur at CO and maintained at the established OVD)

5. Mediotrusion (eliminate mediotrusive tooth contacts that interfere with AG)

6. Laterotrusion (eliminate laterotrusive tooth contacts that interfere with AG)

7. Protrusion (eliminate protrusive tooth contacts that interfere with AG)

8. Polish and reassessment[a]

   [a] Reassessment should verify previous steps and be reconfirmed at subsequent appointments.

growth, which physiologically maintains the OVD at the contracted length of the elevator muscles.[66] During this process, spatial tooth positions relative to both tooth contact in centric relationship or near contact in eccentric relationships becomes a learned repetitive mandibular movement during mastication, deglutition, and speech. A physiologic interocclusal distance occurs in the dentate patient and usually must be reestablished in the partially and completely edentulous patient. The spatial positioning of restored crowns or artificial teeth is often influenced by the patient's neuromusculature and accompanying proprioceptive driven engrams, which serve as a clinical guide.

The most commonly used methods to assess these spatial relationships for either edentulous or dentate patients are the closest speaking space followed by the establishment of an interocclusal distance or space between physiologic rest position (PRP) and MI.[67–77] Before extraction, photographic records and facial proportions are also helpful.[72] Typically, the maxillary incisor length and position are determined by lip profile, tooth display, and contact with the lower lip wet-dry line during fricative formation.[78] Variations occur with lip length, age, gender, malocclusions, and so forth. During sibilant production, the mandible moves downward and forward to the closest speaking space, which is usually less than 1 mm (vertically and horizontally), measured interincisally. This observation provides a clue to vertical and horizontal position of the mandibular incisor. Rarely do the mandibular incisor edges advance anteriorly beyond the maxillary incisor edges during sibilant production. If the chosen maxillary and mandibular incisor lengths or OVD are excessive, the tip of the tongue is not visible during "th" production. When making these assessments, the need for anterior coupling or guidance requiring tooth contact should be considered for the dentate patient, but this may not be desirable for the completely edentulous patient.

Several methods have been suggested to determine the PRP. Some investigators suggest arbitrarily subtracting 3 mm from the PRP to arrive at the proposed OVD for edentulous patients (**Table 1**). However, investigators have found that the vertical dimension at PRP varies significantly after natural tooth contacts are lost, with pain or stress, variant jaw relationships, ridge resorption, and postural body position; these variations may obfuscate the assessment of the PRP and the OVD, which is incorrectly selected.

Table 1
Methods used to determine PRP and interocclusal distance

	Observation
Phonetic Tests	
Fricatives "f"	Maxillary incisal edge to lower lip wet-dry line
Sibilants "s"	The maxillary-mandibular incisal edges approximated during closet speaking space
Thicatives "th"	Lingual dental: tongue should appear between upper and lower incisors
PRP Tests	
Open wide, then lips together	Observe for the presence of ~3 mm of interocclusal space
Swallow	Observe for the presence of ~3 mm of interocclusal space
Hum "m"	Observe for the presence of ~3 mm of interocclusal space
Patient preference	Observe for the presence of ~3 mm of interocclusal space
Rest and peek	Observe for the presence of ~3 mm of interocclusal space

The closest speaking space measured during fricatives and sibilant sounds may be more reliable and consistent than PRP observations. These parameters are subject to many variables (eg, retrognathic patients tend to have greater horizontal movement during testing for the closest speaking space, as well as greater interocclusal distance, when testing for the vertical dimension). Conversely, the prognathic patient has minimal horizontal or vertical movement and less interocclusal space for the same tests. Other growth and developmental anomalies resulting in apertognathia and high or low Frankfort-mandibular angles (FMAs) further obscure these assessments. Patients with a low FMA typically have Angle class II-2 occlusions, with greater AG and increased muscle contraction forces, which limits any attempt to increase the OVD.[79,80] Patients with a high FMA tend toward apertognathic occlusal relationships with decreased muscular forces and less AG or anterior coupling, possibly requiring a reduction of the OVD.

Although an apparent PRP can be observed and an interocclusal distance arbitrarily calculated, its variability and adaptive capacity to change over time renders PRP a questionable and sometimes unreliable point of reference. PRP and OVD computations are difficult maxillomandibular relationships to evaluate because of the confounding patient variables and the associated parameters used for their determination. Because all methods of testing the physiologic rest position are unscientific, the determination of OVD should not be confined to a single technique or consideration.[81,82]

The OVD is limited in range, with inviolate end points; exceeding the elevator muscle contraction length may show this limitation. Indiscriminately increasing the OVD may result in increased muscular forces during mastication. In this situation, the patient's neuromusculature may attempt to return the occlusal interface to the original or physiologic OVD. Conversely, inadequate closing forces occur if the OVD is established too low. Both levels, high or low, have the potential to affect normal tongue function or speech, with altered masticatory muscle function and facial proportions.[83,84]

MANDIBULAR ECCENTRICITY

The opinions regarding the manner in which teeth contact when the mandible is in eccentric positions have been varied, with some preference determined by the position of the tooth within the arch, impending function, and type of restoration/prosthesis being placed. Understanding the accepted terminology and definitions is essential before prescribing a specific eccentric occlusal scheme.

- AG: the influence of the contacting surfaces of anterior teeth on tooth limiting mandibular movements; AG includes right and left laterotrusive and protrusive guidance
- Balanced articulation (BA): the bilateral, simultaneous, anterior, and posterior occlusal contact of teeth in centric and eccentric positions
- Balancing interference: undesirable contact(s) of opposing occlusal surfaces on the nonworking side (mediotrusive side)
- Canine protected articulation: a form of mutually protected articulation, in which the vertical and horizontal overlap of the canine teeth disengages the posterior teeth in the excursive movements of the mandible
- CG: mandibular guidance generated by the condyle and articular disk traversing the contour of the glenoid fossae
- GF: multiple contact relations between the maxillary and mandibular teeth in lateral movements on the working side, whereby simultaneous contact of several teeth acts as a group to distribute occlusal forces

- Mutually protected articulation: an occlusal scheme in which the posterior teeth prevent excessive contact of the anterior teeth in maximum intercuspation, and the anterior teeth disengage the posterior teeth in all mandibular excursive movements; alternatively, an occlusal scheme, in which the anterior teeth disengage the posterior teeth in all mandibular excursive movements, and the posterior teeth prevent excessive contact of the anterior teeth in maximum intercuspation

Mutually Protected Complex

Both D'Amico[85] and Beyron[86,87] separately studied aborigines who had progressive wear of their dentition because of an abrasive diet. This helicoidal wear resulted in a loss of AG and posterior support with an apparent autorotational closure of the mandible and end-on anterior relationship. D'Amico surmised that canine protective articulation was necessary to reduce this destructive process and posterior wear. Beyron also believed that disocclusion was necessary, but that GF was inevitable over time. It was suggested that the long canine root, its position at the corner of the arch, and distance from the joint/muscle (fulcrum) made the canine the ideal tooth to disengage the posterior teeth. Although a greater number of proponents favor canine protective articulation,[88] others report the natural prevalence of GF in the adult dentate population.[89] A low or high FMA has been inversely correlated to canine and GF disocclusion.[80]

AG consists of both the incisal guidance during anteroposterior mandibular movements such as during incising (protrusion), and canine guidance, which occur during posterior closing chewing cycles (laterotrusion) in the dentate patient.[90,91] During lateroprotrusive movements, there may be a crossover or shared involvement of the incisors and canines that disengage the posterior teeth during eccentric mandibular movements. During GF, the posterior buccal cusps may contact in unison with the ipsilateral canines during laterotrusive mandibular movements.[92] In the dentate patient, the lingual fossae of the maxillary anterior teeth are concave, and generally, the AG disocclusion angle is greater in magnitude than the convex CG.

CG includes both horizontal and lateral components, as seen in protrusive and mediolateral mandibular movements, respectively.[93] Other factors include intercondylar distance and side shift variables. The slope of the convex-curvilinear condylar pathway allows the disengagement of the posterior teeth during eccentric mandibular movements; the separation of the jaws allows the presence of cusped teeth without interferences.[94] The lateral CG or inclination is also known as the Bennett angle. This angle affects mediolateral cusp height and may have a slightly greater magnitude in the vertical plane (Fischer angle) than the horizontal condylar inclination.[95,96]

The presence of balancing interferences on the mediotrusive side in the dentate patient is not desirable, because it may create off-axis loading of those posterior teeth involved, and also may distract the nonbraced orbiting condyle-disk complex.[97] However, the patient may tolerate balancing contacts that do not compete with the AG. Posterior mediotrusive contacts may interfere with the AG, thus preventing the disengagement of the posterior teeth during mandibular movements. Electromyographic studies show that the elevator muscles on the mediotrusive balancing side decrease in activity in the presence of a balancing contact, which supports the notion of a protective process.[98-101] Investigations have measured the occlusal forces from anterior to posterior, as well as the threshold sensitivities within the arch. The posterior teeth could sustain greater loading compared with anterior teeth, but anterior teeth had increased sensitivity thresholds at lower levels in contrast to the posterior teeth.[102] The splaying of anterior teeth is a common observation with the loss of posterior occlusal support. These observations support the mutually protective articulation construct, whereby the posterior and anterior teeth perform a function to protect each other, as defined earlier.

Mutually protective articulation Constructs

- Posterior teeth: MI contact only at centric occlusion
- Canines: only contact in laterotrusion, providing posterior disocclusion
- Incisors: only contact in protrusion, providing posterior disocclusion

---

BA

The primary purpose of BA is to stabilize the mucosal supported removable prostheses. Hanau described 9 factors for attaining a BA.[103] Of these 9 factors, 5 are recognized to be important for achieving balance articulation in denture occlusion: inclination of the condyles, incisal guidance, cusp angle, orientation of the occlusal plane, and prominence of the compensating curve. In an edentulous patient and within parameters, 4 of these factors can be modified to achieve a BA. One factor that cannot be physically changed is the patient's condylar inclination. Protrusive and laterotrusive interocclusal records, or axiographic recordings, may be used to program the horizontal condylar inclination and Bennett angle on the semiadjustable or highly adjustable articulators.[104] The articulator may be further adjusted, when conditions warrant, to better simulate the patient's eccentric jaw relationships, thus achieving a BA in the clinical setting.

$$\text{Balanced Articulation} = \frac{\text{Condylar Guidance} \times \text{Incisal Guidance}}{\text{Cusp Angle} \times \text{Compensating Curve} \times \text{Occlusal Plane}}$$

The Thielemann formula provides the algebraic relationship of the 5 BA factors.[105] It is an empirical formula and does not express precise values, but does provide an indicator of the geometric parameters needed to either create or eliminate tooth contact. When the numerator is equivalent to the denominator, then BA should occur, whereby there is simultaneous anterior and posterior occlusal contact of teeth in eccentric positions. In applying the Thielemann formula, when the numerator is greater than the denominator, then an AG should occur. Conversely, if the reverse is true, it results in posterior deflective contacts and a lack of anterior tooth contact in eccentric positions. BA is not absolutely required if the prosthesis is fixed, or supported and stabilized by teeth or implants.

Anterior Coupling and Skeletal Relationships

Dawson[23] proposed the concept of freedom from centric, which allows freedom of movement from CO just before AG disocclusion engages, which is typically less than 0.5 mm. This long centric concept allows the patient to close into both CO and acquired MIP. This construct underscores the importance of not overcontouring or making the maxillary lingual fossae convex when restoring the AG, which can occur by increasing the OVD. Reestablishing the AG requires the ability to create anterior coupling, which becomes difficult when the FMA is high or low, when the maxillomandibular relationship is either retrognathic or prognathic, or when the chosen OVD prevents anterior coupling.[106–109]

- Patients with Angle class II, div 1 occlusions have a significant horizontal overjet, resulting in minimal AG with a concomitant differing anterior and posterior plane of occlusion.[110] These patients typically have horizontal chewing pattern, creating the predisposition for greater posterior deflective occlusal contacts and posterior wear.
- Patients with Angle class II, div 2 commonly have a low FMA and likely have excessive vertical overlap but minimal horizontal overlap, resulting in an immediate disocclusion during eccentric jaw movements. Posterior cusp angles are greater, as is the curve of Spee. The lack of horizontal space creates restriction on the envelope of motion, associated mandibular displacement, and increased anterior forces. The end result is significant frictional wear, which leads to posterior deflective contacts, once the AG has been depleted.
- Angle class III and apertognathic patients essentially have minimal or no AG. A short protrusive may be created but necessitates a shorter posterior cusp angle form, unless the patient has a vertical chewing pattern. The presence of reverse articulations (cross-bite) also may be present in class III patients. The result is atypical working and balancing contacts, which can predispose off-axis loading.
- Apertognathic patients typically have a high FMA and may require reduction of their OVD posterior segments. Treatment may involve surgery, orthodontic, and prosthodontic procedures. Correction of a restricted nasal airway must be considered as a possible secondary cause of excessive posterior tooth eruption, which may create an apertognathia. Also, a determination is necessary if a tongue thrust habit is present and whether it is compensatory. The lip length and ability to achieve lip competency may be compromised in patients with apertognathia, vertical maxillary excess and Angle class II-1 patients.

In these situations, in which patients have discordant growth and developmental skeletal relationships, orthodontic and orthognathic surgery, including reassessment of the OVD and MIP, may be necessary to properly restore anterior coupling and arch alignment (**Tables 2–4**).[111–116]

Table 2
Centric and eccentric tooth relationships

Position	Posterior Tooth Number Contact	Anterior Tooth Number Contact	Repeatable	Pain	Deflection	Facets
CO-MIP			☐	☐	☐	☐
MIP			☐	☐	☐	☐
Protrusion			☐	☐	☐	☐
Right laterotrusion			☐	☐	☐	☐
Left mediotrusion			☐	☐	☐	☐
Left laterotrusion			☐	☐	☐	☐
Right mediotrusion			☐	☐	☐	☐

The centric and eccentric tooth relationships form may be used to record those teeth that contact during various mandibular positions as well as whether the positions are easily repeatable or with pain, deflection of facets beyond age-appropriate wear.

Table 3
Malocclusion classifications

Parameter	Class I	Class II	Class III	Reverse Articulation	Apertognathia
Incisors	☐	☐	☐	☐	☐
Right canine	☐	☐	☐	☐	☐
Right first molar	☐	☐	☐	☐	☐
Left canine	☐	☐	☐	☐	☐
Left first molar	☐	☐	☐	☐	☐

The malocclusion classifications are noted for canine and first molar positions relative to their Angle classification, reverse articulation (cross-bite), and apertognathia.

Shortened Dental Arch and Posterior Occlusal Support

The shortened dental arch typically involves the elimination of 1 or 2 posterior teeth in all 4 quadrants. This concept has been applied in orthodontics when tooth size and arch length discrepancies occur; in removable prosthodontics, to avoid arranging teeth over ridge inclines that might create unstable denture bases; and in implant prosthodontics, to reduce the potential cantilever forces that may exceed the physical properties of the restorative materials and challenge osseointegration. Questions often arise relative to the reduction of masticatory function, or the potential to create increased muscle contraction forces, resulting in greater off-axis forces being applied to the anterior teeth: this condition may further cause tooth migration or loss of occlusal stability. Recent studies have suggested that acceptable mastication may be

Table 4
Cephalometric and occlusal determinants

Parameters	FMA	OP	SNA	SNB	ANB
Angles	<25°>	<10°>	<82°>	<78°>	<2°–4°>
Anterior coupling	0	1	2	3	4
Vertical: horizontal overlap	V:	H:			
Incisal guidance angle					
Canine guidance angle	R:	L:			
Horizontal condylar inclination	R:	L:			
Lateral condylar inclination	R:	L:			
Curve of Spee and Wilson					
Mediolateral arch irregularities					
Facial and dental midline					

The cephalometric and occlusion determinants of interest to the prosthodontist include the frankfort mandibular angle (FMA), occlusal plane angle (OPA), Sella (S) Nasion (A) A point or subspinale (A), B point or supramentale (SNB) and ANB.

Anterior coupling: 0, no contact; 1, cingulum contact; 2, lingual fossa contact; 3, incisal edge-edge contact; 4, reverse articulation.

The measurement of the vertical and horizontal incisor/canine overlap provides some idea as to whether the ratio is 1:1, resulting in a 45°, or 2:1 or 1:2, which may correlate to a 60° or 30° angle, respectively. Other ratios and resultant angles are possible.

The horizontal and lateral condylar inclinations are of importance in magnitude, causing separation of the posterior teeth during eccentric mandibular movements. The anteroposterior and mediolateral occlusal plane curvatures and levels, with the facial and dental midlines, should be recorded.

maintained with 20 occluding dental units.[117,118] When considering a shortened dental arch, each patient must meet the requisites listed in features of occlusal stability.

MANDIBULAR MOVEMENT AND FUNCTIONAL CHANGES WITHIN THE TMJS
Mandibular Movement and Range of Motion

The 3 most likely temporomandibular disorders observed in clinical practice are occlusal-muscle disorders (OMDs) related to parafunction, internal joint derangements (IJDs), and degenerative joint disease (DJD). It is important for the clinician to evaluate each patient for the range of motion (ROM) during mandibular movement and observe signs and symptoms for a variety of the temporomandibular disorders (TMDs) (**Table 5**).[119,120] These evaluations should always take into consideration mediolateral, anterior-posterior and inferior-superior skeletal, arch form, and dental variations, which may skew the measurements and functional mandibular movements.[121,122] It is important to record the most open, protrusive, and right and left laterotrusion measurements. The presence of associated pain, audible sounds, incoordination, hypomobility, hypermobility, or deviation during mandibular movements should be noted (**Fig. 1**). If the ROM recordings are not within normal limits, a diagnosis is needed relative to possible intracapsular or extracapsular causation. Appropriate management should occur before embarking on any procedures that would alter the mandibular position or occlusal interface (**Fig. 2**).[123]

TMDs and Progression

The clinician faces an added dilemma when there is an underlying TMD, and the patient's occlusion needs to be restored, or when teeth need to be replaced (**Tables 6–8**). Arriving at a diagnosis and treatment plan requires a determination of whether there are intracapsular or extracapsular considerations.[119,124–136] Pain of dental origin along with any psychological overlay should be included in the differential diagnosis and management tree.[137–140] In general, treatment that alters the occlusal surfaces is best postponed until there is a clear indication that pain can be relieved and that neuromuscular release and TMJ load stability can be achieved.

Dawson[141] describes occluso-muscle disorders as discomfort or dysfunction from hyperactive, uncoordinated muscle function that is triggered by deflective occlusal interferences to physiologic jaw movements and noxious habits. This dysfunction can be both asymptomatic and within the physiologic adaptive capacity of the patient. It may also range from a subclinical or transient situation to a more overt chief complaint by the patient, such as myofascial pain. Diagnoses that involve the incoordination of the muscles and muscle splinting are typically seen as localized or possibly referred

Table 5						
ROM (in millimeters)						
Position	**Measurement**	**<Hypomobility-Hypermobility>**	**Pain**	**Clicking/Crepitation**	**Reduction**	**Deviation**
Most open	45–55	<45–55>	☐	☐	☐	R-L
Protrusion	8–10	<8–10>	☐	☐	☐	R-L
Right laterotrusion	6–8	<8>	☐	☐	☐	
Left laterotrusion	6–8	<8>	☐	☐	☐	

When evaluating the ROM, the extent of vertical and horizontal movement should be recorded, noting if there is hypomobility or hypermobility, pain, clicking with or without reduction, crepitation. It is also important to correlate any deviation in protrusion and most open position with restricted laterotrusion.

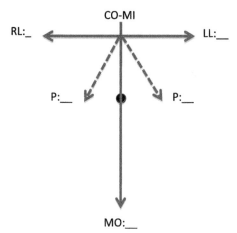

Fig. 1. Wiens ROM pentagram is a chart notation of the ROM, which consists of a horizontal line, representing right and left laterotrusion, and a vertical line, representing the most open position. The intersection of the horizontal and vertical lines represents MI. Restriction on the most open position may indicate muscle spasm, whereas deviations to the right or left may suggest unilateral disk displacement, preventing condylar movement. The circle on the vertical line represents protrusion without deviation. The dashed diagonal lines are used to denote deviation on protrusion, to the right or left. ●, straight protrusion without deviation; LL, left laterotrusion; MO, most open; P, deviation to the right or left in protrusion; RL, right laterotrusion.

muscle pain.[142] Limitation of the ROM in the most open position with normal eccentric jaw movements and an absence of intracapsular disorders is often a benchmark. Extracapsular disorders originating within the musculature may improve with no treatment; patient education and counseling; bruxism/clenching control; occlusal devices; stretch and spray/physical therapy; nonsteroidal antiinflammatory drugs; muscle

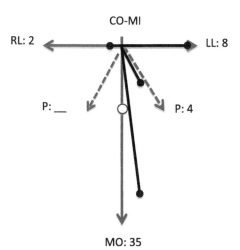

Fig. 2. An example of an ROM pentagram for a patient who presents with left-sided anteriorly displaced disk. Right laterotrusion is obstructed and results in restriction and deviation to the affected left side on protrusion and the most open position. The unaffected right TMJ allows translation and normal range of left laterotrusion.

Table 6
Intracapsular and extracapsular TMDs (American Academy of Orofacial Pain)

Intracapsular	Extracapsular
Congenital or developmental	Myofascial pain disorder
Disk derangement disorders	Local myalgia
Dislocation	Myositis
Inflammatory disorders	Central mediated myalgia
Noninflammatory disorders	Myospasm
Trauma	Myofibrotic contracture

The American Academy of Orofacial Pain divides TMDs into intracapsular and extracapsular categories. A patient may have intracapsular and extracapsular components simultaneously.

relaxants; and possibly occlusal adjustment.[143,144] The value of assessing deflective occlusal contacts, fremitus, mobility, or excessive wear with shifting of tooth positions should not be overlooked. Although occlusal equilibration may create a neuromuscular release to establish a repeatable mandibular closure that facilitates prosthodontic treatment, it may not necessarily eliminate transitory joint clicking that is related to muscle incoordination or in the presence of ongoing parafunctional bruxism and diurnal clenching.[145–149]

Patients presenting with a history of clicking joints, and examination findings of an inability to make unilateral laterotrusion movement, may be accompanied by a deviation in protrusion to the ipsilateral side.[150,151] Intracapsular disorders typically include anterior displaced disks (ADD) that obstruct or impede condylar movement on the affected side. The articular surfaces and interposed disk are subject to systemic, traumatic, and local degenerative processes, which can alter their morphology and physiologic function. These alterations influence spatial mandibular positions and movements, ROM, condylar determinants, and how teeth contact.[152] An ROM assessment with computed tomography or magnetic resonance imaging may be helpful to confirm the intracapsular internal joint derangement diagnosis.[153] Other procedures may be considered to facilitate the outcome of care, such as arthrocentesis with mandibular manipulation or other physical therapy modalities.

Table 7
Research diagnostic criteria for TMDs: Axis I (Dworkin and LeResche)

	Categorization for Clinical Diagnosis
Group I: muscle disorders	Ia. Myofascial pain Ib. Myofascial pain with limitations in aperture
Group II: disk displacement	IIa. Disk displacement with reduction IIb. Disk displacement without reduction and no limitations in aperture IIc. Disk displacement without reduction and with limitations in aperture
Group III: arthralgia, arthritis, arthrosis	IIIa. Arthralgia IIIb. Osteoarthritis of the TMJ IIIc. Osteoarthrosis of the TMJ

Data from Dworkin SF, LeResche L. Research Diagnostic Criteria for Temporomandibular Disorders: Review, Criteria, Examinations and Specifications, Critique. J Craniomandib Disord 1992;6:301–55.

Table 8	
Research diagnostic criteria for TMDs: Axis II	
Categorization for Determining Chronic Pain, Psychological Status, Psychosocial Disability	
Characteristic pain intensity Pain interference score	The average of 0–10 ratings of: 1, pain right now; 2, worst pain; and 3, usual pain
Pain-related disability days	Average of 0–10 ratings of pain-related interference with work, social, and overall activities
Chronic pain grade	Disability days in the previous 6 mo
SCL-90-R scales: mean and age-adjusted and sex-adjusted scores	Scale scores for depression and number of nonspecific physical symptoms

Data from Dworkin SF, Sherman JJ, Mancl L, et al. Reliability, validity, and clinical utility of RDC/TMD Axis II scales: Depression, non-specific physical symptoms, and graded chronic pain. J Orofacial Pain 2002;16:207–20.

Attempts to orthopedically advance the mandible using an occlusal device for patients with ADD may help on a short-term therapeutic basis. Advancing the mandible results in a significantly anterior MIP with limited to no AG and may not resolve the ADD or return of the condyle disks to a stable anterior-superior position. Long-term mandibular advancement may result in TMJ remodeling and changes in the occlusion caused by both intrusion and extrusion of teeth over time.[154] This occurrence may result in the need for continuous use of an occlusal device, orthodontics, or extensive fixed prosthodontic treatment to maintain the established position. In addition, an anterior MIP requires the patient to relearn a new mandibular closure, which may not necessarily be repeatable and likely affects the occlusal interface in an unconventional manner. Should modification of the occlusal surfaces be needed it should be focused toward eliminating overt occlusal trauma, palliation of tooth pain, and achieving a repeatable or uniform closure and gliding tooth contacts.

The inevitable progression from OMD to ADD with reduction, to the loss of the lateral and medial pole attachments, disk perforation, and deformation to end stage of DJD has been questioned.[155] Although various stages of intracapsular disorders have been observed, there is a lack of evidence that confirms that all patients progress from OMD to IJD to DJD.[147,156–169]

Nevertheless, before embarking on procedures that alter the occlusal interface, the clinician should include the management of any intracapsular or extracapsular TMD. The clinician should appreciate that as joint instability and degenerative changes occur, the condylar position and inclination may change, resulting in apertognathia and hyperfunction or deflective occlusal contacts, predominately on the affected side. Close monitoring at regular intervals and treatment flexibility incorporating reversible and limited treatment protocols may be preferred in these situations. Informing the patient of the diagnosis, complexities of treatment, and the prognosis is vital. Because of the limited space in this article, the reader is encouraged to source other information regarding the management of the various intracapsular and extracapsular disorders (see **Tables 6–8**).

SELECTING OCCLUSAL SCHEMES

Selecting the occlusal scheme for dentate patients, or those requiring implant, fixed, or removable prosthodontic care, may vary based on the prevailing patient conditions. The occlusal scheme is challenged by missing teeth, unlevel occlusal planes, skeletal malocclusions, severely worn dentitions, insufficient AG, advanced periodontal disease, and TMDs.

The goal should be to create both occlusal and prosthesis stability, which requires a repeatable closure in CR at an appropriate OVD with stable joints and neuromuscular function, as well as determining the condylar and anterior tooth guidance that determines the occlusal interface during eccentric jaw movements.

In patients with deformed disks, a stable adapted centric posture may be achieved.[170] These patients do not meet the exact criteria of CR, yet a manageable relationship may be achieved, whereby the joints, muscles, and teeth can be loaded without discomfort. The goal for any definitive prosthodontic treatment is to establish an intercuspal position that is comfortable, repeatable, with harmonious tooth guidance, and unchanging.[171,172] The occlusal restoration may be challenging for patients with compromised joints and should be judiciously documented.[173,174]

Canine and incisor guidance is preferred in laterotrusive and protrusive movements that is favorable to the given CG. There should be an absence of posterior deflective or interfering balancing contacts of teeth in mediotrusion, laterotrusion, and protrusion for the dentate patient. GF in laterotrusion that is in unison with the canine guidance represents an alternative occlusion scheme, providing a progressive disocclusion.

Discordant skeletal relationships can result in excessive or minimal AG, which may allow greater or lesser posterior cuspal height, respectively, or change the typical cuspal interface position in MI. Patients with periodontal disease, or insufficient AG (such as missing incisors/canines) benefit by occlusal equilibration to achieve MIP coincident with CO.[175] In these situations, a reduced AG may be required and necessitates a reduction in posterior cuspal height, with narrowing of the occlusal table to reduce the potential for deflective occlusal contacts and to direct occlusal forces down the long axis of the tooth.[176]

A BA occlusal scheme is recommended in situations in which either, or both, arches are restored with removable prostheses. Attempts to further stabilize the removable prostheses may require a shortened dental arch, to avoid placing occlusal loading over an unlevel ridge form, a narrow occlusal table, or a lingualized occlusal scheme as alternatives.

Fixed implant prosthodontics follow similar occlusal schemes and alternatives for fixed prosthodontics; likewise, removable implant prosthodontics should follow the occlusal scheme for removable prosthodontics necessitating a BA. During MI, the natural teeth may intrude 100 μm, which may impose increased occlusal forces on the less intrusive implant restoration. It has been suggested that tooth contacts on a fixed implant restoration require a lighter centric contact (10 μm) than that of a natural tooth, because of the lack of a periodontal ligament surrounding a dental implant and loss of some degree of rebound. However, occlusal overload has been related to implant component failure rather than the loss of osseointegration.

REFERENCES

1. Keshvad A, Winstanley RB. Comparison of the replicability or routinely used centric relation registration techniques. J Prosthodont 2003;12:90–101.
2. Clayton JA. A pantographic reproducibility index for use in diagnosing temporomandibular joint dysfunction: a research report. J Prosthet Dent 1985;54:827–31.
3. Obrez A, Turp JC. The effect of musculoskeletal facial pain on registration of maxillomandibular relationships and treatment planning: a synthesis of the literature. J Prosthet Dent 1998;79:439–45.

4. Linsen SS, Stark H, Samai A. The influence of different registration techniques on condylar displacement and electromyographic activity in stomatognathically healthy subjects: a prospective study. J Prosthet Dent 2012;107:47–52.

5. Obrez A, Stohler C. Jaw muscle pain and its effect on gothic arch tracings. J Prosthet Dent 1996;75:393–8.

6. Bonwill WG. Geometric and mechanical laws of articulation. Transactions of the Pennsylvania Odontological Society. 1885.

7. Balkwill FH. The best form and arrangement of artificial teeth for mastication. Tr Odontol Soc Great Britain 1865-1867;V.

8. Von Spee FG. The condylar path of the mandible in the glenoid fossa. Read at Kiel Germany March 24, 1890.

9. Bonwill WG. Scientific articulation of the human teeth as founded on geometrical, mathematical and mechanical laws. Items Int 1899;21:617–56, 873–80.

10. Monson GS. Occlusion as applied to crown and bridgework. J Am Dent Assoc 1920;7:399–413.

11. Gysi A. Practical application of research results in denture construction. J Am Dent Assoc 1929;16:199–223.

12. Schuyler CH. Factors of occlusion applicable to restorative dentistry. J Prosthet Dent 1953;3:772–82.

13. McCollum BB, Stuart CE. A research project. South Pasadena (CA): Scientific Press; 1955. p. 12–3, 34–86, 91.

14. Mann BS, Pankey LD. Oral rehabilitation: part I. Use of the P-M instrument in treatment planning and in restoring the lower posterior teeth. J Prosthet Dent 1960;10:135–50.

15. Mann BS, Pankey LD. Oral rehabilitation: part II. Restoration of the upper teeth using a functionally generated path technique. J Prosthet Dent 1960;10:151–62.

16. Mann AW, Pankey LD. Concepts of occlusion: the PM philosophy of occlusal rehabilitation. Dent Clin North Am 1963;9:621–39.

17. Guichet NF. Applied gnathology, why and how. Dent Clin North Am 1969;13:687–700.

18. Stuart CE. The contributions of gnathology to prosthodontics. J Prosthet Dent 1973;30:607–8.

19. Guichet NF. Biologic laws governing functions of muscles that move the mandible. Part I. Occlusal programming. J Prosthet Dent 1977;37:648–56.

20. Guichet NF. Biologic laws governing functions of muscles that move the mandible. Part II. Condylar position. J Prosthet Dent 1977;38:35–41.

21. Guichet NF. Biologic laws governing functions of muscles that move the mandible. Part III. Speed of closure–manipulation of the mandible. J Prosthet Dent 1977;38:174–9.

22. Guichet NF. Biologic laws governing functions of muscles that move the mandible. Part IV. J Prosthet Dent 1977;38:301–10.

23. Dawson PE. Evaluation, diagnosis and treatment of occlusal problems. 2nd edition. St Louis (MO): Mosby; 1989.

24. Ramford SP, Ash MM. Occlusion. 3rd edition. Philadelphia: WB Saunders; 1983.

25. Ash MM. Philosophy of occlusion: past and present. Dent Clin North Am 1995;39:233–55.

26. Okeson JP. Management of temporomandibular disorders and occlusion. 4th edition. St Louis (MO): Mosby Year Book; 1998.

27. McNeill C. Science and practice of occlusion. Chicago: Quintessence; 1997. p. 220–32.

28. Zarb GA, Carlsson GE, Sessle BJ, et al. Temporomandibular joint and masticatory muscle disorders. Copenhagen (Denmark): Munksgaard; 1994.
29. Taylor TD, Wiens J, Carr A. Evidence-based considerations for removable and dental implant occlusion: a literature review. J Prosthet Dent 2005;94: 555–60.
30. Pokorny PH, Wiens JP, Litvak H. Occlusion for fixed prosthodontics: a historical perspective of the gnathological influence. J Prosthet Dent 2008;99: 299–313.
31. Tsukiyama Y, Baba K, Clark GT. An evidence-based assessment of occlusal adjustment as a treatment for temporomandibular disorders. J Prosthet Dent 2001;86:57–66.
32. Ash MM. Occlusion: reflections on science and clinical reality. J Prosthet Dent 2003;90:373–84.
33. Ash MM. Occlusion, TMDs, and dental education. Head Face 2007;3:1. Review.
34. Pjetursson BE, Lang NP. Prosthetic treatment planning on the basis of evidence. J Oral Rehabil 2008;35:72–9.
35. Lee D, Wiens JP, Ference J, et al. Assessment of occlusion curriculum in predoctoral dental education: report from ACP task force on occlusion education. J Prosthodont 2012;21(7):578–87.
36. The Academy of Prosthodontics. Glossary of prosthodontic terms, 8th edition. J Prosthet Dent 2005;94:1–95.
37. Ahlgren J. Pattern of chewing and malocclusion of teeth. A clinical study. Acta Odontol Scand 1967;25:3–13.
38. Craddock HL. Occlusal changes following posterior tooth loss in adults. Part 3. A study of clinical parameters associated with the presence of occlusal interferences following posterior tooth loss. J Prosthodont 2008;17:25–30.
39. Tsiggos N, Tortopidis D, Hatzikyriako A, et al. Association between self-reported bruxism activity and occurrence of dental attrition, abfraction, and occlusal pits on natural teeth. J Prosthet Dent 2008;100:41–6.
40. Tallents RH, Macher DJ, Kyrkanides S, et al. Prevalence of missing posterior teeth and intraarticular temporomandibular disorders. J Prosthet Dent 2002; 87:45–50.
41. Kao RT, Chu R, Curtis D. Occlusal considerations in determining prognosis. J Calif Dent Assoc 2000;28:760–9.
42. Berry HM, Hofmann FA. Cineradiographic observations of temporomandibular joint function. J Prosthet Dent 1959;9:31–3.
43. Becker CM, Kaiser DA, Schwalm C. Mandibular centricity: centric relation. J Prosthet Dent 2000;83:158–60.
44. Moss ML. A functional cranial analysis of centric relation. Dent Clin North Am 1975;19:431–42.
45. Posselt U. Terminal hinge movement of the mandible. J Prosthet Dent 1957;7: 787–97.
46. Posselt U. The physiology of occlusion and rehabilitation. Philadelphia: FA Davis; 1962.
47. Johnston LE. Gnathological assessment of centric slides in postretention orthodontic patients. J Prosthet Dent 1988;60:712–5.
48. Celenza FV. The centric position: replacement and character. J Prosthet Dent 1973;30:591–8.
49. Woda A, Vigneron P, Kay D. Nonfunctional and functional occlusal contacts: a review of the literature. J Prosthet Dent 1979;42:335–41.

50. Schuyler CH. Fundamental principles in the correction of occlusal disharmony, natural and artificial. J Am Dent Assoc 1935;22:1193–202.

51. Wassell RW, Adams N, Kelly PJ. The treatment of temporomandibular disorders with stabilizing splints in general dental practice: one-year follow-up. J Am Dent Assoc 2006;137:1089–98.

52. Craddock MR, Parker MH, Cameron SM, et al. Artifacts in recording immediate mandibular translation: a laboratory investigation. J Prosthet Dent 1997;78: 172–8.

53. Clark GT, Tsukiyamka Y, Baba K, et al. Sixty-eight years of experimental occlusal interference studies: what have we learned. J Prosthet Dent 1999; 82:704–13.

54. Rugh JD, Barghi N, Drago CJ. Experimental occlusal discrepancies and nocturnal bruxism. J Prosthet Dent 1984;51:548–53.

55. Tarantola G, Becker I, Gremillion H, et al. The effectiveness of equilibration in the improvement of signs and symptoms of stomatognathic system. Int J Periodontics Restorative Dent 1998;18:595–603.

56. Agerberg G, Sandström R. Frequency of occlusal interferences: a clinical study in teenagers and young adults. J Prosthet Dent 1988;59:212–7.

57. Tsolka P, Morris RW, Preiskel HW. Occlusal adjustment therapy for craniomandibular disorders: a clinical assessment by double-blind method. J Prosthet Dent 1992;68:957–64.

58. Weinberg LA. An evaluation of basic articulators and their concepts. Part II: arbitrary, positional and semi adjustable articulators. J Prosthet Dent 1963;13: 645–63.

59. Taylor TD. Analysis of the lateral condylar adjustments on nonarcon semi adjustable articulators. J Prosthet Dent 1985;54:140–3.

60. Hobo S, Shillinburg HT, Whitsett LD. Articulator selection for restorative dentistry. J Prosthet Dent 1976;36:35–43.

61. Bellanti ND. The significance of articulator capabilities Part I. Adjustable vs. semi adjustable articulators. J Prosthet Dent 1973;29:269–75.

62. Curtis DA, Wachtel HC. Limitations of semi-adjustable articulators with provision for immediate side shift. Part II. J Prosthet Dent 1987;58:569–73.

63. Gracis S. Clinical considerations and rationale for the use of simplified instrumentation in occlusal rehabilitation. Part 2. Setting of the articulator and occlusal optimization. Int J Periodontics Restorative Dent 2003;23: 139–45.

64. Lux CJ, Conradt C, Burden D, et al. Three dimensional analysis of maxillary and mandibular growth increments. Cleft Palate Craniofac J 2004;41:304–14.

65. Heij DG, Opdebeeck H, Steenberghe D, et al. Facial development, continuous tooth eruption, and mesial drift as compromising factors for implant placement. Int J Oral Maxillofac Implants 2006;21:867–78.

66. Turner KA, Missirlian DM. Restoration of the extremely worn dentition. J Prosthet Dent 1984;52:467–74.

67. Niswonger ME. The rest position of the mandible and the centric relation. J Am Dent Assoc 1934;21:1572–82.

68. Silverman MM. The speaking method in measuring vertical dimension. J Prosthet Dent 1953;3:193–9.

69. Swerdlow H. Roentgencephalometric study of vertical dimension changes in immediate denture patients. J Prosthet Dent 1964;14:635–50.

70. Pound E. The mandibular movements of speech and their seven related values. J Prosthet Dent 1966;16:835–43.

71. Atwood DA. A cephalometric study of the clinical rest position of the mandible. Part I: the variability of the clinical rest position following the removal of occlusal contacts. J Prosthet Dent 1956;6:504–9.
72. Boos RH. Intermaxillary relation established by biting power. J Am Dent Assoc 1940;27:1192–9.
73. McGee GF. Use of facial measurements in determining vertical dimension. J Am Dent Assoc 1947;35:342–50.
74. Lytle RV. Vertical relation of occlusion by the patient's neuromuscular perception. J Prosthet Dent 1964;14:12–21.
75. Atwood DA. A critique of research of the rest position of the mandible. J Prosthet Dent 1966;16:848–54.
76. Smith DE. The reliability of pre-extraction records for complete dentures. J Prosthet Dent 1971;25:592–608.
77. Turrell AJ. Clinical assessment of vertical dimension. J Prosthet Dent 1972;28:238–45.
78. Vig RG, Brundo GC. The kinetics of anterior tooth display. J Prosthet Dent 1978;39:502–4.
79. DiPietro GJ, Moergheli JR. Significance of the FMA to prosthodontics. J Prosthet Dent 1976;36:624–35.
80. DiPietro GJ. A study of occlusion as related to the Frankfort-mandibular plane angle. J Prosthet Dent 1977;38:452–8.
81. Desjardins RP. Clinical evaluation of the wax trial denture. J Am Dent Assoc 1982;104:184–90.
82. Woda A, Pionchon P, Palla S. Regulation of mandibular postures: mechanisms and clinical implications. Crit Rev Oral Biol Med 2001;12:166–78.
83. Brown KE. Reconstruction considerations for severe dental attrition. J Prosthet Dent 1980;44:384–8.
84. Rivera-Morales WC, Mohl ND. Relationship of occlusal vertical dimension to the health of the masticatory system. J Prosthet Dent 1991;65:547–53.
85. D'Amico A. Functional occlusion of the natural teeth of man. J Prosthet Dent 1961;11:899–915.
86. Beyron HL. Occlusal relations and mastication in Australian Aborigines. Acta Odontol Scand 1964;22:597–678.
87. Beyron HL. Optimal occlusion. Dent Clin North Am 1969;13:537–54.
88. Thornton LJ. Anterior guidance: group function/canine guidance. A literature review. J Prosthet Dent 1990;64:479–82.
89. Scaife RR, Holt JE. Natural occurrence of cuspid guidance. J Prosthet Dent 1969;22:225–9.
90. Schuyler CH. The function and importance of incisal guidance in oral rehabilitation. J Prosthet Dent 2001;86:219–32.
91. Ross IF. Incisal guidance of natural teeth in adults. J Prosthet Dent 1974;31:155–62.
92. McAdam DB. Tooth loading and cuspal guidance in canine and group-function. J Prosthet Dent 1976;35:283–90.
93. Christensen C. The problem of the bite. D Cosmos 1905;47:1184–95.
94. Ogawa T, Kovano K, Suetsugu T. The influence of anterior guidance and condylar guidance on mandibular protrusive movement. J Oral Rehabil 1997;24:303–9.
95. Bennett NG. A contribution to the study of the movements of the mandible. Proc R Soc Med 1908;1:79–98.
96. Fischer R. Die Offnungsbewegungen des Unterkiefers und ihre Wiedergabe am Artikulator. Schweiz Monatsschr Zahnmed 1935;45:867–99 [in German].

97. Magnusson T, Enbom L. Signs and symptoms of mandibular dysfunction after introduction of experimental balancing-side interferences. Acta Odontol Scand 1984;42:129–35.
98. Williamson EH, Lundquist DO. Anterior guidance: its effect on electromyographic activity of the temporal and masseter muscles. J Prosthet Dent 1983; 49:816–23.
99. Shupe RJ, Mohamed SE, Christensen LV, et al. Effects of occlusal guidance on jaw muscle activity. J Prosthet Dent 1984;51:811–8.
100. Gibbs CH, Mahan PE, Wilkinson TM, et al. EMG activity of the superior belly of the lateral pterygoid muscle in relation to other jaw muscles. J Prosthet Dent 1984;51:691–702.
101. Rugh JD, Graham GS, Smith JC, et al. Effects of canine versus molar occlusal splint guidance on nocturnal bruxism and craniomandibular symptomatology. J Craniomandib Disord 1989;3:203–10.
102. Gibbs CH, Lundeen HC. Jaw movements and forces during chewing and swallowing and their clinical significance. In: Lundeen HC, Gibbs CH, editors. Advances in occlusion. Boston: John Wright; 1982. p. 2–32.
103. Hanau RL. Articulation defined, analyzed and formulated. J Am Dent Assoc 1926;13:1694–709.
104. Tamaki K, Celar AG, Beyrer S, et al. Reproduction of excursive tooth contact in an articulator with computerized axiography data. J Prosthet Dent 1997;78: 373–8.
105. Thielemann K. Die Artikulationsformel, em Hilfsmittel der Hanua-Artikulationslehre, Zahnarzti. Rundshau 1932;41:358–62 [in German].
106. Ambard A, Mueninghoff L. Planning restorative treatment for patients with severe class II malocclusions. J Prosthet Dent 2002;88:200–7.
107. Ngom PI, Diagne F, Aidara-Tambra AW, et al. Relationship between orthodontic anomalies and masticatory function in adults. Am J Orthod Dentofacial Orthop 2007;131:216–22.
108. Brose MO, Tanquist RA. The influence of anterior coupling on mandibular movement. J Prosthet Dent 1987;57:345–53.
109. Lotzmann U, Jablonski F, Scherer C, et al. The neuromuscular effect of anterior guidance on the protrusive movement pattern of the mandible. Observations in the horizontal plane. Schweiz Monatsschr Zahnmed 1990;100:560–4.
110. Angle EH. Treatment of malocclusion of the teeth and fractures of the maxillae, Angle's system. 6th edition. Philadelphia: SS White Dental; 1900.
111. Curtis TA, Langer Y, Curtis DA, et al. Occlusal considerations for partially or completely edentulous skeletal class II patient. Part I: background information. J Prosthet Dent 1988;60:202–11.
112. Curtis TA, Langer Y, Curtis DA, et al. Occlusal considerations for partially or completely edentulous skeletal class II patient. Part II: treatment concepts. J Prosthet Dent 1988;60:334–42.
113. Steiner CC. The use of cephalometrics as an aid to planning and assessing orthodontic treatment. Am J Orthod 1960;46:721–35.
114. Buschang PH, Throckmorton GS, Austin D, et al. Chewing cycle kinematics of subjects with deep bite malocclusion. Am J Orthod Dentofacial Orthop 2007; 131:627–34.
115. Fernandez Sanroman J, Gomez Gonzalez JM, del Hoyo JA. Relationship between condylar position, dentofacial deformity and temporomandibular joint dysfunction: a MRI and CT prospective study. J Craniomaxillofac Surg 1998; 26:35–42.

116. Gross MD, Cardash HS. Transferring anterior occlusal guidance to the articulator. J Prosthet Dent 1989;61:282–5.

117. Eichner K. Recent knowledge gained from long-term observations in the field of prosthodontics. Int Dent J 1984;34:35–40.

118. Kayser AF. Shortened dental arches and oral function. J Oral Rehabil 1981;8:457–62.

119. Mohl ND, Dixon DC. Current status of diagnostic procedures for temporomandibular disorders. J Am Dent Assoc 1994;125:56–64.

120. Sessle BJ, Bryant PS, Dionne RD. Temporomandibular disorders and related pain conditions, Progress in pain research and management, vol. 4. Seattle (WA): IASP Press; 1995.

121. Messerman T, Reswick JB, Gibbs C. Investigation of functional mandibular movements. Dent Clin North Am 1969;13:629–42.

122. Theusner J, Plesh O, Curtis DA, et al. Axiographic tracings of temporomandibular joint movements. J Prosthet Dent 1993;69:209–15.

123. Greene CS. Managing TMD patients: initial therapy is the key. J Am Dent Assoc 1992;123:43–5.

124. Baba KY, Tsukiyama Y, Yamazaki M, et al. A review of temporomandibular disorder diagnostic techniques. J Prosthet Dent 2001;86:184–94.

125. McNeill C, Mohl ND, Rugh JD, et al. Temporomandibular disorders: diagnosis, management, education and research. J Am Dent Assoc 1990;120:253, 255, 257.

126. Magnusson T, Egermark I, Carlsson GE. A longitudinal epidemiologic study of signs and symptoms of temporomandibular disorders from 15 to 35 years of age. J Orofac Pain 2000;14:310–9.

127. Mohl ND, Ohrbach R. Clinical decision making for temporomandibular disorders. J Dent Educ 1992;56:823–33.

128. Just JK, Perry HT, Greene CS. Treating TM disorders: a survey on diagnosis, etiology and management. J Am Dent Assoc 1991;122:55–60.

129. NIH Consensus Development Program. Management of temporomandibular disorders. 1996. Available at: http://www.nlm.nih.gov/medlineplus/. Accessed April 29–May 1, 1996

130. Greene CS, Marbach JJ. Epidemiologic studies of mandibular dysfunction: a critical review. J Prosthet Dent 1982;48:184–90.

131. Mohl ND, Ohrbach R. The dilemma of scientific knowledge versus clinical management of temporomandibular disorders. J Prosthet Dent 1992;67:113–20.

132. Fricton JR, Schiffman EL. The craniomandibular index: validity. J Prosthet Dent 1987;58:222–8.

133. Roda RP, Bagan JV, Bagan JV, et al. Review of temporomandibular joint pathology. Part I: classification, epidemiology and risk factors. Med Oral Patol Oral Cir Bucal 2007;12:E292–8.

134. Roda RP, Bagan JV, Bagan JV, et al. Review of temporomandibular joint pathology. Part II: clinical and radiological semiology. Med Oral Patol Oral Cir Bucal 2008;13:E102–9.

135. Schiffman EL, Truelove EL, Ohrbach R, et al. The research diagnostic criteria for temporomandibular disorders. I: overview and methodology for assessment of validity. J Orofac Pain 2010;24:7–24.

136. Ohrbach R, Turner JA, Sherman JJ, et al. Research diagnostic criteria for temporomandibular disorders: evaluation of psychometric properties of the axis II measures. J Orofac Pain 2010;24:48–62.

137. Rugh JD, Harlan J. Nocturnal bruxism and temporomandibular disorders. Adv Neurol 1988;49:329–41.
138. Rugh JD, Woods BJ, Dahlstrom L. Temporomandibular disorders: assessment of psychological factors. Adv Dent Res 1993;7:127–36.
139. Dworkin SF, Huggins KH, Wilson L, et al. A randomized clinical trial using research diagnostic criteria for temporomandibular disorders–axis II to target clinic cases for tailored self-care TMD treatment program. J Orofac Pain 2002;16:48–63.
140. Herb K, Cho S, Stiles MA. Temporomandibular joint pain and dysfunction. Curr Pain Headache Rep 2006;10:408–14.
141. Dawson PE. Functional Occlusion. St. Louis: Mosby Elsevier; 1997. p. 265–75.
142. Kerstein RB. Disocclusion time measurement studies: a comparison of disocclusion time between chronic myofascial pain dysfunction patients and nonpatients: a population analysis. J Prosthet Dent 1994;72:473–80.
143. Christensen GJ. Treating bruxism and clenching. J Am Dent Assoc 2000;131(2): 233–5.
144. Fricton J. Myogenous temporomandibular disorders: diagnostic and management considerations. Dent Clin North Am 2007;51:61–83.
145. Koh R, Robinson PG. Occlusal adjustment for treating and preventing temporomandibular disorders. Cochrane Database Syst Rev 2003:CD003812.
146. Kirveskari P, Alanen P, Jamsa T. Association between craniomandibular disorders and occlusal interferences. J Prosthet Dent 1989;62:66–9.
147. Seligman DA, Pullinger AG. The role of intercuspal occlusal relationships in temporomandibular disorders: a review. J Craniomandib Disord 1991;5(2): 96–106.
148. Seligman DA, Pullinger AG. The role of functional occlusal relationships in temporomandibular disorders: a review. J Craniomandibular Disord Fac Oral Pain 1991;5:265–79.
149. Kirveskari P, Alanen P, Jamsa T. Association between craniomandibular disorders and occlusal interferences in children. J Prosthet Dent 1992;67:692–6.
150. Tasaki MM, Westesson PL, Isberg AM, et al. Classification and prevalence of temporomandibular joint disk displacement in patients and symptom-free volunteers. Am J Orthod Dentofacial Orthop 1996;109:249–62.
151. Stockstill JW, Mohl ND. Evaluation of temporomandibular joint sounds. Diagnostic analysis and clinical implications. Dent Clin North Am 1991;35: 75–88.
152. Lundeen HC. Mandibular movement recordings and articulator adjustments simplified. Dent Clin North Am 1979;23:231–41.
153. Carr AB, Gibilisco JA, Berquist TH. Magnetic resonance imaging of the temporomandibular joint: preliminary work. J Craniomandib Disord 1987;1: 89–96.
154. Harvold EP. Centric relation. A study of pressure and tension systems in bone modeling and mandibular positioning. Dent Clin North Am 1975;19:473–84.
155. Arnett GW, Milam SB, Gottesman L. Progressive mandibular retrusion–idiopathic condylar resorption. Part I. Am J Orthod Dentofacial Orthop 1996;110: 8–15, 117–27.
156. Pullinger AG, Seligman DA. The degree to which attrition characterizes differentiated patient groups of temporomandibular disorders. J Orofac Pain 1993;7: 196–208.
157. Bates RE, Gremillion HA, Stewart CM. Degenerative joint disease. Part I: diagnosis and management considerations. Cranio 1993;11:284–90.

158. Kahn J, Tallents RH, Katzberg RW, et al. Association between dental occlusal variables and intraarticular temporomandibular joint disorders: horizontal and vertical overlap. J Prosthet Dent 1998;79:658–62.
159. Seligman DA, Pullinger AG. Analysis of occlusal variables, dental attrition, and age for distinguishing healthy controls from female patients with intracapsular temporomandibular disorders. J Prosthet Dent 2000;83:76–82.
160. Pullinger AG, Seligman DA. Quantification and validation of predictive values of occlusal variables in temporomandibular disorders using multifactorial analysis. J Prosthet Dent 2000;83:66–75.
161. Di Paolo C, D'Ambrosio F, Panti F, et al. The condyle-fossa relationship in tempo-romandibular disorders. Considerations on the pathogenetic role of the disc. Minerva Stomatol 2006;55:409–22.
162. John MT, Frank H, Lobbezoo F, et al. No association between incisal tooth wear and temporomandibular disorders. J Prosthet Dent 2002;87:197–203.
163. De Leeuw R, Boering G, Stegenga B, et al. Clinical signs of TMJ osteoarthrosis, and internal derangement 30 years after nonsurgical treatment. J Orofac Pain 1994;8:18–24.
164. Hinton RJ. Adaptive response of the articular eminence and mandibular fossa to altered function of the lower jaw: an overview. In: Carlson DS, McNamara IA, Ribbens KA, editors. Developmental aspects of temporomandibular joint disorders, Craniofacial Growth Series No. 16. Ann Arbor (MI): University of Michigan; 1985. p. 207–34.
165. Luder HU. Articular degeneration and remodeling in human temporomandibular joints with normal and abnormal disc position. J Orofac Pain 1993;7:391–402.
166. Sato J, Goto S, Nasu F, et al. The natural course of disc displacement with reduction of the temporomandibular joint: changes in clinical signs and symptoms. J Oral Maxillofac Surg 2003;61:32–4.
167. Henry CH, Whittum-Hudsnon JA, Tull GT, et al. Reactive arthritis and internal derangement of the temporomandibular joint. Oral Surg Oral Med Oral Pathol Oral Radiol Endod 2007;104:e22–6.
168. Stegenga B, De Bont LG, Boering G, et al. Tissue responses to degenerative changes in the temporomandibular joint: a review. J Oral Maxillofac Surg 1991;49:1079–88.
169. Greene CS. Temporomandibular disorders in the geriatric population. J Prosthet Dent 1994;72:507–9.
170. Dawson PE. New definition for relating occlusion to varying conditions of the temporomandibular joint. J Prosthet Dent 1995;74:619–27.
171. Litvak H, Malament KA. Prosthodontic management of temporomandibular disorders and orofacial pain. J Prosthet Dent 1993;69(1):77–84.
172. Gabler MJ, Greene CS, Palacios E, et al. Effect of arthroscopic temporomandibular joint surgery on articular disc position. J Craniomandib Disord 1989;3:191–202.
173. Ren YF, Isberg A, Westesson PL. Condyle position in the temporomandibular joint. Comparison between asymptomatic volunteers with normal disk position and patients with disk displacement. Oral Surg Oral Med Oral Pathol Oral Radiol Endod 1995;80:101–7.
174. Scapino RP. Histopathology associated with malposition of the human temporomandibular joint disk. Oral Surg Oral Med Oral Pathol 1983;55:382–97.
175. Curtis DA, Wiens J, Plesh O. Canine protected occlusion vs. group disclusion. In: Harpenau L, Kao R, Lundergan W, et al, editors. Hall's Critical Decisions in

Periodontology and Dental Implantology. 5th edition. People's Medical Publishing House-USA; 2013. p. 194–5.

176. Nyman S, Lindhe J, Lundgren D. The role of occlusion for the stability of fixed bridges in patients with reduced periodontal tissue support. J Clin Periodontol 1975;2:53–66.

Gingival Displacement for Impression Making in Fixed Prosthodontics

Contemporary Principles, Materials, and Techniques

Nadim Z. Baba, DMD, MSD[a],*, Charles J. Goodacre, DDS, MSD[b],
Rami Jekki, DDS[b], John Won, DDS, MS[b]

KEYWORDS

- Provisionals • Materials • Definitive impression

KEY POINTS

- Periodontal health and biotype needs to be evaluated and respected in order to preserve gingival position and form.
- Care must be taken not to violate the biologic width during definitive impression making.
- Tissue displacement must be gentle.
- Several techniques for tissue displacement are available.

The clinical success and longevity of indirect restorations depend on the careful and accurate completion of several procedures. One of the challenging procedures is management of the gingival tissues and gingival esthetics. The goal for management of gingival tissues and gingival esthetics is to maintain the normal appearance of healthy gingiva (**Figs. 1** and **2**). Achieving this goal requires optimal health before treatment and minimal trauma during treatment. The best way of optimizing health and minimizing trauma is to avoid contacting the gingiva with restorative materials. However, for esthetic or functional reasons, restoration margins are frequently located within the gingival sulcus.[1] One disadvantage of subgingival margins is that they have the tendency to increase the potential for periodontal problems (gingival inflammation).[2,3] However, periodontal health can be maintained in the presence of subgingival margins but it requires careful execution of the clinical procedures and well-fitting, properly contoured crowns.[4–6] Appropriate, reversible, gingival displacement and tissue management are required,

[a] Hugh Love Center for Research and Education in Technology, Loma Linda University, School of Dentistry, 11092 Anderson Street, Loma Linda, CA 92350, USA; [b] Department of Restorative Dentistry, Loma Linda University, School of Dentistry, Loma Linda, CA, USA
* Corresponding author.
E-mail address: nbaba@llu.edu

Dent Clin N Am 58 (2014) 45–68
http://dx.doi.org/10.1016/j.cden.2013.09.002
0011-8532/14/$ – see front matter © 2014 Elsevier Inc. All rights reserved.

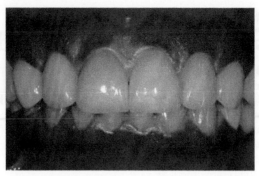

Fig. 1. Normal appearance of healthy gingiva following adequate management of gingival tissues.

which facilitates making the final impression so it accurately records the prepared finish line and some unprepared tooth structure apical to the finish line. The dies will thereby be true replicas of the prepared tooth. This article reviews the factors governing the preservation of gingival position and form along with contemporary and traditional techniques and materials available to obtain a minimally invasive and tissue friendly gingival displacement that preserves periodontal health while facilitating impression making.

FACTORS GOVERNING THE PRESERVATION OF GINGIVAL POSITION AND FORM
Pretreatment Periodontal Health/Periodontal Biotype

Before attempting to perform any gingival displacement technique, it is important to assess the periodontal health of the tooth or teeth involved. Healthy, firm, nonbleeding tissues should be present so there is an optimal intrasulcular environment.[1] Gingiva that is damaged or inflamed is more susceptible to bleeding, which makes it more challenging to obtain optimal accuracy in the impression, especially when a hydrophobic impression material is being used.[7]

The first step in periodontal evaluation of teeth should include an examination of the periapical and/or bitewing radiographs to determine the position of the alveolar crestal bone height and to rule out any pathologic abnormality. Undetected defects in the bone, such as angular bone loss or infrabony pockets, may lead to increased hemorrhage during the procedure and future tissue instability as a result of tissue manipulation in these areas. Therefore, a thorough radiographic examination is an integral component of a pretreatment periodontal evaluation.

The second step is to evaluate the periodontium visually. The color, contour, consistency, position, surface texture, and presence of pain should be evaluated to determine

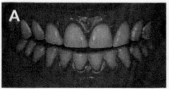
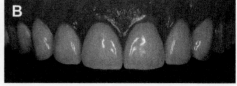

Fig. 2. (A) Preoperative clinical photo of a patient requiring maxillary anterior crowns. (B) Postoperative clinical photo showing a favorable tissue response following adequate management of gingival tissues.

if the gingiva is healthy. The gingival index is a valuable tool in gauging tissue condition.[8] Studies[9–11] found an elevated gingival index in sulci where displacement cords were packed, suggesting injury of the periodontium. All tissue displacement techniques produce trauma to the gingival tissue caused by mechanical or chemical trauma that creates an inflammatory response.[12] In vitro studies[13–15] found that displacement cords combined with chemical displacement agents were cytotoxic to the gingival fibroblasts. However, the injury inflicted by displacement cords is self-limited and reversible.[12,16]

The oral environment of some patients resists the trauma of prosthodontic procedures better than other patients. Slight trauma will usually not produce lasting effects if the gingiva is healthy before the treatment, whereas existing periodontal abnormalities cause exaggerated responses to the slightest tissue insults.

The third step in the pretreatment evaluation is to measure the sulcus depth. Teeth that require gingival displacement procedures will typically have their preparation finish lines located approximately 0.5 to 1.0 mm subgingivally and ideally within the sulcus. An attempt should be made to control the apical extension of the gingival manipulation so as to avoid placing the finish line apical to the base of the gingival sulcus, into the epithelial and connective tissue attachments. Therefore, careful measurement of sulcus depth with a periodontal probe should be made and recorded to calculate how deep the finish line should be placed and how much displacement is possible or necessary to maintain the harmony of the periodontium. Accelerated bone loss could not be documented in a critical evaluation of available evidence because commonly reported changes in probing depths were less than 1 mm, a dimension smaller than the probing accuracy of clinicians.[17] Therefore, subgingival margins most commonly result in negative esthetic changes in the gingiva rather than accelerated bone loss (**Fig. 3**).

When choosing a displacement technique, it is also important to identify the type of tissue being manipulated. Periodontal biotypes were first described by Ochsenbein and Ross in 1969.[18,19] Two biotypes have been described, the thick, flat biotype and the thin, scalloped biotype.[20] They are terms that have been used to describe the tissue thickness and the amount of scalloping of the interdental papilla in different individuals.

In the thick, flat biotype, there is minimal to moderate distance between the location of the midfacial gingival crest and the height of the interproximal papilla (one-half or less of the incisocervical crown dimension). The gingiva is thicker, more fibrotic with an increase in quantity and quality of masticatory mucosa. There is also a greater probing depth and the gingival margin is usually located on enamel. The distance between the cementoenamel junction (CEJ) and the bony crest is about 2 mm. In addition, the underlying bone has limited scalloping and there are usually no bony dehiscences or fenestrations (**Fig. 4**).

The thin, scalloped biotype presents with thin, delicate gingiva, a limited amount of attached gingiva, and the quality of that present is not ideal. The probing depth is

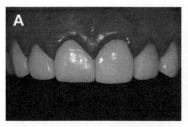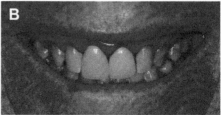

Fig. 3. (*A*) Gingival tissues have negatively responded to overcontoured laminate veneers. (*B*) Gingival tissues have responded negatively to overcontoured crowns.

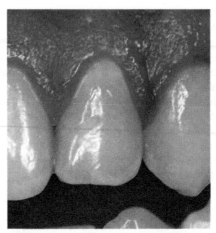

Fig. 4. Appearance of gingival tissue in a thick, flat biotype.

shallow and the gingival margin is frequently not on enamel. It is located at the CEJ or on the root surface with pretreatment recession.[21] There is an increased distance (approximately 4 mm) between the CEJ and the bone. The underlying bone is scalloped, and bony dehiscences and/or fenestrations are often present. One of the characteristics of the thin biotype is that there is a substantial difference between the location of the midfacial gingival crest and the height of the interproximal papilla (a dimension that can equal more than one-half of the incisocervical crown dimension). Thin biotypes present with an acute "gingival angle." This angle is formed by lines connecting the most apical location of facial gingiva and the most coronal papillae heights. In the thin biotype there may be recession present in the absence of any dental restorations, indicating that subgingival restorations are likely to create further recession. It is more difficult to have interdental papilla that fills spaces around both teeth and implants (**Fig. 5**).

A clinical study by Olsson and colleagues[22] evaluated photographically the periodontal characteristics in 113 individuals with varying forms of the maxillary central incisors. They found that individuals with tapered coronal outline forms of maxillary central incisors experienced more gingival recession on facial surfaces. They also

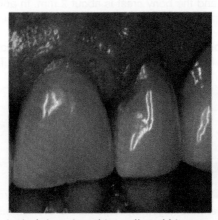

Fig. 5. Appearance of gingival tissue in a thin, scalloped biotype.

determined that maxillary central incisor crown outline form can be used to differentiate between biotypes.

In another study on the relationship between form and clinical features of the gingiva, Olsson and Lindhe[23] examined 108 adolescents between the ages of 16 and 19 lacking any signs of destructive periodontal disease. They found the tapered crown form had greater papilla height and more acute gingival angle (75°–78° vs 87°–97°) than square teeth. Square maxillary central incisor crown forms had significantly wider zones of keratinized gingiva and probing depths were significantly greater. However, they found no significant difference between free gingival thickness and the cervical crown convexity. In the presence of a susceptible environment due to the presence of a thin, scalloped periodontal biotype, it is especially important that oral hygiene be optimized before the initiation of prosthodontic procedures.

Biologic Width

To understand the nature of gingival displacement techniques fully, first the natural state of the periodontium and its relationship with the dentition must be appreciated. To accomplish this, one must understand the components of the physiologic dentogingival complex. It is a proportional relationship between the alveolar bone crest, connective tissue attachment, the epithelial attachment, and the sulcus depth.[24] The alveolar bone crest describes the most coronally positioned portion of the alveolar process. Many connective tissue fibers attach to this portion of bone and it serves as the main bony housing for the teeth. The connective tissue attachment is also referred to as gingival connective tissue and the lamina propria. It consists of 2 layers. The first is the reticular layer, which lies adjacent to the periosteum that connects to the alveolar bone. The second is a papillary layer that is characterized by papillary projections that are woven in between the epithelial rete pegs. The epithelial attachment is the zone of attachment that contains the junctional epithelium and usually ranges from 0.25 to 1.35 mm in length. This type of epithelium regenerates after surgical interventions. It is connected to both enamel and cementum by relatively weak adhesions called hemidesmosomes.[25] The gingival sulcus is the thin, V-shaped space that is found between the free gingiva and the surface of the tooth. The depth of the sulcus is susceptible to change, dependent on the amount of inflammation of gingival tissue. It has been reported that a normal depth of the sulcus falls in the range of 0.5 to 1 mm.

The concept of "biologic width" began with Gargiulo and colleagues[24] in 1961 when they described findings after examining the physiologic dentogingival complex in 30 human cadavers for a total of 287 teeth. It was reported that the average measurement for sulcus depth was 0.69 mm, the epithelial attachment was 0.97 mm, and the connective tissue attachment was 1.07 mm. Thus, it has been commonly stated that based on this research, the biologic width is 2.04 mm. However, other studies have also shown that there is a wide variance in the length of the epithelial attachment, ranging from 1.0 to 9.0 mm.[26] Based on Gargiulo's concept, Cohen coined the term "biologic width" for a lecture discussing the periodontal preparation of the mouth for prosthodontic procedures.[27] Although the exact dimensions of the "biologic width" can be different from person to person, it is widely accepted that restorations should not extend beyond 0.5 to 1.0 mm into the gingival sulcus.[28] It is of integral importance to the maintenance of the healthy periodontium that no restorative effort violates the junctional epithelium or connective tissue fiber apparatus. Furthermore, the authors also suggested maintaining a 3.0-mm safety zone between the crest of the alveolar bone and the margin of a crown. Because it is not possible to detect clinically, through tactile sensation, where the sulcus ends and the junctional epithelium begins, the authors suggested that this zone of safety be recommended.

The consequences of violating the biologic width have been described in the dental literature.[29] If the margins of dental restorations were to extend into the junctional epithelium or beyond, marginal and papillary gingivitis can be observed. Furthermore, this condition can lead to chronic inflammation and progress to periodontitis.

Displacement Cord Positioning Force

Minimally traumatic tissue displacement is necessary to maintain a healthy periodontium that plays an important role in the survival rate of fixed restorations.[9,30] Exerting heavy force to position gingival displacement cord can cause injury to the crevicular epithelium, the junctional epithelium, and the supra-alveolar connective tissue fibers (**Fig. 6**).[1] Heavy forces might also injure the periodontal fibers and disturb the blood supply.[10] Löe and Silness[8] showed that heavy forces during positioning of displacement cord could destroy the uppermost Sharpey fiber. As a result, gingival recession can be observed, and occasionally, loss of attachment.[11,16] Only one study[31] measured the amount of pressure generated by displacement cords or cordless displacement. They found that the pressure generated by displacement cords (5396 KPa) is significantly higher than the one generated by cordless displacement (143 KPa) when using a thick, firm, and viscous paste, containing chloride. Clinicians have the tendency to apply more force when the patient is anesthetized and does not feel any pressure and/or pain during cord placement.[32]

Displacement Time

The amount of time that a cord should be allowed to remain in the sulcus is an important factor. The goal of the clinician is to leave the cord long enough to create adequate displacement of the gingiva for impression making. However, to preserve periodontal health, it is also important not to leave the cord in the sulcus too long. Studies[11,16,33–39] demonstrated no prolonged harmful effects of the epithelial attachment when the cords are placed in the sulcus in a careful manner for a reasonable time, and healthy gingival tissues will heal in a few days. Anneroth and Nordenram[40] showed that dry cords placed in the sulcus adhere to the crevicular epithelium. When the cord is removed before

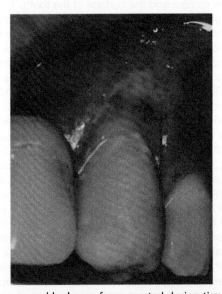

Fig. 6. Gingival recession caused by heavy force exerted during tissue displacement.

impression making, the crevicular epithelium is torn and removed, thereby inducing a wound-healing reaction.

The amount of time needed for cords to remain in the sulcus has been evaluated by several authors and was found to range from 1 minute to 30 minutes.[16,33–36,41] Fischer[34] recommended the use of a cord impregnated with ferric sulfate (FS) for 1 minute to provide the amount of displacement needed. Baharav and colleagues[36] tested a 2-cord technique for tissue displacement and concluded that the cords need to stay in the sulcus for 4 minutes before impression-making to produce sufficient crevicular width expansion. Benson and colleagues[33] found that 10 to 20 minutes of gingival displacement will allow the clinician enough time (30 minutes) to make multiple impressions. In a dog study, Harrison concluded that nonmedicated cord was safely used for up to 30 minutes.[16] There is no long-term damage to the periodontal tissue when short placement times are used, provided the healing process is not disturbed. Ramadan and colleagues[35] showed that cords placed no longer that 3 minutes in the sulcus will allow the clinician to get adequate healing. Several studies[11,16,32,38,39,41–43] demonstrated that displacement cords cause destruction of the junctional epithelium that takes between 5 and 14 days to heal. Although precise time recommendations are not available, the above studies reveal the importance of reducing gingival displacement as much as possible.

Based on the total time of retraction, it is important to consider the protocol to be used carefully when a large number of teeth are being prepared in the presence of a thin biotype. It might be prudent to prepare one tooth to completion with cord present, then remove the cord and move to the next tooth. After all the teeth are prepared, then repack the previously prepared teeth rather than leave the cord in the sulcus of the first prepared teeth while the remainder is being prepared.

MATERIALS FOR TISSUE DISPLACEMENT
Displacement Cords

The use of displacement cord is the most popular method for tissue displacement in fixed prosthodontics.[30,33] In a 1985 survey of North American dentists, Donovan and colleagues[44] showed that 95.55% of them use displacement cords routinely in their practice. A more recent survey of 1246 prosthodontists regarding their current methods used to expose their margin preparation revealed that 98% of respondents use displacement cords and 48% use a 2-cord technique for more than half of their impressions.[30]

Different types of cords have been advocated for tissue displacement (unwaxed floss, 2/0 untreated surgical silk, twisted cords, synthetic material). However, 2 types have become the primary ones used clinically: braided and knitted cords (**Fig. 7**).[9,11,45–47] There is a lack of standardization in cord size and clinical efficacy, making the choice of displacement cord based on the personal preference of the clinician. The cords

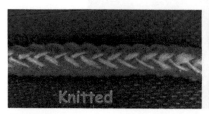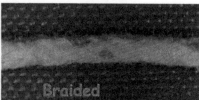

Fig. 7. Primary type of retraction cords used clinically.

can be dispensed from a container (which could lead to cross-contamination), a clicker, or precut and individually wrapped (which eliminates guessing the length of the cord needed for each tooth) (**Fig. 8**).

Braided cords have been described as having a consistent and tight weave. The braiding makes them resistant to separation during placement and therefore they are considered to be easy to manipulate and pack into place.[48] Regardless of the configuration, these cords absorb the medicaments efficiently and do not split or tear during placement. A clinical study aimed at comparing the performance of 3 types of displacement cords found that the braided cords were ranked better than the twisted ones.[49] Both serrated or smooth packing instruments can be used with braided cords without any concern to the clinician. Several packing instruments are available to purchase from manufacturers and vary in design and angulation. The choice of the instrument depends on the clinician's preference.

Knitted cords have substantially increased in popularity in recent years due to their ease of placement and their ability to expand when wet, making them easy to insert in the sulcus.[50] They are also available in different diameters and colors and similarly to the braided cords they lack standardization among manufacturers. Their design requires the use of thin, smooth, and nonserrated instruments. Serrated instruments can lift loosely woven cords out of the sulcus. It is suggested to start the cord placement in the interproximal area where tissue is more easily displaced. The authors think that a periodontal probe can be effectively used when the gingiva is thin and delicate and there is minimal sulcus depth (**Fig. 9**).

Hemostatic Medicaments

Questionnaires (1246 of 2436) reviewing the current methods used by prosthodontists to expose the finish line showed that 81% of prosthodontists soak their cords in a hemostatic agent before placing them into the sulcus. Fifty-five percent used aluminum chloride (AC), 23% used FS or ferric subsulfate, and 70% used an additional agent after the cord is placed. For that purpose, FS in an infuser syringe was most commonly used.[30] Several medicaments (aluminum potassium sulfate [Alum], aluminum sulfate, AC) have been shown to provide sufficient tissue displacement without any iatrogenic effect on the soft tissue.[44]

Several hemostatic medicaments are available to be used in conjunction with displacement cords and many have been substantially studied.[35,44,51–54]

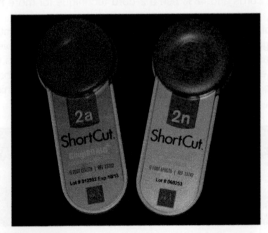

Fig. 8. Clicker cord dispenser.

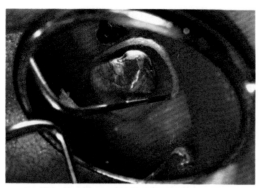

Fig. 9. Use of a periodontal probe for cord placement in the case of thin gingiva with minimal sulcus depth.

Epinephrine

In the 1980s it was determined that 55% to 79% of dentists used displacement cords impregnated with epinephrine.[55] A recent survey indicated that the percentage of dentists using epinephrine for tissue displacement decreased when compared with previous years.[30] Epinephrine is known to cause adverse cardiovascular problems (hypertension, increased heart rate)[56,57] and/or other symptoms such as anxiety, increased respiratory rate, tachycardia, and, in rare instances, death.[33,44,58–62]

Human and animal studies[44,58,60,63–65] evaluating the effect of epinephrine absorbed from displacement cords packed in the gingival sulcus expressed some concerns about the adverse health effects of this medicament. There is approximately 50 times more epinephrine in 1 inch of displacement cord than in 1 carpule of 1:100.000 epinephrine.[66] Under certain conditions, epinephrine is absorbed systematically when used in conjunction with a displacement cord. Reducing the concentration and the contact time of epinephrine with the gingiva seemed to reduce the adverse effects. Of 495 surveyed dentists, 396 used displacement cords with epinephrine. Twenty percent of these dentists had patients with significant systemic side effects. A 3% increase in their patient's pulse and 9% increase in blood pressure were recorded. They concluded that dentists have equally effective agents available on the market for them to use with no systemic side effects.[44] A histologic study on the effect of several displacement materials on the gingival sulcus epithelium showed that an extended contact of epinephrine with the crevicular epithelium could cause necrosis.[16] The use of epinephrine can expose the underlying connective tissue and setup a wound-healing response that could result in a less that ideal gingival response for some patients.

Other studies[44,64] showed that a low concentration of epinephrine could safely be used in displacement cords without concerns for side effects. However, there is a general consensus that epinephrine should be avoided for tissue displacement given the significant number of complications that can occur specifically in patients with cardiovascular problems[44,53,67,68] in addition to a pronounced vasoconstrictor effect.[33,44,65,69]

Several studies[12,49,51,57] compared the effectiveness of epinephrine to other medicaments available for tissue displacement. In a blind study, Jokstad[49] found that neither the students nor the faculty members that participated in the experiment could tell the difference between gingival displacement obtained by epinephrine or aluminum sulfate. He concluded that no clinical benefit could be recognized between an epinephrine- or an AC-containing cord. Similarly to the previous study, Weir and Williams[51] found that epinephrine did not produce superior displacement to AC. In another study, no practical difference was found between potassium aluminum sulfate, epinephrine, and AC.[12] In addition, Pelzner and colleagues[57] found that epinephrine-impregnated cords produce an unsatisfactory amount of tissue displacement and lead to 60% of impression remake.

Astringents

Astringents are metal salts that cause contraction of the gingival tissue by contracting small blood vessels. They precipitate tissue and blood proteins that physically inhibit bleeding by decreasing exudation and making the surface of the gingival tissue tougher.[66,70] These hemostatic agents do not penetrate the cells; they only affect the superficial layer of the mucosa.[70] However, an extended duration of contact with the gingival tissues can cause delayed healing or tissue damage.[50,71,72] The pH of the hemostatic agents differs from one company to the other.[73] Some studies demonstrated that they are highly acidic and their use removes the smear layer,[61,74–76] a potential cause of postoperative sensitivity and an adverse effect on the bonding mechanism of adhesive cements.[76,77]

Hemostatic agents are available in liquids or gels and the most commonly used are aluminum sulfate, AC, Alum, FS, and nasal and ophthalmic decongestants.[33,41,44,62] Recently, manufacturers introduced hemostatic agents in the form of pastes or foam (Expasyl, Gingitrac, Magic foam cord, Racegel, Traxodent).[31,32,43]

Liquids/Gels

One of the popular hemostatic agents is AC with a concentration ranging from 20% to 25% (**Fig. 10**). Studies showed that a 5% to 10% AC solution along with a displacement cord is safe and effective.[35,58] However, if used with in concentrations higher that 10%, AC can be irritating and may cause damage to the gingival tissue.[72] Buffered AC was introduced to prevent irritation of the gingival tissue. Reiman[41] found that AC is least irritating with no permanent damage to gingival tissue when the solution is left in the sulcus for up to but not exceeding 15 minutes. Several authors recommend soaking the displacement cords in AC to enhance hemostasis and avoid laceration of the gingival tissue.[33,51] Runyan and colleagues[54] studied the effect of soaking displacement cords in AC on moisture absorption. They concluded that doing so has no effect on the cord's ability to absorb fluid.

Several studies[78–81] evaluated the effect of hemostatic agents on the polymerization of poly(vinyl siloxane) (PVS) impression material. One study[78] found that hemostatic agents interfered with the quality of surface detail reproduction of the PVS due to the presence of sulfur in these agents. In contract, other studies[79–81] concluded that hemostatic medicaments showed no inhibitory potential over PVS.

Another popular hemostatic agent is FS with a concentration ranging from 12.7% to 20% (**Fig. 11**). At high concentration FS is highly acidic and an irritant to the gingival tissues.[61,62,66,74] For optimal results, FS can be rubbed into the bleeding area using a soaked cotton pellet or an even better technique is to use a dento-infuser syringe tip to burnish the gingival surface with the FS (**Fig. 12**). Due to its high iron content, FS can cause a brown-to-black staining of dentin under porcelain crowns[82] and similarly of the gingival tissues.[39] Fumed silica is added to Viscostat to limit the acid activity, making it kinder to hard and soft tissue.

When FS is used as a hemostatic agent, Machado and Guedes[80] found it to affect the accuracy of surface detail reproduction of PVS. Thus, it is important to rinse and remove all remnants of the FS on hard and soft tissue with a pumice and water paste to create a dentin smear layer before impression making.[78] The authors of this article have found that cotton pellets soaked in AC can be used to remove the FS from a tooth's surface and the AC can subsequently be rinsed away with water.

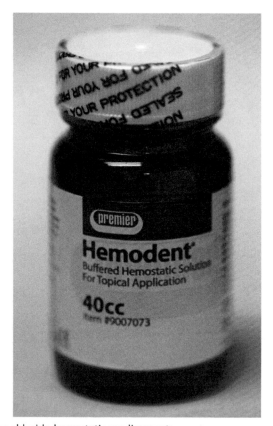

Fig. 10. Aluminum chloride hemostatic medicaments.

Alum and aluminum sulfate have also been suggested as hemostatic medicaments. They are not widely used due their limited properties and irritating effect. However, studies[44,51,65] found that they are safe hemostatic agents with no systemic effects when used properly. A cord impregnated with Alum can be safely left the sulcus for as long as 20 minutes without any adverse effects.[33] In a 100% concentration Alum was shown to be only slightly less effective in shrinking the gingival tissues than epinephrine with less inflammatory changes in the gingival tissue.[12]

Recently, sympathomimetic amines like tetrahydrozoline (Visine) or oxymetazoline hydrochloride (visine LR), used in ophthalmic or nasal decongestants, have been suggested as hemostatic agents. They produce local vasoconstriction with minimal side effects[62] and can be purchased over the counter. In an animal study[83] the use of tetrahydrozoline solution had fewer adverse effects on epithelial cells than a 25% AC solution. Sabio and colleagues[79] studied the effect of these solutions on the tensile strength and inhibition of polymerization of 4 types of impression materials. They found that they affected neither the tensile strength nor the polymerization of the tested impression materials.

Pastes/Foam/Gel

Cordless displacement materials (CDM) have been recently introduced as an alternative to the liquid hemostatic medicaments. They are available in different forms (paste, foam, or gel) and meant to be injected or packed into the sulcus **(Fig. 13)**.[31,32,43,47,84,85]

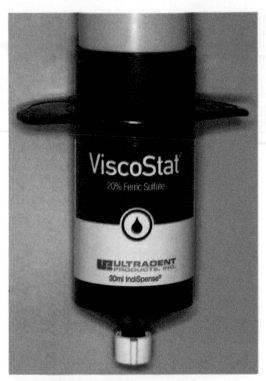

Fig. 11. Ferric sulfate hemostatic medicaments.

CDM in the form of pastes are thick, firm, and viscous and contain 15% AC along with 85% fillers (mostly a Kaolin matrix) in addition to water and some modifiers.[86] Bennani and colleagues[31] showed that their viscosity decreased with increasing shear stress demonstrating a typical pseudoplastic behavior. This high concentration of AC (>10%) can cause local tissue damage, transient ischemia,[32,44,66] and tooth sensitivity.[32] In contrast, it has been determined that CDM are less traumatic to the gingival tissue than conventional displacement cords, less painful to the patient, and quicker to deliver.[43,87,88] After making an impression using CDM, studies showed that gingival tissues recovered within a week.[32,43] Yang and colleagues[88] compared epinephrine-impregnated cords to CDM and found that they demonstrate clinically insignificant tissue recession.

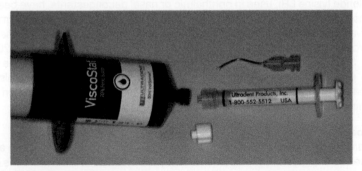

Fig. 12. Viscostat Dento-infuser system.

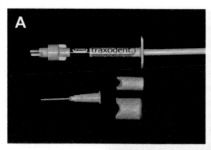
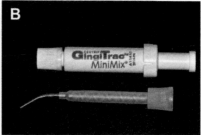
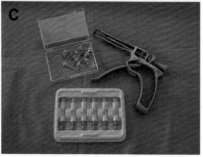

Fig. 13. Cordless displacement materials. (*A*) Traxodent system. (*B*) GingiTrac system. (*C*) Expasyl system.

They are preferred for tissue displacement around cement-retained implant prostheses and for Computer-aided design/Computer-aided manufacturing digital impressions.[89] The amount of displacement obtained with this material can be very limited especially in deeply positioned implants and with deep subgingival margins preparations.[85,89] CDM generated 37.7 times less pressure at placement than displacement cord.[31]

Another form of CDM paste is also available but does not contain any hemostatic agent. It is a PVS paste that works by generating hydrogen and expanding in the sulcus[89] and can also be used in conjunction with a compression cap to enhance the displacement effects of the material. Hemostasis must be obtained before applying the paste and the compression cap. Similar to the previously discussed paste, studies showed that gingival tissues recovered within a week following the use of these CDM impression pastes.[32,43]

Experimental CDM strips were also introduced in 1996.[47] This soft material called Merocel (Merocel Co, Mystic, CT, USA) is a synthetic polymer, spongelike in texture, cut into 2-mm strips. The strips are easily shaped and adaptable to the sulcus. Merocel displacement material is extensively used in medicine[90] and very effective for absorption of fluids, blood, and saliva. When placed in the sulcus, the material swells and effectively expands the gingival tissue away from the finish line.[47] Following impression making, the soft tissue completely recovered within 24 hours. Similarly to the other CMD, this material works best when the gingival margins are not too subgingival.[47]

TECHNIQUES FOR TISSUE DISPLACEMENT
Mechanochemical Tissue Displacement

The single cord technique
The single cord technique is indicated when making an impression for a small number of abutments with healthy tissues and no hemorrhage. It is the easiest technique to

accomplish and is useful when the prepared margins are juxta or supragingival or when the sulcus depth is not deep enough for a second cord to be located apical to the finish line. A single cord presoaked with hemostatic medicament is packed in the sulcus. The cord can be removed right before making the final impression or left in the sulcus to control bleeding and tissue fluids if the finish line is completely visible and the cord is positioned below the finish line with unprepared tooth structure present occlusal to the cord. Excellent results are obtained when the soft tissue maintains its lateral displacement and the finish line is visible after tissue displacement. If the tissues collapse over the packed cord and prevent visual access to the prepared finish lines, a less than accurate final impression can be obtained with possible tear of the impression material in that area. In such a case, some clinicians[91–93] recommend using electrosurgery (ES) or a soft tissue laser to excise the collapsed tissue obstructing access to the prepared finish line.

The double cord technique

The double cord technique is indicated when making an impression for single or multiple abutments. Even though the technique takes additional time to place a second cord and the gingival displacement associated with 2 cords has the potential to induce more gingival trauma, many clinicians have used it very successfully in their practices. A survey of 1246 prosthodontists regarding their current methods used to expose their margin preparation revealed that 48% of respondents use a 2-cord technique for more than half of their impressions.[30]

This technique is beneficial when the finish line is located sufficiently below the gingival margin that 2 cords can be placed into the sulcus. It is also effective when the soft tissue encompasses the first cord and does not maintain lateral tissue displacement. A small diameter cord, presoaked with hemostatic medicament, is positioned at the base of the gingival sulcus to prevent hemorrhage and seepage. The finish line must be visible after the first small cord is placed into the sulcus. A second cord, larger in diameter and also impregnated with hemostatic medicament, is placed into the sulcus on top of the first cord. The small diameter cord remains in place at the time the impression is made to reduce the collapse of the gingival tissue, control hemorrhage, and reduce the tearing of the impression material.[39] Before making the final impression, the second cord is removed while the smaller diameter cord is left in place.

The authors of this article suggest that the sulcus and the cords not be desiccated but all surface moisture be removed using compressed air. Desiccation causes the second cord to adhere to the soft tissue and when removed bleeding is more likely to occur. Likewise, the impression material is more likely to adhere to the first smaller diameter cord when the area is desiccated, causing adherence of the impression material to the smaller cord and greater potential for impression material tearing when the impression is removed because the cord often becomes incorporated into the polymerized impression material. It is most ideal when the impression is removed and the first, smaller diameter cord remains in the sulcus.

Surgical Tissue Displacement

ES

ES, also referred to as tissue dilation or troughing, has been used alone or as an adjunct to mechanochemical tissue displacement.[91,92,94,95] ES is mostly used to reduce hyperplastic tissues, expose the gingival margins, and prevent bleeding (**Fig. 14**).[91,94,96] It is also used to widen the gingival sulcus without reducing the height of the gingival margin so the impression material gains access to the prepared finish line and records some

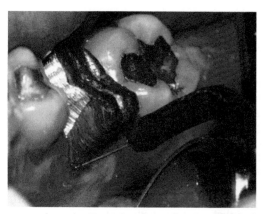

Fig. 14. Electrosurgery used on the lingual surface of a mandibular first molar to obtain tissue displacement.

tooth structure apical to the finish line. It also facilitates removal of the impression after polymerization without tearing of the marginal material.

The purpose of ES is to remove several layers of cells from the inner lining of the gingival sulcus, creating tissue displacement.[92] Careful patient selection and a thorough review of the medical history are required when ES is planned. Even though the new generation of pacemakers and implanted cardioverter defibrillators are protected by electric filters and shunting systems designed to detect and direct inappropriate current flow away from them,[97,98] the use of ES is strongly contraindicated in patients with pacemakers and implanted cardioverter defibrillators. The electromagnetic interference created in patients that are pacemaker dependent can be life threatening.[97] In addition, ES should be used with caution in esthetically sensitive areas because healing is unpredictable following the removal of the gingival tissue.

Different types of electrode scalpels are available for use with a fully rectified, undamped high-frequency alternating current.[91,92] Maness and colleagues[99] compared tissue alteration produced by several electrosurgical machines with varying frequencies and waveforms. They found that the full-wave rectification machines with high frequency and a continuous-output waveform produced less tissue alteration than the other type of machines they used. The most effective electrode for tissue displacement is a 0.5-mm diameter electrode used with constant motion.[100] Concerns were raised on the effect of ES on the pulp when the electrodes are in contact with a metallic restoration. Several authors found that there will be adverse effects on the pulpal and periodontal tissue if the electrodes are in contact with the metallic restoration for an extended period of time.[101–103] Other complications related to the inappropriate selection and use of an electrode include gingival recession, tissue necrosis, and/or loss of cellular definition. When used safely, ES has no adverse effects on wound healing.[104–107] Studies found that there is no significant difference in wound healing between a surgical scalpel and ES.[105–107] However, when used for a deep gingival resection, damage to the deep tissue layers (cementum or bone) and retarded healing were observed.[96,107,108] Repeated use of the electrode in the same area caused severe tissue damage.[96] Hence, it is strongly recommended to confine the use of ES to the free gingival tissue.

Most studies agree that soft tissues return to their normal appearance between 7 and 10 days[94,96,104,106] with no significant loss of gingival height.[96,102] Postoperatively, patients could experience a small reduction in the gingival margin (0.5–1.0 mm)[100,104] and some pain following the use of ES. The most painful areas are the palatal of the maxillary anterior sextant and the area of the third molars.[100] Severity of pain could range from slight to severe and the use of over-the-counter analgesics is recommended.

Rotary gingival curettage

Rotary gingival curettage (RGC) has been advocated by some clinicians as an alternative tissue displacement to ES. When selecting this technique, it is important to have an attached gingiva free of inflammation with an acceptable width of marginal gingiva and a high degree of keratinization.[109] RGC, similarly to ES, removes the inner epithelium of the gingival sulcus along with some of the underlying connective tissue.[100,110] The results after healing are not predictable. However, when compared with ES, RGC showed no significant difference in tissue response both clinically and histologically.[46,111] Complete tissue healing was obtained after 10 days. In contrast, another study showed that curettage with a rotary instrument is more likely to produce gingival recession than ES (gingival recession greatest with rotary instrument, minimal with ES, none with retraction cord).[3] The authors of this article do not recommend gingival curettage as a technique for tissue displacement in any area where changes in gingival position would produce a negative esthetic result.

Laser tissue sculpting for tissue displacement

Laser tissue sculpting for tissue displacement has offered the practitioner an alternative surgical technique for tissue displacement (see **Fig. 13**). Laser is an acronym from *Light amplification by stimulated emission of radiation*. It is a device that generates an intense (high energy) beam of coherent monochromatic light converted into thermal energy (heat) when it enters the soft tissue. The result is the vaporization or ablation of the targeted tissue, hence a controlled coagulation that increases hemostasis. Diode lasers are most commonly used for tissue displacement because of their low wavelength (near infrared spectrum). Other types of lasers can also be used for tissue displacement: Neodynium-doped yttrium aluminum garnet (Nd:YAG) and Erbium-doped yttrium aluminum garnet. The use of a laser results in minimal or no postoperative pain and can sometimes be used selectively without anesthesia. They displace gingival tissues and the result is less hemorrhage and gingival recession.[112,113] Abdel Gabbar and Aboulazm[113] compared mechanochemical to laser tissue displacement. They found that the laser resulted in less hemorrhage and less inflammation with a faster, painless gingival healing. In a recent study, Gherlone and colleagues[93] compared the diode laser, Nd:YAG laser, and the double-cord technique when used for gingival displacement in fixed prosthodontics. They found that lasers are more effective than conventional methods in obtaining hemostasis. However, they run at a higher operating cost. They also concluded that the diode lasers exhibited better hemostasis than the double-cord technique and the Nd:YAG lasers.

Although there is potential for the use of lasers in dentistry, Christensen[114] indicated that removing soft tissue with a surgical scalpel or ES is faster than cutting it with a laser.

SULCUS INSPECTION FOR RETAINED FOREIGN MATERIALS

Following injection of impression material into the gingival sulcus and removal of the tray after final material polymerization, a thorough inspection should be performed to insure that no impression material or retraction cords have been retained in the gingival sulcus. Several cases of swelling, pain, and periodontal inflammation have been reported following the retention of impression materials in the sulcus (see

Fig. 6).[115–118] Follow-up reports[119] showed that a healthy gingival complex was obtained following the removal of the retained material.

In addition, the sulcus should be inspected for any remnants of provisional cement that could be left in the sulcus following cementation of the provisional crown/prosthesis. Fragments of cements can cause gingival inflammation and possible tissue recession.

PROVISIONAL PROSTHESIS

Following tissue displacement and impression making, a provisional prosthesis needs to be fabricated to serve for a limited period of time, after which it is to be replaced by a definitive prosthesis. The provisional prosthesis will have a biologic, mechanical, and esthetic role. Felton and colleagues[120] found a direct relationship between the degree of marginal discrepancy of a crown margin and the severity of periodontal inflammation. To prevent any periodontal complications and reverse the mechanical insults that occur as a result of tooth preparation and gingival displacement, the clinician should avoid provisionals that are rough, ill fitting, and overcontoured.[121–124] Wilson and Maynard[1] found that overextended provisionals can cause and maintain a periodontal lesion. Waerhaug and colleagues[125] showed that poor provisional contours, marginal adaptation, and surface roughness lead to plaque accumulation and as a consequence poor periodontal health. Many clinicians prefer the straightforwardness of the direct technique. Whether the indirect or direct technique is used for the fabrication of a provisional prosthesis, marginal discrepancies vary with the type of resinous material used.[126,127] Tjan and colleagues[128] evaluated the vertical marginal discrepancy of provisional crowns fabricated with a direct method and found that there are significant differences between resinous materials. Barghi and Simmons[129] showed that provisional crowns fabricated with the direct technique did not demonstrate well-adapted margins unless they were relined after their initial polymerization. Relined resin crowns exhibited a smaller increase in gap size, compared with non-relined ones. Relining of provisional crowns may reduce increases in the marginal gap size that facilitate dissolution of provisional luting cements and encourage plaque accumulation.[130] Other studies[126,131–133] evaluated the indirect fabrication of provisionals and found that this technique yields a significant marginal improvement over prostheses made by direct fabrication. The advantages of the indirect fabrication when compared with the direct fabrication of provisionals are that there are reduced chair time and occlusal adjustments, optimal control of axial contours and occlusal morphology, and reduced pulpal trauma from chemicals and temperature changes associated with direct provisional restoration fabrication. A clear disadvantage of the indirect fabrication technique is the additional laboratory steps and fees.[134] The trauma that can be caused by the heat of the direct technique of provisional fabrication along with the free monomer can be devastating to the pulpal tissues and varies according to the type of matrix, the type of resin, and the method of cooling of the polymerizing resin.[134–139]

Regardless of the provisional material used (methyl methacrylate, ethyl methacrylate, bis-GMA composite, visible light-polymerized composite, polycarbonate resin), it is extremely important to have a very smooth surface on the provisional prosthesis before cementation. Methyl and ethyl methacrylate can be polished with a flour of pumice followed by any buffing agent. Smoothness of composite resin can be achieved by an application of a resin glaze. In a clinical study using 3 types of provisional crowns placed subgingivally, MacEntee and colleagues[140] found no detectable change in gingival tissue over a 3-week period.

REFERENCES

1. Wilson RD, Maynard G. Intracrevicular restorative dentistry. Int J Periodontics Restorative Dent 1981;1:34–49.
2. Silness J. Periodontal conditions in patients treated with dental bridges. 3. The relationship between the location of the crown margin and the periodontal condition. J Periodontal Res 1970;5:225–9.
3. Valderhaug J, Ellingsen JE, Jokstad A. Oral hygiene, periodontal conditions and carious lesions in patients treated with dental bridges. A 15-year clinical and radiographic follow-up study. J Clin Periodontol 1993;20:482–9.
4. Richter WA, Mahler DB. Physical properties vs. clinical performance of pure gold restorations. J Prosthet Dent 1973;29:434–8.
5. Koth DL. Full crown restorations and gingival inflammation in a controlled population. J Prosthet Dent 1982;48:681–5.
6. Brandau HE, Yaman P, Molvar M. Effect of restorative procedures for a porcelain jacket crown on gingival health and height. Am J Dent 1988;1:119–22.
7. Sorensen JA, Doherty FM, Newman MG, et al. Gingival enhancement in fixed prosthodontics: Part I. Clinical findings. J Prosthet Dent 1991;65:100–7.
8. Löe H, Silness J. Tissue reactions to string packs used in fixed restorations. J Prosthet Dent 1963;13:318–23.
9. Azzi R, Tsao TF, Carranza FA, et al. Comparative study of gingival retraction methods. J Prosthet Dent 1983;50:561–5.
10. Xhonga FA. Gingival retraction techniques and their healing effect on the gingiva. J Prosthet Dent 1971;26:640–8.
11. Ruel J, Schuessler PJ, Malament K, et al. Effect of retraction procedures on the periodontium in humans. J Prosthet Dent 1980;44:508–15.
12. de Gennaro GG, Landesman HM, Calhoun JE, et al. A comparison of gingival inflammation related to retraction cords. J Prosthet Dent 1982;47:384–9.
13. Liu CM, Huang FM, Yang LC, et al. Cytotoxic effects of gingival retraction cords on human gingival fibroblasts in vitro. J Oral Rehabil 2004;31:368–72.
14. Nowakowska D, Saczko J, Kulbacka J, et al. Cytotoxic potential of vasoconstrictor experimental gingival retraction agents – in vitro study on primary human gingival fibroblasts. Folia Biol (Praha) 2012;58:37–43.
15. Kopac I, Batista U, Cvetko E, et al. Viability of fibroblasts in cell culture after treatment with different chemical retraction agents. J Oral Rehabil 2002;29:98–104.
16. Harrison JD. Effect of retraction materials on the gingival sulcus epithelium. J Prosthet Dent 1961;11:514–21.
17. Knoernschild KL, Campbell SD. Periodontal tissue responses after insertion of artificial crowns and fixed partial dentures. J Prosthet Dent 2000;84:492–8.
18. Ochsenbein C, Ross S. A reevaluation of osseous surgery. Dent Clin North Am 1969;13:87–102.
19. Weisgold AS. Contours of full crown restoration. Alpha Omegan 1977;70:77–89.
20. Seibert JS, Lindhe J. Esthetics and periodontal therapy. In: Lindhe J, editor. Textbook of clinical periodontology. 2nd edition. Copenhagen (Denmark): Munksgaard; 1989. p. 477–514.
21. Claffey N, Shanley D. Relationship of gingival thickness and bleeding to loss of probing attachment in shallow sites following nonsurgical periodontal therapy. J Clin Periodontol 1986;13:654–7.
22. Olsson M, Lindhe J, Marinello CP. On the relationship between crown form and clinical features of the gingiva in adolescents. J Clin Periodontol 1993; 20:570–7.

23. Olsson M, Lindhe J. Periodontal characteristics in individuals with varying form of the upper central incisors. J Clin Periodontol 1991;18:78–82.
24. Gargiulo AW, Wentz F, Orban B. Dimensions and relations of the dentogingival junction in humans. J Periodontol 1961;32:261–7.
25. Schroeder HE, Listgarten MA. Fine structure of the developing epithelial attachment of human teeth. Monogr Dev Biol 1971;2:1–134.
26. Vacek JS, Gher ME, Assad DA, et al. The dimensions of the human dentogingival junction. Int J Periodontics Restorative Dent 1994;14:154–65.
27. Ingber JS, Rose LF, Coslet JG. The "biologic width" – a concept in periodontics and restorative dentistry. Alpha Omegan 1977;70:62–5.
28. Nevins M, Skurow HM. The intracrevicular restorative margin, the biologic width, and the maintenance of the gingival margin. Int J Periodontics Restorative Dent 1984;4:30–49.
29. Maynard JG Jr, Wilson RD. Physiologic dimensions of the periodontium significant to the restorative dentist. J Periodontol 1979;50:170–4.
30. Hansen PA, Tira DE, Barlow J. Current methods of finish-line exposure by practicing prosthodontists. J Prosthodont 1999;8:163–70.
31. Bennani V, Aarts JM, He LH. A comparison of pressure generated by cordless gingival displacement techniques. J Prosthet Dent 2012;107:388–92.
32. Al Hamad KQ, Azar WZ, Alwaeli HA, et al. Aclinical study on the effects of cordless and conventional retraction techniques on the gingival periodontal health. J Clin Periodontol 2008;35:1053–8.
33. Benson BW, Bomberg TJ, Hatch RA, et al. Tissue displacement methods in fixed prosthodontics. J Prosthet Dent 1986;55:157–292.
34. Fischer DE. Tissue management: a new solution to an old problem. Gen Dent 1987;35:178–82.
35. Ramadan FA, El-Sadeek M, Hassanein ES. Histopathologic response of gingival tissues to hemodent and aluminum chloride solutions as tissue displacement materials. Egypt Dent J 1972;18:337–52.
36. Baharav H, Kupershmidt I, Laufer BZ, et al. The effect of sulcular width on the accuracy of impression materials in the presence of an undercut. Int J Prosthodont 2004;17:585–9.
37. Anneroth G, Goeransson P. Exposing the gingival margin by taking impressions with elastic material – some clinical and histopathological aspects. Odontol Tidskr 1965;73:394–409.
38. Löe H, Theilade E, Jensen SB. Experimental gingivitis in man. J Periodontol 1965;36:177–87.
39. Wassell RW, Barker D, Walls AW. Crowns and other extra-coronal restorations: impression materials and technique. Br Dent J 2002;192:679–90.
40. Anneroth G, Nordenram A. Reaction of the gingiva to the application of threads in the gingival pocket for taking impressions with elastic material. An experimental histologic study. Odontol Revy 1969;20:301–10.
41. Reiman MB. Exposure of subgingival margins by nonsurgical gingival displacement. J Prosthet Dent 1976;36:649–54.
42. Feng J, Aboyoussef H, Weiner S, et al. The effect of gingival retraction procedures on periodontal indices and crevicular fluid cytokine levels: a pilot study. J Prosthodont 2006;15:108–12.
43. Phatale S, Marawar PP, Byakod G, et al. Effect of retraction materials on gingival health: a histopathological study. J Indian Soc Periodontol 2010;14:35–9.
44. Donovan TE, Gandara BK, Nemetz H. Review and survey of medicaments used with gingival retraction cords. J Prosthet Dent 1985;53:525–31.

45. Fisher DW. Conservative management of the gingival tissue for crowns. Dent Clin North Am 1976;20:273–84.
46. Tupac RG, Neacy K. A comparison of gingival displacement with gingitage technique. J Prosthet Dent 1981;46:509–15.
47. Ferrari M, Cagidiaco MC, Ercoli C. Tissue management with a new gingival retraction material: a preliminary clinical report. J Prosthet Dent 1996;75:242–7.
48. Kumbuloglu O, User A, Toksavul S, et al. Clinical evaluation of different gingival retraction cords. Quintessence Int 2007;38:91.e92–8.
49. Jokstad A. Clinical trial of gingival retraction cords. J Prosthet Dent 1999;81:258–61.
50. Morgano SM, Malone WF, Gregoire SE, et al. Tissue management with dental impression materials. Am J Dent 1989;2:279–84.
51. Weir DJ, Williams BH. Clinical effectiveness of mechanical-chemical tissue displacement methods. J Prosthet Dent 1984;51:326–9.
52. Nowakowska D, Saczko J, Kulbacka J, et al. Dynamic oxidoreductive potential of astringent retraction agents. Folia Biol (Praha) 2010;56:236–8.
53. Kellam SA, Smith JR, Scheffel SJ. Epinephrine absorption from commercial gingival retraction cords in clinical patients. J Prosthet Dent 1992;68:761–5.
54. Runyan DA, Reddy TG Jr, Shimoda LM. Fluid absorbency of retraction cords after soaking in aluminum chloride solution. J Prosthet Dent 1988;60:676–8.
55. Shaw DH, Krejci RF. Gingival retraction preference of dentists in general practice. Quintessence Int 1986;17:277–80.
56. Vernale C. Cardiovascular response to local dental anesthesia with epinephrine in normotensive and hypertensive subjects. Oral Surg Oral Med Oral Pathol 1960;13:942–52.
57. Pelzner RB, Kempler D, Stark MM, et al. Human blood pressure and pulse rate response to racemic epinephrine retraction cord. J Prosthet Dent 1978;39:287–92.
58. Woycheshin FF. An evaluation of the drugs used for gingival retraction. J Prosthet Dent 1964;14:769–76.
59. Houston JB, Appleby RC, DeCounter L, et al. Effect of r-epinephrine-impregnated retraction cord on the cardiovascular system. J Prosthet Dent 1970;24:373–6.
60. Forsyth RP, Stark MM, Nicholson RJ, et al. Blood pressure responses to epinephrine-treated gingival retraction strings in the rhesus monkey. J Am Dent Assoc 1967;78:1315–9.
61. Csillag M, Nyiri G, Vag J, et al. Dose-related effects of epinephrine on human gingival blood flow and crevicular fluid production used as a soaking solution for chemo-mechanical tissue retraction. J Prosthet Dent 2007;97:6–11.
62. Hilley MD, Milam SB, Giescke AH Jr, et al. Fatality associated with the combined use of halothane and gingival retraction cord. Anesthesiology 1984;60:587–8.
63. Land MF, Couri CC, Johnston WM. Smear layer instability caused by hemostatic agents. J Prosthet Dent 1996;76:477–82.
64. Bowles WH, Tardy SJ, Vahadi A. Evaluation of new gingival retraction agents. J Dent Res 1991;70:1447–9.
65. Buchanan WT, Thayer KE. Systemic effects of epinephrine-impregnated retraction cord in fixed partial denture prosthodontics. J Am Dent Assoc 1982;104:482–4.
66. Felpel LP. A review of pharmacotherapeutics for prosthetic dentistry: Part I. J Prosthet Dent 1997;77:285–92.

67. Bader JD, Bonito AJ, Shugars DA. A systematic review of cardiovascular effects of epinephrine on hypertensive dental patients. Oral Surg Oral Med Oral Pathol Oral Radiol Endod 2002;93:647–53.

68. Yagiela JA. Adverse drug interactions in dental practice: interactions associated with vasoconstrictors. Part V of a series. J Am Dent Assoc 1999;130:701–9.

69. Meechan JG, Jastak JT, Donaldson D. The use of epinephrine in dentistry. J Can Dent Assoc 1994;60:825–34.

70. Mohan M, Gupta A, Shenoy V, et al. Pharmacological agents in dentistry: a review. Br J Pharmaceut Res 2011;1:66–87.

71. Akca EA, Yildirim E, Dalriz M, et al. Effects of different retractions medicaments on gingival tissue. Quintessence Int 2006;37:53–9.

72. Ciancio SG, Bourgault PC. Clinical pharmacology for dental professionals. 3rd edition. Chicago: Year Book Medical Publishers; 1989. p. 316.

73. Woody RD, Miller A, Staffanou RS. Review of the pH of hemostatic agents used in tissue displacement. J Prosthet Dent 1993;70:191–2.

74. Land MF, Rosenstiel SF, Sandrik JL. Disturbance of the dentinal smear layer by acidic hemostatic agents. J Prosthet Dent 1994;72:4–7.

75. Kuphasuk W, Harnirattisai C, Senawongse P, et al. Bond strengths of two adhesive systems to dentin contaminated with a hemostatic agent. Oper Dent 2007; 32:399–505.

76. Ayo-Yusuf OA, Driessen CH, Botha AJ. SEM-EDX study of prepared human dentin exposed to gingival retraction fluids. J Dent 2005;33:731–9.

77. O'Keefe KL, Pinzon LM, Rivera B, et al. Bond strength of composite to astringent-contaminated dentin using self-etching adhesives. Am J Dent 2005;18:168–72.

78. O'Mahony A, Spencer P, Williams K, et al. Effect of 3 medicaments on the dimensional accuracy and surface detail reproduction of polyvinyl siloxane impressions. Quintessence Int 2000;31:201–6.

79. Sabio S, Franciscone PA, Mondelli J. Effect of conventional and experimental gingival retraction solutions on the tensile strength and inhibition of polymerization of four types of impression materials. J Appl Oral Sci 2008;16:280–5.

80. Machado CE, Guedes CG. Effects of sulfur-based hemostatic agents and gingival retraction cords handled with latex gloves on the polymerization of polyvinyl siloxane impression materials. J Appl Oral Sci 2011;19:628–33.

81. de Camargo LM, Chee WW, Donovan TE. Inhibition of polymerization of polyvinyl siloxanes by medicaments used on gingival retraction cords. J Prosthet Dent 1993;70:114–7.

82. Conrad HJ, Holtan JR. Internalized discoloration of dentin under porcelain crowns: a clinical report. J Prosthet Dent 2009;101:153–7.

83. Kopac I, Sterle M, Marion L. Electron microscopic analysis of the effects of chemical retraction agents on cultured rat keratinocytes. J Prosthet Dent 2002;87:51–6.

84. Labban N. A simple technique to reduce the risk of irreversible gingival recession after the final impression. J Prosthodont 2011;20:649–51.

85. Beier US, Kranewitter R, Dumfahrt H. Quality of impressions after use of the Magic FoamCord gingival retraction system – a clinical study of 269 abutment teeth. Int J Prosthodont 2009;22:143–7.

86. Poss S. An innovative tissue-retraction material. Compend Contin Educ Dent 2002;23(Suppl 1):13–7.

87. Manolakis A, Bartsch N, Hahn P. Clinical comparison of a gingiva retraction paste and impregnated cords (abstract 1837). Paper presented at: International

Association for Dental Research/American Association for Dental Research/Canadian Association for Dental Research 82nd General Session. Honolulu, March 12, 2004.

88. Yang JC, Tsai CM, Chen MS, et al. Clinical study of a newly developed injection-type gingival retraction material. Chin Dent J 2005;24:147–52.

89. Bennani V, Schwass D, Chandler N. Gingival retraction techniques for implants versus teeth. J Am Dent Assoc 2008;139:1354–63.

90. Aldridge T, Brennan PA, Crosby-Jones A, et al. Use of a polyvinyl acetyl sponge (Merocel®) nasal pack to prevent kinking of the endotracheal tube used during laser excision. Br J Oral Maxillofac Surg 2013;51(3):268.

91. La Forgia A. Mechanical-chemical and electrosurgical tissue retraction for fixed prosthesis. J Prosthet Dent 1964;14:1107–14.

92. Podshadley AG, Lundeen HC. Electrosurgical procedures in crown and bridge restorations. J Am Dent Assoc 1968;77:1321–6.

93. Gherlone EF, Maiorana C, Grassi RF, et al. The use of 980-nm diode and 1064-nm Nd:YAG laser for gingival retraction in fixed prostheses. J Oral Laser Appl 2004;4:183–90.

94. Malone WF, Manning JL. Electrosurgery in restorative dentistry. J Prosthet Dent 1968;20:417–25.

95. Lampert SH. Combined electrosurgery and gingival retraction. J Prosthet Dent 1970;23:164–72.

96. Noble WH, McClatchey KD, Douglass GD. A histologic comparison of effects of electrosurgical resection using different electrodes. J Prosthet Dent 1976;35:575–9.

97. Dawes JC, Mahabir RC, Hillier K, et al. Electrosurgery in patients with pacemakers/implanted cardioverter defibrillators. Ann Plast Surg 2006;57:33–6.

98. Stone KR, McPherson CA. Assessment and management of patients with pacemakers and implantable cardioverter defibrillators. Crit Care Med 2004;32:S155–65.

99. Maness WL, Roeber FW, Clark RE, et al. Histologic evaluation of electrosurgery with varying frequency and waveform. J Prosthet Dent 1978;40:304–8.

100. Coelho DH, Cavallaro J, Rothschild EA. Gingival recession with electrosurgery for impression making. J Prosthet Dent 1975;33:422–6.

101. Krejci RF, Reinhardt RA, Wentz FM, et al. Effects of electrosurgery on dog pulps under cervical metallic restorations. Oral Surg 1982;54:575–82.

102. Robertson PB, Lüscher B, Spangberg LS, et al. Pulpal and periodontal effects of electrosurgery involving cervical metallic restorations. Oral Surg Oral Med Oral Pathol 1978;46:702–10.

103. D'Souza R. Pulpal and periapical immune response to electrosurgical contact of cervical metallic restorations in monkeys. Quintessence Int 1986;17:803–8.

104. Klug RG. Gingival tissue regeneration following electrical retraction. J Prosthet Dent 1966;16:955–62.

105. Eisenmann D, Malone WF, Kusek J. Electron microscopic evaluation of electrosurgery. Oral Surg Oral Med Oral Pathol 1970;29:660–5.

106. Aremband D, Wade AB. A comparative wound healing study following gingivectomy by electrosurgery and knives. J Periodontal Res 1973;8:42–50.

107. Glickman I, Imber LR. Comparison of gingival resection with electrosurgery and periodontal knives – A biometric and histologic study. J Periodontol 1970;41:142–8.

108. Nixon KC, Adkins KF, Keys DW. Histological evaluation of effects produced in alveolar bone following gingival incision with an electrosurgical scalpel. J Periodontol 1975;46:40–4.

109. Brady WF. Periodontal and retorative considerations in rotary gingival curettage. J Am Dent Assoc 1982;105:231–6.

110. Kamansky FW, Tempel TR, Post AC. Gingival tissue response to rotary curettage. J Prosthet Dent 1984;52:380–3.

111. DeVitre R, Galburt RB, Maness WJ. Biometric comparison of bur and electrosurgical retraction methods. J Prosthet Dent 1985;53:179–82.

112. Scott A. Use of an erbium laser in lieu of retraction cord: a modern technique. Gen Dent 2005;53:116–9.

113. Abdel Gabbar F, Aboulazm SF. Comparative study on gingival retraction using mechanochemical procedure and pulsed Nd-YAG laser irradiation. Egypt Dent J 1996;41:1001–6.

114. Christensen GJ. Is the current generation of technology facilitating better dentistry? J Am Dent Assoc 2011;142:959–63.

115. Price C, Whitehead FI. Impression materials as foreign bodies. Br Dent J 1972;133:9–14.

116. O'Leary TJ, Standish SM, Bloomer RS. Severe periodontal destruction following impression procedures. J Periodontol 1973;44:43–8.

117. Blankenau RJ, Kelsey WP, Cavel WT. A possible allergic response to polyether impression material: a case report. J Am Dent Assoc 1984;108:609–10.

118. Shapiro N. Severe gingival damage after polysiloxane impression procedures. A case report. J Periodontol 1988;59:769–70.

119. Glenwright HD. Bone regeneration following damage by polysulphide impression material. A case report. J Clin Periodontol 1975;2:250–2.

120. Felton DA, Kanoy BE, Bayne SC, et al. Effect of in vivo crown margin discrepancies on periodontal health. J Prosthet Dent 1991;65:357–64.

121. Waerhaug J. Effect of rough surfaces upon gingival tissue. J Dent Res 1956;35:323–5.

122. Chiche G. Improving marginal adaptation of provisional restorations. Quintessence Int 1990;21:325–9.

123. Orkin DA, Reddy J, Bradshaw D. The relationship of the position of crown margins to gingival health. J Prosthet Dent 1987;57:421–4.

124. Dragoo MR, Williams GB. Periodontal tissue reactions to restorative procedures, part II. Int J Periodontics Restorative Dent 1982;2:34–45.

125. Waerhaug J, Zander HA. Reaction of gingival tissues to self-curing acrylic restorations. J Am Dent Assoc 1957;54(6):760–8.

126. Richards ND, Mitchell RJ. Effects of materials and techniques on accuracy of temporary fixed partial dentures [abstract 1484]. J Dent Res 1984;63:336.

127. Koumjian JH, Holmes JB. Marginal accuracy of provisional restorative materials. J Prosthet Dent 1990;63:639–42.

128. Tjan AH, Castelnuovo J, Shiotsu G. Marginal fidelity of crowns fabricated from six proprietary provisional materials. J Prosthet Dent 1997;77:482–5.

129. Barghi N, Simmons W. The marginal integrity of the temporary acrylic resin crown. J Prosthet Dent 1976;36:274–7.

130. Zwetchkenbaum S, Weiner S, Dastane A, et al. Effects of relining on long-term marginal stability of provisional crowns. J Prosthet Dent 1995;73:525–9.

131. Crispin BJ, Watson JF, Caputo AA. The marginal accuracy of treatment restorations: a comparative analysis. J Prosthet Dent 1980;44:283–90.

132. Monday JJ, Blais D. Marginal adaptation of provisional acrylic resin crowns. J Prosthet Dent 1985;54:194–7.
133. Ehrenberg DS, Weiner S. Changes in marginal gap size of provisional resin crowns after occlusal loading and thermal cycling. J Prosthet Dent 2000;84: 139–48.
134. Tjan AH, Grant BE, Godfrey MF. Temperature rise in the pulp chamber during fabrication of provisional crowns. J Prosthet Dent 1989;62:622–6.
135. Driscoll CF, Woosley G, Ferguson WM. Comparison of exothermic release during polymerization of four materials used to fabricate interim restorations. J Prosthet Dent 1991;65:504–6.
136. Moulding MB, Teplinsky PE. Intrapulpal temperature during direct fabrication of provisional restorations. Int J Prosthodont 1990;3:299–304.
137. Moulding MB, Loney RW. The effect of cooling techniques on intrapulpal temperature during direct fabrication of provisional restorations. Int J Prosthodont 1991;4:332–6.
138. Fleisch L, Cleaton-Jones P, Forbes M, et al. Pulpal response to a bis-acryl-plastic (Protemp) temporary crown and bridge material. J Oral Pathol 1984;13:622–31.
139. Grajower R, Shaharbani S, Kaufman E. Temporary rise in pulp chamber during fabrication of temporary self-curing resin crowns. J Prosthet Dent 1979;41: 535–40.
140. MacEntee MI, Bartlett SO, Loadholt CB. A histologic evaluation of tissue response to three currently used temporary acrylic resin crowns. J Prosthet Dent 1978;39:42–6.

Removable Partial Dentures
Clinical Concepts

David M. Bohnenkamp, DDS, MS

KEYWORDS

- Classification systems • Clasp assemblies • Computer-aided design
- Laboratory work authorization • Partially edentulous patient
- Removable partial denture

KEY POINTS

- Although classic theories and rules for removable partial dentures (RPDs) designs have been presented and should be followed, excellent clinical care for partially edentulous patients may also be achieved with computer-aided design (CAD)/computer-aided manufacturing (CAM) technology and unique blended designs.
- These nontraditional RPD designs and fabrication methods provide for improved fit, function, and esthetics using CAD software, composite resin for contours and morphology of abutment teeth, metal support structures for long edentulous spans and collapsed occlusal vertical dimensions, and flexible nylon thermoplastic material for metal-supported clasp assemblies.

RATIONALE AND INDICATIONS FOR RPDS

The primary reason often cited for the fabrication and delivery of an RPD for dental patients is the replacement of missing teeth in a cost-effective manner.[1] Most clinicians also choose an RPD for a partially edentulous patient if they need to restore lost residual ridge, achieve appropriate esthetics, increase masticatory efficiency, and improve phonetics but are unable to do so with dental implants or fixed partial dentures due to financial constraints or patient desires (**Figs. 1–4**).

In certain situations, RPDs are indicated as a choice of treatment of partially edentulous patients when the length of the edentulous span contraindicates a fixed partial denture, there is a need for residual ridge support for mastication, or a patient has a guarded prognosis for their periodontal condition (**Figs. 5–8**).[2] Other indications for RPDs are excessive loss of residual ridge, a requirement for a denture base flange, obtaining proper tooth position not achievable due to the biomechanics of dental

The author has nothing to disclose.
Department of Prosthodontics, University of Iowa College of Dentistry and Dental Clinics, 801 Newton Road, Iowa City, IA 52242, USA
E-mail address: david-bohnenkamp@uiowa.edu

Dent Clin N Am 58 (2014) 69–89
http://dx.doi.org/10.1016/j.cden.2013.09.003
0011-8532/14/$ – see front matter © 2014 Elsevier Inc. All rights reserved.

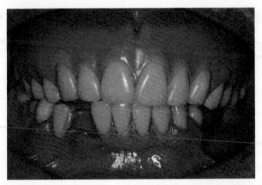

Fig. 1. Frontal view of rebased maxillary complete denture opposing defective interim mandibular RPD. (*From* Bohnenkamp DM. Clinical Patient Scenarios. In: Jones JD, Garcia LT, editors. Removable Partial Dentures: A Clinician's Guide. Ames, Iowa: Wiley-Blackwell; 2009; with permission.)

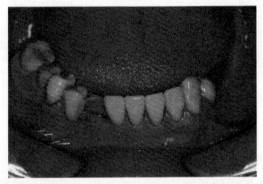

Fig. 2. Occlusal view of mandibular arch of patient with deficient residual ridges. (*From* Bohnenkamp DM. Clinical Patient Scenarios. In: Jones JD, Garcia LT, editors. Removable Partial Dentures: A Clinician's Guide. Ames, Iowa: Wiley-Blackwell; 2009; with permission.)

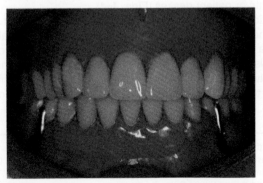

Fig. 3. Frontal view of new maxillary complete denture opposing mandibular bilateral distal extension RPD. (*From* Bohnenkamp DM. Clinical Patient Scenarios. In: Jones JD, Garcia LT, editors. Removable Partial Dentures: A Clinician's Guide. Ames, Iowa: Wiley-Blackwell; 2009; with permission.)

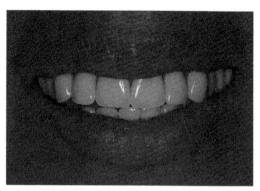

Fig. 4. Extraoral view of a patient wearing new affordable removable prostheses that provide improved esthetics, phonetics, and function. (*From* Bohnenkamp DM. Clinical Patient Scenarios. In: Jones JD, Garcia LT, editors. Removable Partial Dentures: A Clinician's Guide. Ames, Iowa: Wiley-Blackwell; 2009; with permission.)

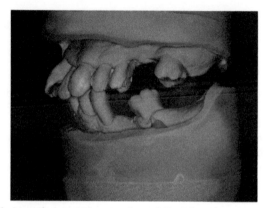

Fig. 5. Left lateral view of mounted casts of partially edentulous a patient with guarded periodontal condition. (*From* Bohnenkamp DM. Clinical Patient Scenarios. In: Jones JD, Garcia LT, editors. Removable Partial Dentures: A Clinician's Guide. Ames, Iowa: Wiley-Blackwell; 2009; with permission.)

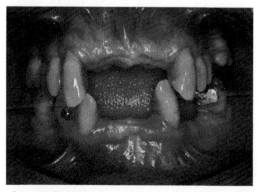

Fig. 6. Frontal view of a partially edentulous patient postextraction of periodontally compromised teeth. (*From* Bohnenkamp DM. Clinical Patient Scenarios. In: Jones JD, Garcia LT, editors. Removable Partial Dentures: A Clinician's Guide. Ames, Iowa: Wiley-Blackwell; 2009; with permission.)

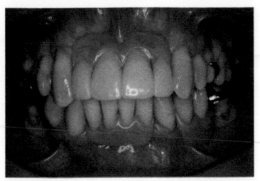

Fig. 7. Frontal view of new maxillary and mandibular RPDs to stabilize remaining periodontally weakened teeth. (*From* Bohnenkamp DM. Clinical Patient Scenarios. In: Jones JD, Garcia LT, editors. Removable Partial Dentures: A Clinician's Guide. Ames, Iowa: Wiley-Blackwell; 2009; with permission.)

implants, patient dexterity and oral hygiene issues, and a large maxillofacial defect requiring cross-arch stabilization.

COMMUNICATING RPD DESIGNS TO THE LABORATORY

In the United States, individual state dental boards mandate that dentists complete a laboratory work authorization form for the fabrication of an RPD by a dental laboratory. This work authorization form is actually a prescription to a dental laboratory for this service and should be completed accurately with as much attention to detail as possible. In most states, because it is considered a legal document, dentists must also keep a copy of the signed authorization form on file for several years.

As with prescriptions for medications, there are certain items that should be included on a laboratory work authorization in addition to a dentist's signature and license number, date, and patient name and address. Most important is a description of

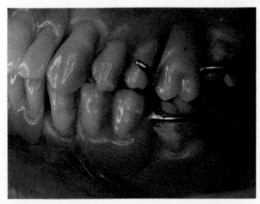

Fig. 8. Left lateral view of a patient with tooth-borne maxillary and mandibular RPDs to help stabilize periodontally compromised teeth. (*From* Bohnenkamp DM. Clinical Patient Scenarios. In: Jones JD, Garcia LT, editors. Removable Partial Dentures: A Clinician's Guide. Ames, Iowa: Wiley-Blackwell; 2009; with permission.)

the kind and type of laboratory service desired as well as details of the design and the materials to be used for the RPD (**Fig. 9**).

Dentists should accurately describe the following features and components of an RPD on the laboratory work authorization form:

1. Major connector
2. Type of metal and acrylic resin
   a. Framework only
   b. Fully fabricate
      i. Shade, mold, and type of material for artificial teeth must be included
      ii. Denture base color and characterization
3. Tooth numbers
   a. Type of clasps
   b. Amount and location of retentive undercuts
   c. Type and location of metal rests

In order to enhance communication with the dental laboratory, the definitive RPD design can be drawn in color on the laboratory work authorization form (**Fig. 10**). A key for success is to make sure that the color-coded design drawn on the work authorization is the same as the description written on the form. If not, then sometimes the best advice for dentists is to listen to the laboratory technician for feedback on what changes are necessary in order to fabricate an RPD in the laboratory to restore form, function, and esthetics as prescribed by the clinician. As an example, note how the design drawn in **Fig. 10** shows replacement of teeth 3, 4, 5, 13, and 14 with a Kennedy class III maxillary RPD design, but space limitations allowed the laboratory to place only 3 denture teeth, instead of the 5 requested by the clinician (**Fig. 11**).

REVIEW OF RPD THEORIES AND CLASSIC DESIGNS

In 1925, Dr Edward Kennedy proposed 4 distinct categories to classify maxillary and mandibular partially edentulous arches—classes I, II, III, and IV—in an attempt to suggest principles of design for a particular situation.[3] Each of the 4 Kennedy classifications refers to a single edentulous area, except class I, which refers to bilateral posteriorly extended edentulous areas. In 1954, Dr Oliver C. Applegate proposed

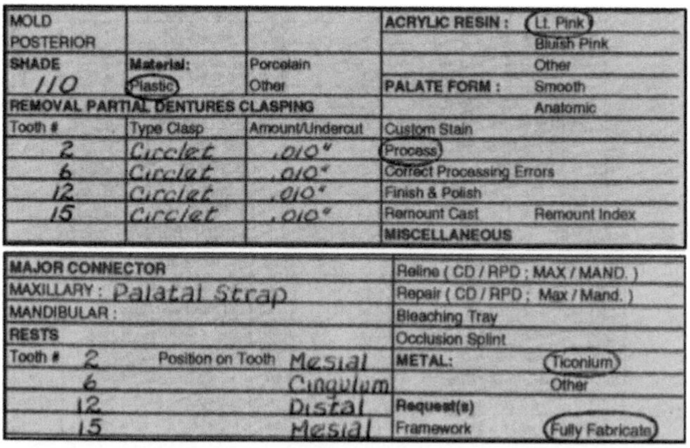

MOLD POSTERIOR			ACRYLIC RESIN :	Lt. Pink
				Bluish Pink
SHADE	Material:	Porcelain		Other
110	Plastic	Other	PALATE FORM :	Smooth
REMOVAL PARTIAL DENTURES CLASPING				Anatomic
Tooth #	Type Clasp	Amount/Undercut	Custom Stain	
2	Circlet	.010"	Process	
6	Circlet	.010"	Correct Processing Errors	
12	Circlet	.010"	Finish & Polish	
15	Circlet	.010"	Remount Cast	Remount Index
			MISCELLANEOUS	

MAJOR CONNECTOR			Reline (CD / RPD ; MAX / MAND.)	
MAXILLARY : Palatal Strap			Repair (CD / RPD ; Max / Mand.)	
MANDIBULAR :			Bleaching Tray	
RESTS			Occlusion Splint	
Tooth # 2	Position on Tooth	Mesial	METAL:	Ticonium
6		Cingulum		Other
12		Distal	Request(s)	
15		Mesial	Framework	Fully Fabricate

Fig. 9. Items that can be included on a laboratory authorization form to insure proper fabrication of metal and acrylic resin components of an RPD.

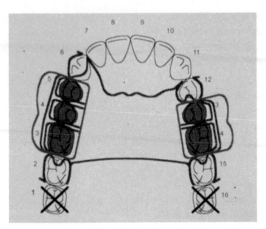

Fig. 10. Color-coded drawing of maxillary RPD design showing replacement of teeth 3, 4, 5, 13, and 14.

additional edentulous areas within each arch, referred to as "modification spaces," for applying the Kennedy classification method (**Fig. 12**).[4]

In his textbook, Applegate described 8 rules for classification of modification spaces. His most important rule to remember is, "the most posterior edentulous area(s) being restored always determine(s) the classification." Modification spaces under rule 8 are not allowed for a Kennedy class IV partially edentulous arch, because it is an anterior partially edentulous space bounded posteriorly by natural dentition (**Figs. 13** and **14**).

Most classic designs for the 4 Kennedy classifications of RPDs are based on 3 fundamental principles: support, stability, and retention.[5] Because class III RPDs are completely tooth-borne and do not receive support from the underlying edentulous residual ridge; the retentive clasping concepts are much more simplified than class I and II RPDs, which are both tooth-borne anteriorly and tissue-supported posteriorly. It is understood that a class III RPD is afforded maximum rigidity and stability in function with Akers cast circumferential clasps. A Roach clasp, however, such as

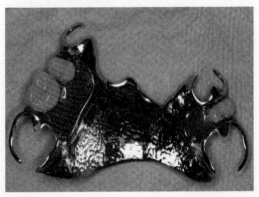

Fig. 11. Fully fabricated maxillary RPD with replacement of teeth 3, 4, and 13 only due to space limitations.

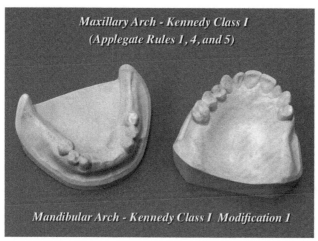

Fig. 12. Kennedy classifications and Applegate rules for maxillary and mandibular partially edentulous arches.

the I-bar clasp, or finger clasp, may engage undercuts on a class III RPD when esthetics is a major factor (**Figs. 15** and **16**).

In certain circumstances, a reverse Akers cast circumferential clasp may be used to engage a distofacial undercut on a more stable abutment tooth when the most posterior abutment tooth for a class I or II distal extension RPD is periodontally compromised and may be lost in the future. This clasp assembly should minimize torquing of the abutment tooth and allow for the RPD to be repaired with the addition of an acrylic resin denture tooth at the time of tooth loss without remaking the prosthesis (**Fig. 17**).

Fundamental design considerations for an RPD require that support be derived from the remaining teeth, the hard and soft tissues of the residual ridge, or both. Knowing that healthy teeth can be displaced by as much as 0.2 mm and the soft tissue overlying residual bone can be displaced by 1.0 mm or more, dentists should carefully choose

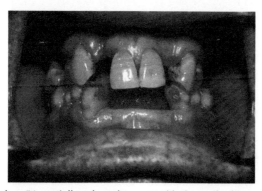

Fig. 13. Kennedy class IV partially edentulous mandibular arch. (*From* Bohnenkamp DM, Garcia LT. The use of a rotational-path design for a mandibular removable partial denture. Compend Contin Educ Dent 2004;25(7):552–67; with permission.)

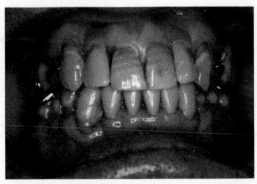

Fig. 14. Mandibular anterior edentulous space restored with a rotational path RPD. (*From* Bohnenkamp DM, Garcia LT. The use of a rotational-path design for a mandibular removable partial denture. Compend Contin Educ Dent 2004;25(7):552–67; with permission.)

the direct and indirect retentive components that prevent displacement of an RPD away from and toward the teeth and soft tissues.[6]

The choice of direct retainers made by clinicians for RPDs can be either suprabulge (cast circumferential clasp and wrought wire clasp) or infrabulge (I-bar or T-bar). Both cast circumferential and wrought wire clasps engage a retentive undercut on an RPD abutment tooth by traversing across the height of contour of the tooth from an occlusal to gingival direction. Both I-bar and T-bar clasps engage a retentive undercut on an RPD abutment tooth by approaching the tooth from a gingival direction underneath the height of contour of the tooth.

In addition to different clasp assemblies for retention and reciprocation, there are different thoughts about the design of RPDs for bilateral and unilateral distal extension Kennedy classifications based on support and stability for the abutment teeth. Each of these designs addresses the need to minimize the torquing forces on the abutment teeth by the clasp assemblies when the RPD moves during function.

The 3 most common designs chosen by dentists and dental laboratories for distal extension RPDs include I-bar, T-bar, or round wire clasps. The Kratochvil design

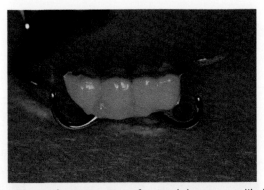

Fig. 15. Composite resin tooth components of a tooth-borne mandibular RPD with I-bar finger clasps. (*From* Bohnenkamp DM. Clinical Patient Scenarios. In: Jones JD, Garcia LT, editors. Removable Partial Dentures: A Clinician's Guide. Ames, Iowa: Wiley-Blackwell; 2009; with permission.)

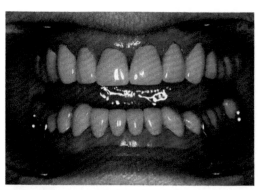

Fig. 16. Intraoral frontal view of mandibular RPD with I-bar clasps for a Kennedy class III partially edentulous arch. (*From* Bohnenkamp DM. Clinical Patient Scenarios. In: Jones JD, Garcia LT, editors. Removable Partial Dentures: A Clinician's Guide. Ames, Iowa: Wiley-Blackwell; 2009; with permission.)

(1963) uses a mesial or cingulum rest, distal guide plate, and I-bar clasp with a .01 in. midfacial retentive undercut location (**Figs. 18** and **19**). The Roach design (1934) uses a distal or cingulum rest, distal guide plate, lingual reciprocation, and a T-bar or 1/2 T-bar clasp with a .01 in. distofacial retentive undercut location (**Figs. 20** and **21**). The Applegate design (1955) uses a distal or cingulum rest, distal guide plate, lingual reciprocation, and a wrought wire or platinum-gold-palladium clasp with a .02 in. mesiofacial retentive undercut (**Figs. 22** and **23**).

The dental literature shows that the design of a clasp assembly affects the magnitude of movement of abutment teeth adjacent to a distal extension base but does not affect the direction of movement.[7] It has also been stated that the stability of the denture base seems of greater importance than the type of clasp retainer in terms of abutment tooth mobility.[8] Thus, for the support and stability of abutment teeth, there seems to be no conclusive evidence that one design theory is superior to the others. Ideally, clinicians choose and prescribe the clasp assembly for a distal extension RPD based on avoiding occlusal interference from metal rests, the location of retentive

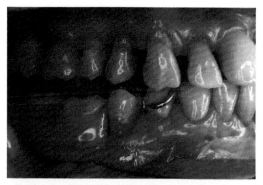

Fig. 17. Mandibular distal extension RPD with a reverse circlet clasp adjacent to periodontally involved tooth. (*From* Bohnenkamp DM. Clinical Patient Scenarios. In: Jones JD, Garcia LT, editors. Removable Partial Dentures: A Clinician's Guide. Ames, Iowa: Wiley-Blackwell; 2009; with permission.)

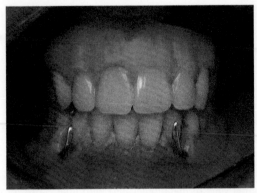

Fig. 18. Mandibular bilateral distal extension RPD with I-bar infrabulge retentive clasps. (*From* Garcia LT, Bohnenkamp DM. The Use of Composite Resin in Removable Prosthodontics. Compend Contin Educ Dent Dentistry 2003;24:688–96, with permission.)

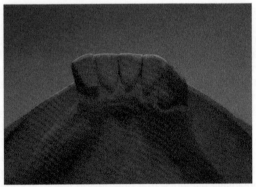

Fig. 19. Master cast showing composite resin cingulum rest seats on the lingual surfaces of mandibular canines. (*From* Garcia LT, Bohnenkamp DM. The Use of Composite Resin in Removable Prosthodontics. Compend Contin Educ Dent Dentistry 2003;24:688–96, with permission.)

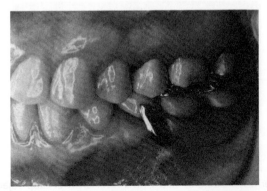

Fig. 20. Mandibular unilateral distal extension RPD with 1/2 T-bar infrabulge retentive clasp. (*From* Bohnenkamp DM. Clinical Patient Scenarios. In: Jones JD, Garcia LT, editors. Removable Partial Dentures: A Clinician's Guide. Ames, Iowa: Wiley-Blackwell; 2009; with permission.)

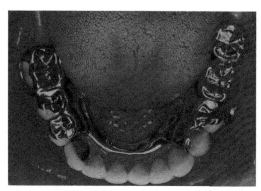

Fig. 21. Occlusal view of mandibular unilateral distal extension RPD for Kennedy class II partially edentulous arch. (*From* Bohnenkamp DM. Clinical Patient Scenarios. In: Jones JD, Garcia LT, editors. Removable Partial Dentures: A Clinician's Guide. Ames, Iowa: Wiley-Blackwell; 2009; with permission.)

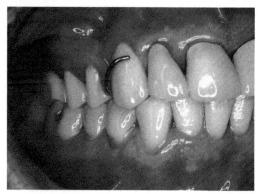

Fig. 22. Maxillary bilateral distal extension RPD with 19-gauge cast round suprabulge retentive clasp. (*From* Bohnenkamp DM. Clinical Patient Scenarios. In: Jones JD, Garcia LT, editors. Removable Partial Dentures: A Clinician's Guide. Ames, Iowa: Wiley-Blackwell; 2009; with permission.)

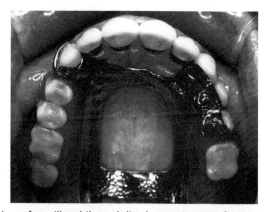

Fig. 23. Occlusal view of maxillary bilateral distal extension RPD for Kennedy class I partially edentulous arch. (*From* Bohnenkamp DM. Clinical Patient Scenarios. In: Jones JD, Garcia LT, editors. Removable Partial Dentures: A Clinician's Guide. Ames, Iowa: Wiley-Blackwell; 2009; with permission.)

undercuts, and the esthetic demands of patients. In simple terms, let patient desires for esthetics and comfort, hard and soft tissue anatomy, and occlusal relations dictate which design and clasp assembly is indicated, prescribed by the dentist, and fabricated by the dental laboratory.

COMPUTER-AIDED RPD DESIGNS

The concept of using computer-aided technology to design and fabricate RPD metal frameworks has been studied for almost a decade by several investigators.[9] Techniques have been described in dental and in engineering literature for fabricating patterns for RPD frameworks using CAD/CAM technology to survey 3-D scanned dental casts.[10,11] In 2009, an investigation by Chinese researchers documented the fit of a computer-designed metal framework for a partially edentulous patient.[12] As the first step in CAD/CAM design of an RPD, the master stone cast of a patient was scanned. The computer software and rapid prototyping technology was then used to develop a sacrificial pattern that was sprued, cast in chromium-cobalt alloy, finished, and polished using conventional laboratory methods. The metal framework was adjusted to fit the patient intraorally. After trial fitting, the metal framework was judged clinically acceptable.

As recently as 2010, several prosthodontists reported on a method to digitally survey and create virtual patterns for fabricating RPD metal frameworks.[13] In this study, researchers used proprioceptive software to create a virtual design for each component of the RPD frameworks on a digital scan of partially edentulous stone casts. The metal RPD frameworks were then fabricated using a selective laser melting technique.

From these reports, the advantages of CAD/CAM designs for RPDs seem to be improved fit, decreased time for fabrication, less labor required, and fewer sources of error. Although the initial investment costs and training associated with CAD/CAM is of concern, once the learning curve is reached, the time and efficiency of fabricating RPDs with this new technology will improve. In the future, most of the restorative disciplines may be fully revised and the design and fabrication methods evolved to an extent where dentistry can be performed by computer-assisted methods with optimum safety, simplicity, and reliability.[14]

In contrast to fixed prosthodontic and implant applications, the removable side of the dental laboratory business has lagged behind, usually forced to fabricate full and partial dentures conventionally. That all has changed, however, with the new 3-D scanners and denture design software modules recently introduced to the market and integrated with 3-D printing technology (**Figs. 24** and **25**).[15]

As reported in dental laboratory journals, a few companies have helped to further the production of digitally designed RPDs, which are printed in wax and then cast and fabricated conventionally. These open-architecture scanners with powerful new denture design software capabilities will open the door for dental laboratory technicians to create a fully digital, machine-produced partial-denture product (**Figs. 26** and **27**). An additional advantage of a digitally produced RPD or full denture is that the machines can reproduce the exact same product again from a file stored on the laboratory's server. This is especially helpful for the elderly or for Alzheimer patients who tend to lose or misplace their removable prostheses.

With the advent of digital dentistry embracing high-precision scanners, CAD/CAM software, and 3-D printers combined with industrial casting and finishing techniques, a solution is finally available that can cut time and labor by more than half. The design and fabrication process has evolved and eliminates multiple time-consuming steps to create well-fitted, esthetic, and functional restorations. Dental laboratories continue to

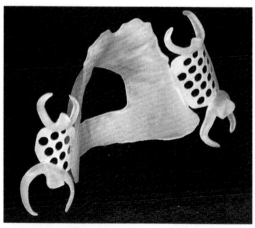

Fig. 24. Computer-designed polycarbonate RPD framework. (*From* Lanier D. CAD/CAM dentures? Inside Dental Technology 2011;2(3); with permission.)

fine tune the scanning, digital designing, 3-D printing, investing, and casting of RPDs with a completely digital RPD process as noted in industry publications.[16,17]

For additional information from evidence-based dental literature on CAD for RPDs, see article "A critically appraised topic (CAT) review of CAD/CAM removable partial denture frameworks" by Drs Lisa Lang and Ibrahim Tulunoglu elsewhere in this issue.

UNIQUE AND BLENDED RPD DESIGNS

Dental laboratory technicians continue to improve fabrication processes by testing combinations of old and new materials and techniques. One such combination uses flexible nylon polyamide denture base resin with conventional heat-polymerized polymethyl methacrylate acrylic resin denture bases. A laboratory technician processes, finishes, polishes, and adjusts a flexible nylon polyamide denture base resin framework with mesh retention in the edentulous areas on the master model. Then, a

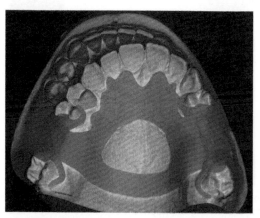

Fig. 25. Polycarbonate RPD framework on the master cast. (*From* Lanier D. CAD/CAM dentures? Inside Dental Technology 2011;2(3); with permission.)

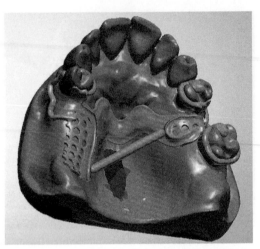

Fig. 26. Digital design of maxillary unilateral RPD framework. (*From* Kreyer R. Digital partial design and manufacturing: using 3D printing technology to fabricate removable partial denture frameworks. Inside Dental Technology. 2012;3(7); with permission.)

laboratory technician processes and finishes the acrylic resin denture base edentulous areas and denture teeth to the flexible retentive mesh material using a heat-polymerized conventional technique.[18]

For those partially edentulous patients who prefer no metal in their RPD framework and/or clasps, the entire framework and essential components can be fabricated using flexible nylon polyamide denture base resin. As seen in the photographs of a partially edentulous patient (**Fig. 28**), teeth 8, 13, 21, and 28 are clasped with esthetic, flexible nylon retentive clasps after processing the entire RPD in the Valplast material. Unfortunately, these RPD designs do not have vertical displacement components

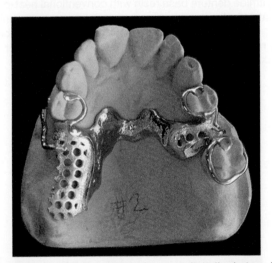

Fig. 27. Conventional metal RPD framework that was digitally designed, printed in wax, cast, and finished for trial fitting in patient's mouth. (*From* Kreyer R. Digital partial design and manufacturing: using 3D printing technology to fabricate removable partial denture frameworks. Inside Dental Technology. 2012;3(7); with permission.)

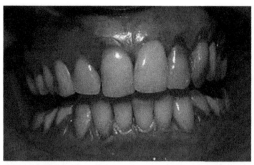

Fig. 28. Maxillary and mandibular Valplast RPDs with anterior flexible nylon clasps. (*Courtesy of* Zahntechnik.)

(metal rests) and must rely on the soft tissue for support. There are, however, dental laboratories that can provide vertical support by fabricating a conventional metal framework supported RPD with anterior flexible nylon clasps (**Fig. 29**). This combination of nylon clasps with a metal framework not only improves the esthetics of a traditional RPD but also ensures the rigidity of the major connector and provides vertical support with metal occlusal rests.[19]

Another unique esthetic RPD innovation that clinicians may use is to modify the morphology of mandibular canines with composite resin for vertical support and retention of a mandibular distal extension RPD. In these cases, modification of the lingual surfaces of the mandibular canines with composite resin to form cingulum rest seats can be done to avoid using unesthetic distoincisal metal rests for vertical support of the metal framework. In some situations, the facial surfaces on a patient's mandibular canines can also be modified with composite resin to provide .01 in. midfacial undercuts for I-bar clasp retention for the Kennedy class I RPD (**Figs. 30–33**). If the composite resin rest seats wear or fracture, the lingual tooth surfaces can be etched and bonded and the cingulum rest seats reformed to the original shape recorded in the intaglio surface of the metal RPD framework.

When there are both functional and esthetic demands due to significant loss of anterior residual ridge support for a conventional RPD or a heavily worn dentition with loss of significant vertical of dimension, then the treatment of choice may be either a

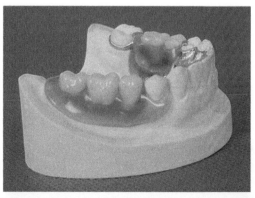

Fig. 29. Blended RPD design using a cast metal framework with conventional metal clasps in the posterior and flexible nylon polyamide retentive clasps in the anterior. (*Courtesy of* French Alibaba.)

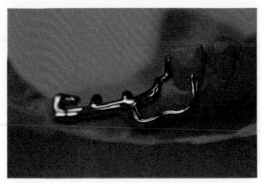

Fig. 30. Composite resin added to mid-facial of abutment tooth to provide .01 in. undercut for I-bar retentive clasp.

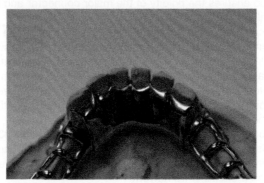

Fig. 31. Composite resin cingulum rest seats added to lingual of mandibular canines for metal framework support.

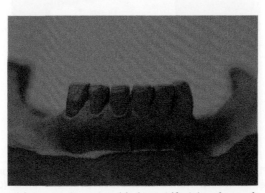

Fig. 32. Master cast with composite resin added to midfacial surfaces of mandibular canines.

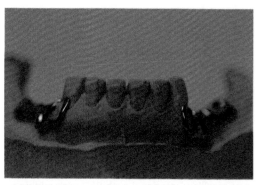

Fig. 33. Metal framework seated on master cast with I-bar retentive clasps and .01 in. under-cut on mandibular canines.

rotational path RPD with a runner bar to support the acrylic resin denture teeth and the denture base material (**Figs. 34–36**) or an overlay RPD to restore lost tooth structure (**Figs. 37** and **38**). Without the runner bar added during the wax-up of the metal frame-work, there is a risk that the denture base flange and/or denture teeth may fracture off a conventional RPD due to lack of rigidity and flexure of the metal lattice work retentive element.

RULES FOR RPD DESIGNS

In 1988, several investigators proposed alternate framework designs uniquely different from the classic designs for RPDs. Their article reviewed the factors associ-ated with the prognosis of treatment with RPDs. Furthermore, the article described framework designs applied in different clinical situations and compared them with more conventional designs. It seems important to these investigators to consider a framework design that places a premium on comfort, esthetics, and oral hygiene of patients rather than to follow mechanical rules that are entirely theoretic and have not been confirmed scientifically or clinically.[20]

The clinical concepts provided in this article represent only a small amount of the knowledge required to treat partially edentulous patients with an RPD. As an aid to design and fabricate RPDs, the following rules of engagement are provided to help

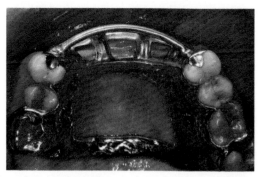

Fig. 34. Occlusal view of try-in of maxillary rotational path RPD framework with runner bar cast to framework. (*Courtesy of* Dr Whit Pharr.)

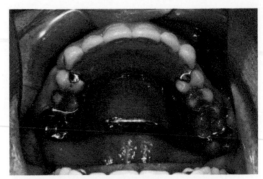

Fig. 35. Occlusal view of maxillary rotational path RPD with additional support for acrylic resin denture base and denture teeth. (*Courtesy of* Dr Whit Pharr.)

dentists and dental laboratory technicians communicate better and achieve the best results.

Major Connectors in the Maxillary Arch

1. Borders should be placed a minimum of 6 mm from the gingival margin or on the lingual surfaces of teeth.
2. Borders should follow the valleys between the crests of the rugae on the anterior palate.
3. Borders should cross the midline at right angles.
4. Palatal strap should not be less than 8 mm wide.

Major Connectors in the Mandibular Arch

Lingual bar

1. Superior border should be 3 mm from the gingival margin and the bar itself 5 mm wide.
2. Total depth of 8 mm should be available on the lingual surface of the mandible—"If you don't have eight, then you must plate."

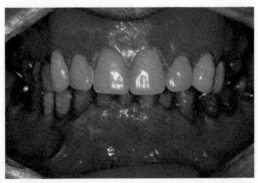

Fig. 36. Frontal view of maxillary rotational path RPD with improved strength and rigidity from runner bar. (*Courtesy of* Dr Whit Pharr.)

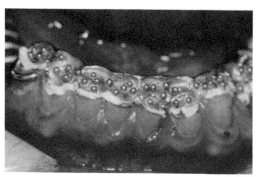

Fig. 37. Mandibular overlay RPD metal framework with bead retentive elements being fitted to the occlusal and incisal surfaces of mandibular teeth.

Lingual plate

1. Use if planning to extract compromised teeth and add replacement teeth to metal framework in future
2. Should be scalloped interproximally and cover the cingulum
3. Should be supported bilaterally by a rest located no further posterior than mesial fossae of the first premolars
4. Use drop-offs when loss of tissue height interproximally has occurred or when the teeth are widely spaced.

Retentive elements for distal extension denture bases

1. Maxillary arch should extend the entire length of the residual ridge over the tuberosity.
2. Mandibular arch should extend two-thirds the length of the edentulous ridge and never extend onto or cover the retromolar pad.
3. Use open latticework with one strut between each tooth for attachment of denture base to framework.
4. Request a metal tissue stop on all distal extension designs (add acrylic resin stop if metal frame can be displaced toward tissue at try-in).

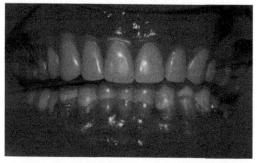

Fig. 38. Mandibular overlay unilateral distal extension RPD with tooth-colored acrylic resin processed to the metal framework to restore lost vertical dimension of occlusion and provide acceptable esthetics and function for the patient.

Rest seats

1. Occlusal rest seat preparation for posterior teeth. One-third to one-half the mesio-distal diameter and half the facial-lingual width measured from cusp tip to cusp tip. Floor of the rest seat angled downward toward center of tooth. Tooth reduction should be at least 1.0 mm and may need 1.5 mm at the marginal ridge for an adequate thickness of metal.
2. Lingual or cingulum rest for maxillary canine
3. Incisal rest for mandibular canine. Small V-shaped notch located 1.5–2 mm from the proximal-incisal angle of the tooth. Cingulum rest fabricated on mandibular canine with bonded composite resin if metal rest on incisal is unaesthetic or interferes with occlusion.

Clasps

1. .01 in.—Amount of retentive undercut needed for cast metal half-round circumferential clasps
2. .02 in.—Amount of retentive undercut needed for wrought wire or cast metal round clasps
3. Circumferential—suprabulge half round cast clasp needs .01 in. mesiofacial or distofacial undercut; contraindicated for Kennedy class I or II distal extension arches
4. Reverse circumferential—suprabulge half round cast clasp may engage a .01 in. distofacial undercut of an abutment tooth adjacent to the Kennedy class I or II distal extension edentulous space
5. T-bar or 1/2 T-bar—infrabulge cast clasp needs .01 in. distofacial undercut; contraindicated if deep soft or hard tissue undercut present
6. I-bar—infrabulge clasp needs .01 in. midfacial undercut; contraindicated if deep tissue undercut present
7. Wrought wire—suprabulge clasp needs .02 in. mesiofacial undercut; contraindicated if esthetics is major concern
8. Only one-third of end of a retentive clasp should be in the undercut; enamelplasty indicated if approach arm of clasp is below height of contour on abutment tooth
9. Reciprocal clasp must be located above the survey line, close to the height of contour, but no higher than the middle third of the tooth preferably at the junction of the gingival and middle third of the tooth.

SUMMARY

This article provides a review of the traditional clinical concepts for the design and fabrication of RPDs. Although classic theories and rules for RPD designs have been presented and should be followed, excellent clinical care for partially edentulous patients may also be achieved with CAD/CAM technology and unique blended designs. These nontraditional RPD designs and fabrication methods provide for improved fit, function, and esthetics by using CAD software, composite resin for contours and morphology of abutment teeth, metal support structures for long edentulous spans and collapsed occlusal vertical dimensions, and flexible nylon thermoplastic material for metal-supported clasp assemblies.

REFERENCES

1. Stefanac N. Treatment planning in dentistry. 2nd edition. St Louis (MO): Mosby Elsevier; 2007. p. 53–67, 208.

2. Stewart KL, Rudd KD. Stabilizing periodontally weakened teeth with removable partial denture. J Prosthet Dent 1968;19(5):465–82.
3. Kennedy E. Partial denture construction. Dent Items Interest 1925;47:23–5.
4. Applegate OC. Essentials of removable partial prosthesis. 1st edition. Philadelphia: Saunders; 1954.
5. Carr AB, Brown DT. McCracken's removable partial prosthodontics. 12th edition. St Louis (MO): Mosby Elsevier; 2011. p. 3, 10, 179–81, 232.
6. Phoenix R, Cagna DR, DeFreest CF, et al. Stewart 's clinical removable partial prosthodontics. 4th edition. Chicago: Quintessence Publishing Co., Inc; 2008. p. 14.
7. Browning JD, Medros LW, Eick JD. Movement of three removable partial denture clasp assemblies under occlusal loading. J Prosthet Dent 1986;55(1):69–74.
8. Barco MT, Flinton RJ. An overview of four removable partial denture clasps. Int J Prosthodont 1988;1(2):159–64.
9. Williams RJ, Bibb R, Rafik T. A technique for fabricating patterns for removable partial denture frameworks using digitized casts and electronic surveying. J Prosthet Dent 2004;91(1):85–8.
10. Williams RJ, Bibb R, Eggbeer D. CAD/CAM in the fabrication of removable partial denture frameworks: a virtual method of surveying 3-dimensionally scanned dental casts. Quintessence J Dent Technol 2004;2(3):268–76.
11. Bibb R, Eggbeer D, Williams R. Rapid manufacture of removable partial denture frameworks. Rapid Prototyp J 2006;12(2):95–9.
12. Yan G, Liao W, Dai N, et al. The computer-aided design and rapid prototyping fabrication of removable partial denture framework. 2nd IEEE International Conference Publication. August, 2009. p. 266–8.
13. Han J, Wang Y, Lü PJ. A preliminary report of designing removable partial denture frameworks using a specifically developed software package. Int J Prosthodont 2010;23(4):370–5.
14. Azari A, Nikzad S. The evolution of rapid prototyping in dentistry: a review. Rapid Prototyp J 2009;15(3):216–25.
15. Lanier D. CAD/CAM Dentures? Inside Dent Tech 2011;2(3):2–5. Available at: www.dentalaegis.com/idt.
16. Snyder R, Tagliarino C. An inside look at the rpd process through the eyes of a digital dental laboratory. Inside Dent Tech 2012;3(7):2–5. Available at: www.dentalaegis.com/idt.
17. Kreyer R. Digital Partial Design and Manufacturing–Using 3D printing technology to fabricate removable partial denture frameworks. Inside Dent Tech 2012;3(7):2–5. Available at: www.dentalaegis.com/idt.
18. Kolbeck J. Fabricating a Flexi-Combo Partial Denture. NADL J Dent Tech 2013;3:1–15.
19. Ito M, Wee AG, Miyamoto T, et al. The combination of a nylon and traditional partial removable dental prosthesis for improved esthetics: a clinical report. J Prosthet Dent 2013;109(1):5–8.
20. Budtz-Jorgensen E, Bochet G. Alternate framework designs for removable partial dentures. J Prosthet Dent 1998;80(1):58–66.

Alternatives to Traditional Complete Dentures

Norma Olvera, DDS, MS*, John D. Jones, DDS

KEYWORDS

- Flangeless • Denture • Palateless • Removable prosthesis • Modified denture
- Edentulous • Ridge preservation

KEY POINTS

- The flangeless and palateless denture has been a controversial treatment modality because of the uncertainties surrounding its effectiveness on retention.
- Retention, border molding, diagnosis, and treatment planning are important in this treatment.
- The scrupulous detail and meticulous attention to protocol throughout the course of treatment with the flangeless denture cannot be overemphasized.
- Although alternatives to traditional complete dentures are not routinely used to make complete dentures, they have been successfully used for the treatment of edentulous patients.
- Alternatives to traditional complete dentures provide valuable prosthodontic treatment that should be considered in treating select edentulous patients.

INTRODUCTION

Alternative designs in traditional complete denture therapy have been controversial because of the uncertainties surrounding the effectiveness of retention of the prosthesis. The importance of retention for a maxillary complete denture has been well recognized in the literature. As early as the mid-twentieth century, crucial aspects of retention including atmospheric pressure, intimate tissue contact, and peripheral seal were identified.

Hardy and Kapur[1] and others[2–6] reported on the posterior palatal seal and its advantages related to placement and location. More recent publications[7–9] have discussed specifics of the palatal seal such as clinical determination, location, adaptation, anatomic structures, and the value of border molding to create a retentive seal. Border molding in the fabrication of complete dentures has been described by several investigators,[10–12] but the question remains as to how much a limited flange or a denture flange that is not border molded in the anterior vestibule truly affects the seal.

Department of Comprehensive Dentistry, University of Texas Health Science Center at San Antonio, 7703 Floyd Curl Drive, San Antonio, TX 78229-3900, USA
* Corresponding author.
E-mail address: OlveraN@uthscsa.edu

Dent Clin N Am 58 (2014) 91–102
http://dx.doi.org/10.1016/j.cden.2013.09.004
0011-8532/14/$ – see front matter © 2014 Elsevier Inc. All rights reserved.

dental.theclinics.com

The purpose of this article is to help answer this question through a literature update on specific alternative prostheses,[13–15] and to show how these alternatives are effectively used to treat edentulous patients (**Boxes 1** and **2**).

MODIFIED PALATELESS AND FLANGELESS REMOVABLE PROSTHESIS

After World War II, the evolution of autopolymerizing resins allowed the repair and modification of complete dentures and removable partial dentures without cumbersome processing techniques. Depending on the number and position of remaining teeth, a removable prosthesis can be made palateless. Removable partial dentures (RPDs) have been used for many years with flangeless tooth replacements.[16–19]

A key indication for a modified extension of prosthesis is when a labial flange is not needed because there is sufficient bone and lip support. In these instances, adding a buccal flange can distort the facial support and muscles of facial expression, limit function, and compromise aesthetics.

RPDs are designed with metal bases and reinforced acrylic pontics, tube teeth, and/or braided posts that typically do not incorporate a denture base flange; the denture teeth are set directly against the residual alveolar ridge or are placed directly on the metal base. In essence, there is no flange because the physiologic function and residual ridge does not require any additional support.

In these scenarios, the length of artificial teeth depends on the amount of existing interocclusal space. The width of artificial teeth varies from the perspective of facial/lip support.

Box 1
Chronologic importance of maxillary complete denture retention

1950s
  Stamoulis: atmospheric pressure, intimate tissue contact, peripheral seal
  Hardy: Posterior palatal seal; advantages, placement, location

1960s
  Laney, Gonzalez: palatal relief and posterior palatal seal

1970s
  Silverman: dimensions and displacement of posterior palatal seal

1980s
  Ettinger: posterior palatal seal, a review
  Calomeni: posterior palatal seal, location and preparation

1990s
  Sykora: adaptation and shape

2000s
  Kim: relining and dimensional accuracy
  Rashedi: current concepts for determination

2010s
  Perry: anatomy and physiology

> **Box 2**
> **Chronologic development of the modified prosthesis: palateless and flangeless denture**
>
> 1700s: porcelain teeth
>
> 1800s: vulcanite
>
> 1930s: acrylic resin
>
> 1940s: autopolymerizing acrylic resin
>
> Flangeless denture introduced in PubMed: 1965, 1980, 2002
>
> Future developments with digital dentures

The tooth position must support the movement of the lips and facial muscles during normal movements of facial expression. The basic rules of aesthetics must be followed (**Figs. 1** and **2**).

DIAGNOSIS AND TREATMENT PLANNING

Diagnosis and careful treatment planning is essential and vital to a successful outcome. The American College of Prosthodontists[20] categorizes the severity of different oral entities in the Prosthodontic Diagnostic Index classification system.

Use of a diagnostic-driven evaluation includes the following: psychological classification, frena and muscle attachments, tongue position, sublingual fold, tori, ridge relation, lateral throat form, palatal form, soft-tissue quality of the palate, and bony undercuts.

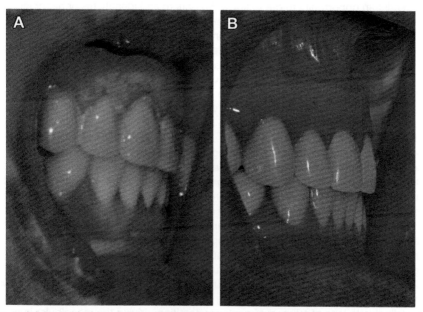

Fig. 1. (*A*) Sagittal view of the anterior teeth in maximum intercuspation, illustrating the complete extension and thickness of the labial flange. (*B*) Sagittal view of the anterior teeth in maximum intercuspation, illustrating the design without the complete extension of the labial flange.

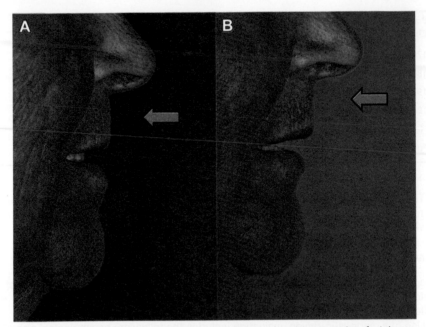

Fig. 2. (*A*) Conventional denture with buccal flange showing excessive facial support (*arrow*). (*B*) Flangeless denture illustrating ideal lip support (*arrow*).

As standard protocol for complete denture fabrication, the initial interview provides the dentist an opportunity to get to know the patient and identify his or her chief concerns. Treatment expectations can be determined by both patient and dentist.

The health history includes, but is not limited to, review of past medical conditions, systems review, allergies, and current medications, all of which are mandatory elements for each patient needing prosthodontic care. The dental history should include how, why, and when the teeth were lost; whether the patient has had previous experience with a removable partial denture or complete denture prosthesis; and the patient's prosthetic experience with or without a flange. A preexisting prosthesis allows the dentist to evaluate the denture and flanges, and to assess patient function with the preexisting prosthesis.

As part of standard protocol, a thorough clinical and radiographic examination is also included in the fabrication of complete denture prosthesis to obtain diagnostic data in formulating a treatment plan. Radiographs may show the size and trabecular pattern of the bone and position of the genial tubercles, sinuses, and mental foramen. In addition, any radiographic evidence of abnormality, residual teeth, and root tips is documented and addressed. Clinical examination often reveals anterior bony undercuts that pose unusual difficulties in complete denture construction. In fabrication of a maxillary complete denture, it is not unusual to see a prominent maxillary residual ridge with a severe anterior labial undercut.

The maxilla often presents with a protruding trajectory before any tooth extraction, producing the appearance of a protruding upper lip. The trajectory of the premaxilla is generally due to loss of support of posterior dentition, driving the mandibular incisors against the lingual aspects of the maxillary anterior teeth.

When the mandibular anterior teeth are in stable solid Type 1 bone and the maxillary anterior teeth are surrounded by Type 2 to 3 bone, the maxillary anterior teeth are generally displaced buccal to their original position based on general occlusal function. Aesthetically, on extraction of the buccally displaced maxillary anterior teeth, the residual ridge is already in position to support the upper lip.

In addition, with osseous bone-graft procedures becoming more of a standard of care in immediate extraction sites, loss of the remaining maxillary alveolar ridge is minimized. If a denture base extension is placed in the premaxilla, two-thirds of the upper lip will be severely distorted from the base of the nose to the edge of the upper lip, specifically the wet-dry line.

Assuming the premaxilla buccal undercut does not require preprosthetic surgery, the flangeless maxillary complete denture is indicated to meet aesthetic requirements and ideal support of the upper lip. By maintaining undercuts in the premaxilla, additional retention is potentially available. Undercuts of the residual alveolar maxillary ridge should be scrutinized carefully, and not removed indiscriminately (**Fig. 3**).

PRELIMINARY IMPRESSIONS

Alginate impression material[21] is readily used for preliminary impressions, but can be poorly managed; it is extremely accurate to the 75-μm level. The water to powder ratio may be varied to desired stiffness, but the impressions must be poured soon after to ensure accuracy of the material. Accurate diagnostic impressions are made to replicate the patient's vestibule, capture the mucosa, and develop the appropriate contours.

The impressions are poured in a type III dental stone and trimmed to specified dimensions, and the landmarks are drawn on the resulting cast. Alginate serves as an excellent material when making preliminary impressions for a modified denture.

FINAL IMPRESSIONS

Final impressions are made using custom resin impression trays. These impression trays must be adjusted to give 1 to 2 mm to allow for the proper extension of

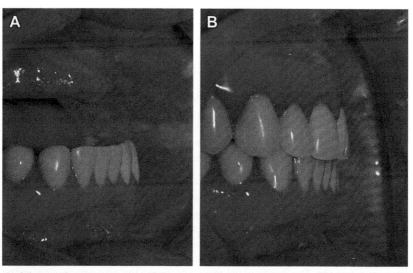

Fig. 3. (*A*) Note the 45° trajectory of the premaxilla in relation to mandibular tooth position. (*B*) Flangeless denture showing relationship of maxillary artificial denture teeth to mandibular tooth position. Note that additional acrylic into the labial vestibule is not needed as for a full-length labial flange.

thermoplastic material or border-molded impression material. When planning for a flangeless denture, this is followed by a wash of impression material. The anterior vestibule should be recorded appropriately using established standard-protocol border-molding procedures. Different impression materials are used as final impressions in the fabrication of complete dentures. There are many variables that affect selection of impression material. When undercuts are present that limit a conventional flange, a modification of the flange may be indicated.

Although most alveolar bony undercuts are not desirable, there are times when surgical modification of undesirable bony undercuts is not possible and must be managed clinically. In these instances, a resilient, elastomeric impression material is used. The impression is managed under standard-protocol boxing and pouring techniques.

JAW RELATION RECORDS

Normally, jaw relation records begin with well-fitting, stable record bases that typically fill the entire vestibule from the resulting impressions. The resulting record bases must be comfortable and stable on the master casts without displacement or rocking. If rocking exists and the record base does not fit the cast, it will not fit well intraorally. After the record base is made, occlusion rims are made using specific dimensions and are adapted to the base.

During the jaw relation record appointment, the maxillary occlusion wax rim is contoured following aesthetic and phonetic clinical parameters. The occlusal wax rim is contoured to achieve the best profile for the patient by viewing the nasolabial folds and the position of the philtrum. On evaluating the fullness of the upper lip, appropriate support of the upper lip must be determined before assessing the length of the occlusal wax rim. The relaxed position of the lip must allow the patient to bring the lips together and to wipe the upper lip with the tongue, and on smiling the "curtain of tissue" of the upper lip should be raised and lowered comfortably without any visible distortion.

The best way to determine correct lip position and function is to evaluate the appearance in the sagittal view. The length of the buccal flange is determined to meet the previously noted aesthetic, functional patient expectations. The key difference in the maxillary occlusal wax rim for the flangeless complete denture is that there is no flange on the occlusal wax rim.

In conventional dentures, frequently the anterior flange of the rim protrudes, creating a full appearance under the nose, making it feel distorted to the patient. The advantage of a modified flange is that by eliminating the labial flange, the patient's profile appears more natural and comfortable. The anterior artificial teeth are still set in an ideal relationship. Correct position of the denture teeth aids in retention from the perspective of load distribution, and mechanical, biological, and physical factors of denture retention as described by Fish,[22] Pound,[23] Schiesser,[24] and Beresin.[25]

If the denture teeth are placed correctly, the modified flange is not detectable. When the patient smiles, the upper lip rests at the cervical one-third of the denture teeth, and the border of the modified flange is not visible.

The remaining denture design and fabrication procedures follow the standard clinical protocol. The midline, the corners of the mouth, and the high lip line are marked on the occlusion wax rim. The length of the rim is shortened based on phonetics using the fricatives "f" and "v." The length of the occlusal wax rim is also determined using aesthetics, and is approximately 1 to 2 mm incisally located, depending on whether the patient is male or female and on the length of the upper lip. The mandibular occlusal wax rim is used to support the lower lip and to assist in assuring that the edge of the maxillary occlusal wax rim from a sagittal view splits the lower lip in half.

Vertical dimension of rest is recorded by measuring the proper jaw separation of the mandible to the maxilla by marks made using a pen or adhesive tape on the tip of the nose and the most prominent part of the chin; and measuring the distance between the marks and having the patient pronounce "m" or "Emma." The maxillary and mandibular occlusal wax rims are reduced at the anterior edge until the rims measure 2 to 3 mm less than the vertical dimension of rest (**Figs. 4** and **5**).

AESTHETIC TRY-IN

The aesthetic try-in resembles evaluation procedures performed during the jaw relation appointment. It begins with the evaluation of the patient's profile and the position of the upper lip. If the lip support is inadequate, modification of the flange can be made for the final denture. Aesthetics is then viewed in repose and smiling positions. Phonetics such as "f" and "v," "s," "th," "ch," and "j" are used during this appointment. The posterior occlusion must be stable, and the centric relation position is verified to obtain optimal occlusion. The complete denture occlusion can be designed based on occlusal schemes ranging from anatomic,[26] lingualized,[27] to monoplane,[28] depending on previous conditions and other patient factors.

Good communication with the dental laboratory technician is critical when prescribing the design and when processing the modified complete denture. The modified complete denture must be discussed before processing to eliminate the perceived correction needed to fill the vestibule to accommodate conventional fabrication of denture flange. In addition, the thickness of the denture border in the modified flange area is often increased to facilitate processing and reduced after processing to create the desired thickness.

DENTURE PROSTHESIS INSERTION APPOINTMENT

Just as in the jaw relation appointment, the fullness and profile is evaluated along with length of the teeth, the midline, and plane of occlusion. During the jaw relation appointment, thicker and bulky occlusal wax rims limit the clinical evaluation phonetically, so careful clinical evaluation can be refined at the prosthesis insertion appointment. At the trial denture appointment, the patient may perceive an enhanced clinical appearance, although there are still limitations if the blocked-out denture base causes lip protrusion or fullness.

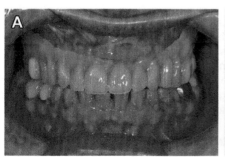
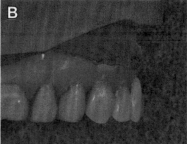

Fig. 4. (*A*) Aesthetic try-in with flangeless trial denture. (*B*) Trial denture on maxillary master cast.

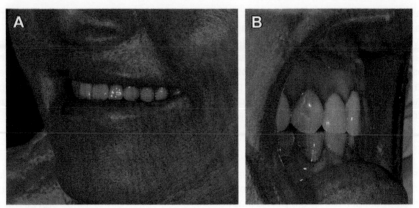

Fig. 5. (*A*) Final flangeless maxillary denture with full smile. (*B*) Sagittal view of final flangeless maxillary denture in maximum intercuspation.

The patient with a stable denture base will have a better opinion of the final result, with aesthetics and phonetics being easier to evaluate. Even if the complete dentures are made to almost the exact specifications of the previous prosthesis, the design will still be different, with a consequent significant learning adjustment for the patient. An important aspect of the placement appointment is teaching the patient how to care for dentures. Addressing expectations for chewing, speaking, and wearing the denture cannot be overemphasized.

Teaching individuals how to physically care for their prosthesis and their investment in their oral health is one of best services a dentist can offer to patients. Patients need to be cautioned that dentures do not replace natural teeth and have significant limitations. Patients must be instructed on how to clean their prostheses and review their use, and to remove the prosthesis for at least 8 hours a day to provide rest to the supporting tissues. One important aspect of the flangeless denture is that if the decision is made that a flange is not desirable for a patient, this must not occur at the placement appointment, but should be determined at the treatment-planning phase before processing and manufacture of the prosthesis.

POSTPLACEMENT CARE

The importance of the postplacement appointment must be understood by patients. Patients should return to the dentist the next day to address any immediate concerns. A crucial aspect of this appointment is to evaluate how the patient is managing the prosthesis without a labial denture flange.

Similar to previous appointments, evaluation includes assessment of comfort, function, retention, and facial support. A disadvantage of the flangeless denture occurs when there has been facial alveolar bone loss and a flange is needed for additional support of the upper lip. The next-day appointment addresses problems and prevents potential complications from becoming bigger issues, thus preventing significant discomfort and unnecessary psychological damage.

SUBSEQUENT TREATMENT AND MAINTENANCE

Future maintenance appointments are critical to the successful wearing of a flangeless maxillary denture. A prosthesis without a flange does not necessarily mean there are

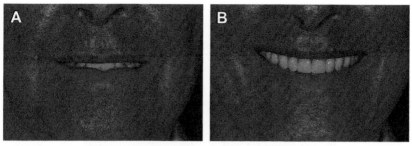

Fig. 6. Flangeless maxillary denture and mandibular complete denture. (*A*) Frontal view of the patient in repose. (*B*) Final view of patient in smiling position.

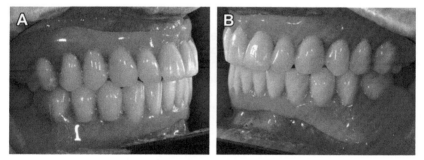

Fig. 7. Completed flangeless maxillary and mandibular complete dentures in maxillary intercuspation. (*A*) Right frontal view. (*B*) Left frontal view.

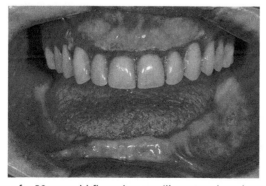

Fig. 8. Frontal view of a 20-year-old flangeless maxillary complete denture.

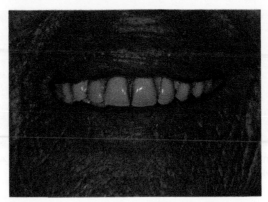

Fig. 9. Facial view of a 20-year-old flangeless maxillary denture.

fewer postinsertion appointments, but these future appointments provide additional time to reinforce education and home-care instructions. Some patients may think that once they receive their new dentures they no longer require future dental appointments.

Maintenance and refitting procedures are necessary for all patients. Not all patients may need refitting or relining procedures for their prosthesis, but the supporting hard and soft tissues change and denture teeth wear over time. Patients are tempted to simply use some adhesive to keep the dentures in place, but without refitting the dentures in these situations, wearing ill-fitting dentures can be extremely destructive to both a conventional denture and a flangeless designed denture (**Figs. 6–9**).

INDICATIONS

Existing lip support does not require additional flange thickness or length to create the illusion of normalcy.

Residual anterior mandible and premaxillae are at a 45° angle.

Adding excessive acrylic resin in the vestibule distorts desired lip support.

ADVANTAGES

There is no distortion of desired aesthetic facial support.

No additional surgical intervention is required to remove osseous residual ridge.

With thorough understanding and patient education, there is general patient acceptance of aesthetic results.

LIMITATIONS

Bony contour of residual ridge may not yield sufficient lip support, requiring additional labial flange length and bulk acrylic to meet aesthetic goals.

SUMMARY

Although the flangeless complete denture is not used routinely, it has been successfully used for the treatment of edentulous patients. The importance of retention, border molding, diagnosis, and treatment planning in treating such patients is reviewed herein. The scrupulous detail and meticulous attention to protocol throughout the course of treatment with the flangeless denture is emphasized and the advantages, indications, and limitations described.

The modified maxillary denture is a valuable treatment modality that should be considered when treating select edentulous patients.

ACKNOWLEDGMENTS

Dr Dan Bakko is acknowledged for his assistance with the photography.

REFERENCES

1. Hardy IR, Kapur KK. Posterior border seal—its rationale and importance. J Prosthet Dent 1958;8:386–97.
2. Silverman SI. Dimensions and displacement patterns of the posterior palatal seal. J Prosthet Dent 1971;25(5):470–88.
3. Laney WR, Gonzalez JB. The maxillary denture: its palatal relief and posterior palatal seal. J Am Dent Assoc 1967;75(5):1182–7.
4. Ettinger RI, Scandrett FR. The posterior palatal seal, a review. Aust Dent J 1980; 25:197–200.
5. Calomeni AA, Feldmann EE, Kuebker WA. Posterior palatal seal location and preparation on the maxillary complete denture cast. J Prosthet Dent 1983; 49(5):628–30.
6. Sykora O, Sutow EJ. Posterior palatal seal adaptation: influence of processing technique, palate shape and immersion. J Oral Rehabil 1993;20(1):19–31.
7. Rashedi B, Petropoulos VC. Current concepts for determining the postpalatal seal in complete dentures. J Prosthodont 2003;12(4):265–70.
8. Kim Y, Michalakis KX, Hirayama H. Effect of relining method on dimensional accuracy of posterior palatal seal. An in vitro study. J Prosthodont 2008;17(3):211–8 Epub 2007 Jan 11.
9. Perry JL. Anatomy and physiology of the velopharyngeal mechanism. Semin Speech Lang 2011;32(2):83–92 Epub 2011 Sept 26.
10. Sharry JJ. Complete denture prosthodontics. 3rd edition. St. Louis (MO): McGraw-Hill; 1974.
11. Zarb GA, Bolender CL, Carlsson GE. Boucher's prosthodontic treatment for edentulous patients. 11th edition. St. Louis (MO): Mosby; 1985.
12. Rahn AO, Ivanhoe JR, Plummer KD. Textbook of complete dentures. 6th edition. Philadelphia: Williams and Wilkins, Media; 2009.
13. Kinsel RP. Development of gingival esthetics in the edentulous patient prior to dental implant placement using a flangeless removable prosthesis: a case report. Int J Oral Maxillofac Implants 2002;17(6):866–72.
14. Reynolds TJ. The flangeless fixed denture. J Oral Implantol 1980;9(1):45–55.
15. Freeman SP. Technique: a flangeless immediate denture technique. J Conn State Dent Assoc 1965;39:11–3.
16. Phoenix RD, Cagna DR, DeFreest CF. Stewart's clinical removable partial prosthodontics. 4th edition. Carol Stream (IL): Quintessence; 2008.
17. Jones JD, Garcia LT. Removable partial dentures: a clinician's guide. Ames (IO): Wiley-Blackwell; 2009.
18. Carr AB, Brown DT. McCracken's removable partial prosthodontics. 9th edition. St. Louis (MO): Mosby; 2010.
19. Grasso JE, Miller EL. Removable partial prosthodontics. 3rd edition. St. Louis (MO): Mosby; 1991.

20. McGarry TJ, Nimmo A, Skiba JF, et al. Classification system for partial edentulism. J Prosthodont 2002;11(3):181–93.
21. Rudd KD, Morrow RM, Strunk RR. Accurate alginate impressions. J Prosthet Dent 1969;22(3):294–300.
22. Fish SF. Principles of full denture prosthesis. 6th edition. Springfield (IL): C.C. Thomas; 1964.
23. Pound E. Personalized denture procedures: dentist's manual. Anaheim, CA: Denar Corp; 1973.
24. Schiesser FJ. The neutral zone and polished surfaces in complete dentures. J Prosthet Dent 1964;14(5):854–65.
25. Beresin VE. The neutral zone in complete dentures. J Prosthet Dent 2006;95(2): 93–101.
26. Jordan LG. Arrangement of anatomic-type artificial teeth into balanced occlusion. J Prosthet Dent 1978;39(5):484–94.
27. Lang BR. Complete denture occlusion. Dent Clin North Am 2004;48(3):641–65.
28. Jones PM. The monoplane occlusion for complete dentures. J Am Dent Assoc 1972;85(1):94–100.

Geriatric Prosthodontic Care

Mary Norma Partida, DDS, MPH

KEYWORDS

- Geriatrics • Oral health • Trends • Prosthodontics

KEY POINTS

- The geriatric population size is increasing.
- In the 65-years and older cohort there is an increase in certain medical conditions that affect oral health.
- The utilization of dental services by the elderly depends on many factors, such as insurance, socioeconomic status, ethnicity, education, access, and perceived needs.
- A trend seen in the delivery of dental services to older people is an increased need for prosthodontic treatment.
- In the oral health care of geriatric patients there are multifactorial issues that must be taken into account. These are not only limited to dental techniques but also include risks, nutrition, quality of life, and psychosocial needs.

INTRODUCTION

The geriatric population is growing at a faster pace than any group globally. Common medical conditions have dental implications. Although edentulism rates are declining, there are still higher rates of tooth loss in the elderly due to caries, periodontal disease, and ability of the patient to perform oral hygiene care.

There is much diversity in lifestyles and beliefs of the elderly population. Because of this diversity, the delivery of geriatric prosthodontic care must consider several factors in the diagnosis, treatment planning, and delivery of dental treatment. Some barriers exist for the geriatric patient in access to care.

AGING TRENDS

Baby boomers are a cohort that was born between the years of 1946 and 1964. The first baby boomers turned 65 years in 2011. It is estimated there will be 71.5 million people age 65 years and older by the year 2030.[1] Currently, 1 in every 8, or 13.1% of the population, is an older American.[2] Persons reaching age 65 have an average life expectancy of 83.8 years with women outliving men.[2] Of geriatric populations, the 85 and older cohort is the fastest growing segment. With this increase in the 65

Department of Comprehensive Dentistry, The University of Texas Health Science Center, San Antonio Dental School, 7703 Floyd Curl Drive, San Antonio, TX 78257, USA
E-mail address: PARTIDAM@uthscsa.edu

Dent Clin N Am 58 (2014) 103–112
http://dx.doi.org/10.1016/j.cden.2013.09.005
0011-8532/14/$ – see front matter © 2014 Elsevier Inc. All rights reserved.

and older population there will continue to be oral health care needs. The demand for dental professionals knowledgeable in geriatric dentistry will be necessary.

With the aging population there is much diversity in education and socioeconomic status. As the baby boomers continue to migrate to geriatric cohorts there will be changes in the labor workforce. There is a higher educational attainment in the baby boomer age group. The average person in latter baby boomer years was employed 78% of the weeks from age 18 to 46.[3] **Fig. 1** shows the percentage of weeks employed by educational attainment during years 1978 to 2010. There is a higher tendency for women who have attained higher educational levels to work more weeks. Men with higher educational attainment also worked more weeks. Educational attainment of less than high school diploma showed the fewest weeks employed for men and women.

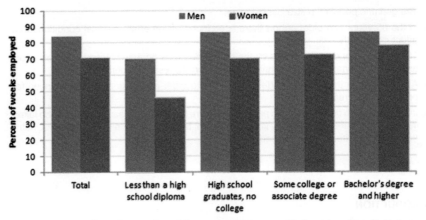

Fig. 1. Percentage of weeks employed from age 18 to age 46, by educational attainment and sex, 1978–2010. (*From* Bureau of Labor Statistics, U.S. Department of Labor. The Editor's Desk: Labor market attachment of baby boomers by educational attainment on the Internet. Available at http://www.bls.gov/opub/ted/2012/ted_20120807.htm.)

With higher educational attainment levels, this will affect dental economics and what baby boomers consider important. A dentist who is keen on understanding population changes will certainly be more in tune to the needs of the elderly. A recent trend seen in the elderly is the use of Internet and social networking. According to the Pew Foundation, persons 65 years and older had an increase in Internet usage from 1% in 2006 to 33% elderly persons using the Internet in 2011.[4] Internet sites visited most often were search engines, news, and government sites. Patient education is important in dentistry. If the geriatric population were increasingly using the Internet, this would be an excellent means to create dental educational web sites for geriatric patients.

COMMON MEDICAL CONDITIONS

Despite higher educational attainment levels, geriatric populations have higher rates of comorbid diseases compared with younger cohorts. The most common medical conditions in the elderly are coronary heart disease, hypertension, cancer, arthritis, dementia, and traumatic injuries such as falls. **Fig. 2** graphs the chronic medical conditions in the elderly according to ethnicity.[5]

There is increasing scientific evidence in the medical and dental professions that oral health and systemic diseases are related.[6] Periodontal disease induces an elevated systemic inflammatory status. Studies have shown that there is a relationship

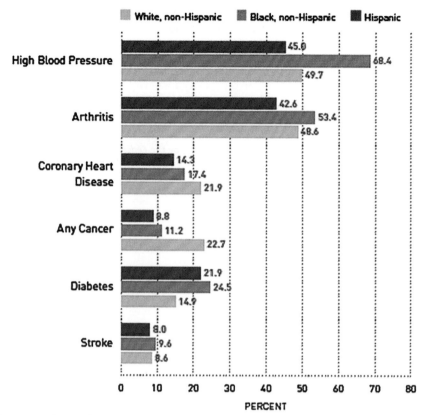

Fig. 2. Prevalence of chronic conditions among adults +65 years and varied by race/ethnicity in 2002–2003. (*From* CDC, National Center for Health Statistics, National Health Interview Survey, 2006.)

between periodontal disease and atherosclerotic disease, especially stroke.[7] Diabetes is a risk factor for periodontal disease. Uncontrolled periodontal disease can aggravate diabetic complications. Controlled periodontal disease can improve glycemic control.[8,9] Dental professionals should intercollaborate with medical professionals when systemic conditions influence oral health care.

Globally and nationally, the health of geriatric populations is a priority. The Department of Health and Human Services has recognized oral health and access to care as a leading indicator for overall health in the Healthy People 2020 objectives. The oral health section of Healthy People 2020 takes into account age, gender, educational attainment, socioeconomic status, race, and access to health insurance.

A new and major goal of Health People 2020 is to improve the health, function, and quality of life of older adults. Objectives very relevant to the elderly are

- Increase awareness of the importance to overall health and well-being
- Increase acceptance and adoption of effective prevention interventions
- Reduce disparities in access to effective preventive and dental treatment services.

The Fédération Dentaire Internationale World Dental Federation has collaborated with the World Health Organization and the International Association of Dental

Research to review and revise global oral health goals, objectives, and targets. Like Healthy People, the target year is 2020. The objectives focus on reducing mortality from oral-facial disease, developing evidence-based policies and programs developing cost-effective prevention programs, and reducing oral health disparities. **Box 1** summarizes the priority target conditions selected for the global oral health 2020.

Box 1
Global oral health 2020: priority target conditions

Global Oral Health: priority target conditions selected by the Fédération Dentaire Internationale, World Health Organization, and International Association of Dental Research

- Pain
- Infectious diseases
- Oral HIV infection
- Trauma
- Dental caries
- Periodontal diseases
- Salivary gland disorders
- Health care services
- Functional disorders
- Oropharyngeal cancer
- Noma
- Craniofacial anomalies
- Developmental anomalies
- Oral mucosal diseases
- Tooth loss
- Health care information

As people become older, the correlation between oral health and general health is notable. Oral diseases have manifestations related to chronic systemic conditions. With age, there is an increase in medical conditions that require medication usage. The combination of systemic disease and medications can have a pronounced effect that can increase susceptibility to oral health disease. Another major factor is that with age it may become increasingly difficult to maintain good oral hygiene especially with medical conditions such as stroke or arthritis.

DENTAL UTILIZATION BY THE ELDERLY

There is a range of dental utilization in the elderly due to the diversity of the population. With the increase in geriatric population size and longevity, there is an increased need for dental services. Factors that influence dental utilization are

- Socioeconomic status
- Educational attainment
- Insurance
- Health, health beliefs, and/or perceived needs

The elderly populations have increased rates of tooth loss, dental caries, periodontal disease, xerostomia, and oral cancer.[10] Tooth loss or edentulism increases with age. In the 75-years and older cohort, approximately one-third are edentulous.[11] Tooth loss or edentulism can result in psychosocial changes in a person's life. Psychological conditions related to edentulism are depression, anxiety, and fear.[12] The effects of edentulism play a major role in quality of life. Impact of edentulism in the elderly includes

- Speech
- Esthetics
- Function
- Nutritional deficiencies
- Psychological issues, self-image
- Quality of life

Frail elderly in long-term facilities can have difficulty obtaining dental services or access to services. As a result, oral health neglect is higher for institutionalized geriatric people that lead to increased tooth loss.

As the geriatric population increases, there are declining rates of edentulism. In 1971 the edentulism rate was approximately 50% for the elderly.[13] In 2004, the edentulism rate had decreased to 23% of the elderly being edentulous. Higher rates of edentulism are found in Native Americans, followed by African Americans, then Caucasians, with Asians and Hispanics having the lowest edentulism rates.[14]

With the increase in tooth retention is seen an increase of dental service utilization. In a 10-year longitudinal study, dentists 40 years and older benefited from an increase of 30.3% to 64.3% in patient visits, service, and expenditures.[15] Healthy community-dwelling geriatric people have the largest increase in relative health spending.[16] In 2010 dental service spending increased 2.3%.[17] Out-of-pocket spending accounts for 40% of dental spending. Out-of-pocket spending in 2010 increased only 0.5%.[17] In 2009, the average dental out-of-pocket expense was $873 and exceeded the average out-of-pocket prescription costs of $700.[18] The 85-years and older cohort has the highest increased rates of dental prevention visits.[19]

TRENDS IN DENTAL SERVICES FOR THE ELDERLY

Dental services for geriatric patients are influenced by costs of the dental services, dental insurance, access to the dental office, debt owed, and perceived needs. The national rate of dental insurance coverage is 60%.[18] Elderly patients without dental insurance are more likely to delay dental treatment than those having dental insurance.[18] Having dental insurance coverage decreased the chance of experiencing financial hardship because of costs.[18]

The 65-years and older population is diverse and will continue to be as the population increases. Most senior adults are living in a community and are functionally independent. Of geriatric people, only 5% to 10% live in a long-term care facility because of their inability to perform activities of daily living.[20] Baby boomers have higher educational attainment levels than their parents. They are more educated, have higher socioeconomic levels, and value good health care.[21] Many are concerned with esthetics and maintaining good health. **Table 1** is a comparison of 1988 to 1998 of the increasing trend by elderly persons on private practice patient load, services rendered, and patient expenditure.[21]

It is estimated that with the geriatric population growth and retiring older persons maintaining their dental insurance that dentists in the United States will continue to increase practice income by customary dental procedures.[22]

Table 1		
Private practitioner reports on patients in practice		
Case Load	1988	1998
% 65+	16.4	19.9
% Total services	13.6	17.5
% Total patient expenditures	18.0	22.0

Data from Meskin L, Berg R. Impact of older adults on private dental practices, 1988–1998. J Am Dent Assoc 2000;131:1188–95.

With increased age there is an increased need for major prosthodontics services inclusive of fixed crowns and bridges, and complete and partial dentures. Current trends in prosthodontics practices indicate a slight decrease in fixed prosthodontics.[23] Over a 6-year period from 2001 to 2007 there was an increase in treatment time of implant placement and implant restorations.[23] **Fig. 3** shows a mean percentage of time by selected dental procedure in years 2002, 2004, and 2007.

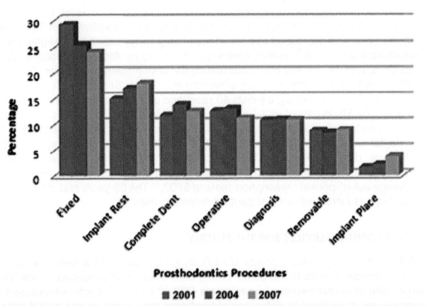

Prosthodontics Procedures

■ 2001 ■ 2004 ■ 2007

Fig. 3. Mean percentage of time by selected type of procedure, 2001, 2004, and 2007. (*From* Nash K, Pfiefer D, Sadowsky S, et al. Private practice of prosthodontists: current conditions of practice in the United States. J Prosthodont 2010;19:175–86; with permission.)

The trend for practice in Prosthdontics is an increase in fixed procedures and replacement of missing teeth with increased patient interest in implants. For complete denture wearers, the ideal treatment is a 2-implant retained mandibular overdenture. Patient quality of life is improved as well as bite force.[24] With the decline of edentulism and a more dentate elderly population, the need for prosthodontics will continue to rise.

CONSIDERATIONS TO ORAL HEALTH PLANNING AND DELIVERY

There cannot be enough emphasis on the aging population being a very diverse one in health, socioeconomic levels, education, and health beliefs. Although many older adults are living well independently, it may be that in the future this can change. Health conditions can occur and the ability to perform the activities of daily living can decline. With increasing age, especially in the 85-years and older cohort, there is an increase in dementia. Currently 5.3 million Americans have Alzheimer disease and this number is expected to more than double by 2050.[25]

Consequently, in the oral health treatment planning of geriatric patients, there are many considerations to be made.

Patient education in dental facts should be life-long for everyone. If private practice dentists give their patient constant educational facts on their oral health and changes in life, then patients can understand better the importance of prevention and maintaining regular dental visits. Because Internet usage is increasing in the elderly, legitimate web sites should be given to patients on prevention and dental facts recommended by not only dentists but also organizations such as the American Association of Retired Persons, Centers for Disease Control and Prevention, American Dental Association, American Nurses Association, and American Medical Association.

More education on interprofessional learning is needed in medical, health professions, and dental schools. Because oral health is a part of general well-being and health, medical and health care professions need more interaction with dentistry to be educated, value oral health, and understand the relation to total health.[21] Health care providers in long-term care facilities need constant updated education on providing oral health care and the importance for function and nutrition and well-being of the elderly individual.

Patient perceptions of self and their needs influence their decisions on accepting dental treatment. These health beliefs can be barriers or motivators in the elderly seeking dental treatment (**Box 2**).[21,26]

Box 2
Health beliefs, behaviors, and attitudes

- People seek dental care if they perceive the need is important and fear the condition will worsen without treatment
- People must have confidence that treatment will improve their health
- People with lower education attainment and income levels have lower expectations
- Some elderly think dental problems are a part of aging
- Some elderly believe teeth have social meaning and stigma
- Many elderly have the desire to look and stay attractive
- Many elderly think oral health is a psychological factor

Understanding a patient's health beliefs and attitudes is crucial in the diagnostic phase and in the treatment planning stages. If wearing a removable prosthesis has a negative connotation, then the patient will have difficulty adjusting to the prosthesis regardless how well it is made.[12,27] Dental professionals are more focused on the function and the technical aspect of dental treatment and tend to overlook the psychosocial factors. Dental education has emphasized the art and science of dentistry. To serve the geriatric patient better, dental schools need to educate dental students in the humanities and psychosocial factors.[28]

Dental education should strive to expand teaching in geriatric patient care.[29]

Prevention is of key importance in geriatric oral health. Geriatric prosthodontics necessitates treatment planning with this in mind. Dental check-ups may need to be

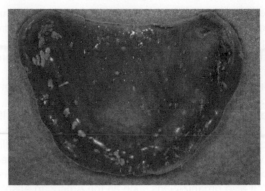

Fig. 4. Microorganism growth on denture.

scheduled more frequently and oral hygiene reinforced. Patients that wear removable partial dentures have a higher risk of root caries.[30] Incorporating the use of a combination of fluoride and chlorhexidine for at least 1 year has proven a useful intervention in tooth loss.[31] Microorganisms can breed successfully on denture materials, as shown in **Fig. 4**.

SUMMARY

Geriatric prosthodontic care encompasses many aspects and requires in-depth knowledge of the aging population. As the 65 and older populations increase, so will the demand and need for dental services. Prosthodontic dental services will continue to be sought by the elderly. The health of geriatric patients is related to oral health.

Geriatric patients are influenced by personal beliefs, behaviors, and attitudes to health care. The practicing dentist must understand this realm as well as the functional and technical aspects of dentistry. To ensure the best geriatric patient care, dental schools must educate dental students on interprofessional learning as well as expand geriatric training.

REFERENCES

1. Federal Interagency Forum on Aging Related Statistics. Older Americans 2004: Key Indicators of Well-being. Available at: http://www.aoa.gov/agingstatsdotnet/Main_Site/Data/2004_Documents/entire_report.pdf. Accessed November 1, 2012.
2. A Profile of Older Americans: 2011. Available at: http://www.aoa.gov/aoaroot/aging_statistics/Profile/2011/2.aspx. Accessed November 2, 2012.
3. TED: The Editor's Desk. Labor market attachment of baby boomers by educational attainment. Available at: http://www.bls.gov/opub/ted/2012/ted_20120807.htm. Accessed November 16, 2012.
4. Pew Internet and American Life Project. Presentation: older adults and social networking. Mary Madden, Project GOAL Panel. National Press Club; 2011. Available at: pewinternet.org/~/media/Files/Presentations/2011/Oct/Older Adults and Social Media pdf - 10 17 11.pdf. Accessed November 16, 2012.
5. CDC: The State of Aging and Health in America. Report 2007. Available at: http://apps.nccd.cdc.gov/SAHA/Default/Default.aspx. Accessed December 3, 2012.
6. Ferguson DA, Steinberg B, Schwien T. Dental economics and the aging population. Compend Contin Educ Dent 2010;31(6):418–20.

7. Joshipura K, Zevallos JC, Ritchie CS. Strength and evidence relating periodontal disease and atherosclerotic disease. Compend Contin Educ Dent 2009;30(7): 430–9.

8. Mealey BL, Oates TW. Diabetes mellitus and periodontal disease. J Periodontol 2006;77(8):1289–303.

9. Mealy BL, Ocampo GL. Diabetes and periodontal disease. Periodontol 2000 2007;44:127–53.

10. Schou L. Oral health, oral health care, and oral health promotion among older adults: social and behavioral dimensions. In: Cohen LK, Gift HC, editors. Disease prevention and oral health promotion. Copenhagen (Denmark): Munksgaard; 1995. p. 213–58.

11. Chen X, Clark J, Naorungrol S. Length of tooth survival in older adults with complex medical, functional, and dental backgrounds. J Am Dent Assoc 2012;143(6): 566–78.

12. Sowmya MK, Vinaya B, Krishna Prosad D. Psychological impact of edentulousness. JIADS 2011;2(1):34–6. Available at: http://jiads.net/Archives/new-issues/7.pdf. Accessed December 18, 2012.

13. Shay K. Older dental patients: myths and realities. August 2010. Available at: http://www.dentalcare.com/en-US/dental-education/continuing-education/ce6/ce6.aspx. Accessed November 13, 2012.

14. Liang W, Plassman BL, Remle C, et al. Edentulism trends among middle-aged and older adults in the United States: comparison of five racial/ethnic groups. Community Dent Oral Epidemiol 2012;40:145–53.

15. Meskin L, Berg R. Impact of older adults on private dental practices, 1988-1998. J Am Dent Assoc 2000;131:1188–95.

16. Kramarow E, Lubitz J, Lentzner H, et al. Trends in the health of older Americans, 1970-2005. Health Aff 2007;26(5):1417–25.

17. National Health Expenditures 2010 Highlights. Available at: http://www.cms.gov. Accessed November 4, 2012.

18. Pryor C, Prottas J, Lottero B, et al. The Cost of Dental Care and the Impact of Dental Insurance Coverage. Published August 2009: The Access Project. Available at: http://www.rwjf.org/en/research-publications/find-rwjf-research/20. Accessed November 7, 2012.

19. Skaar D, O'Connor H. Dental service trends for older U.S. adults, 1998-2006. Spec Care Dentist 2012;32(2):42–8.

20. Dolan T, Atchison K, Huynh T. Access to dental care among older adults in the United States. J Dent Educ 2005;69(9):961–74.

21. Kiyak HA, Reischmuth M. Barriers to and enablers of older adults' use of dental services. J Dent Educ 2005;69(9):975–86.

22. Eklund S, Pittman J, Smith R. Trends in per-patient gross income to dental practices. J Am Dent Assoc 1998;129:1559–65.

23. Nash K, Pfiefer D, Sadowsky D, et al. Private practice of prosthodontists: current conditions of practice in the United States. J Prosthodont 2010;19(3): 175–86.

24. Geckili O, Bilhan H, Mumcu E, et al. Comparison of patient satisfaction, quality of life, and bite force between elderly edentulous patients wearing mandibular two implant-supported overdentures and conventional complete dentures after 4 years. Spec Care Dentist 2012;32(4):136–41.

25. Centers for Disease Control and Prevention. Report on Dementia/Alzheimer's Disease. Available at: http://www.cdc.gov/mentalhealth/basics/mental-illness/dementia.htm. Accessed December 12, 2012.

26. Colussi C, Torres De Freitas S, Marino M. The prosthetic need WHO index: a comparison between self-perception and professional assessment in an elderly population. Gerodontology 2009;26:187–92.
27. Graham R, Mihaylov S, Jepson N, et al. Determining need for removable partial denture: a qualitative study of factors that influence dentist provision and patient use. Br Dent J 2006;200(3):155–8.
28. MacEntee M. The educational challenge of dental geriatrics. J Dent Educ 2010; 74(1):13–9.
29. Ettinger R. Meeting oral health needs to promote the well-being of the geriatric population: educational research issues. J Dent Educ 2010;74(1):29–35.
30. Preshaw PM, Walls A, Jakubovics N, et al. Association of removable partial denture use with oral and systemic health. J Dent 2011;39:711–9.
31. Hujoel PP, Powell L, Kiyak HA. The effects of simple interventions on tooth mortality: findings in one trial and implications in future studies. J Dent Res 1997;76(4): 867–74.

Latest Biomaterials and Technology in Dentistry

Roya Zandparsa, DDS, MSc, DMD

KEYWORDS

- Dental • Biomaterials • Technology • Implant • Navigation • Laser
- Nanotechnology • Tissue engineering

KEY POINTS

- In oral and maxillofacial surgery, navigation technology is applied with particular success in arthroscopy of the temporomandibular joint, in the surgical treatment of posttraumatic deformities of the zygomatic bone, in orthognathic surgery, and for distractions, osteotomies, tumor surgery, punctures, biopsies, and removal of foreign bodies.
- The use of laser beams for caries removal allows the preservation of the natural shape of decayed cavities without the need for preventive extension of prepared cavities.
- With nanodentistry, it is possible to maintain comprehensive oral health care by involving the use of nanomaterials, biotechnology, and ultimately dental nanorobotics. Nanorobots induce oral analgesia, desensitize teeth, manipulate the tissue to realign and straighten an irregular set of teeth, and improve the durability of teeth. They can also be used for preventive, restorative, and curative procedures.
- Strategies to engineer tissue can be categorized into 3 major classes: conductive, inductive, and cell transplantation approaches.
- Several populations of cells with stem cell properties have been isolated from different parts of the tooth. These populations include cells from the pulp of both exfoliated (children's) and adult teeth, from the periodontal ligament that links the tooth root with the bone, from the tips of developing roots, and from the tissue (dental follicle) that surrounds the unerupted tooth.

Replacement of missing tooth structure has been challenging. A long-term goal of dentistry was the ability to anchor a foreign material into the jaw to replace a tooth.[1,2]

DENTAL IMPLANTS

It is thought that the history of dental implants dates back to the ancient Egyptians around 3000 BC, because they used to hammer trimmed seashells into the jaw to replace missing teeth. Dental implants require the optimization of several important variables to enhance the chances of success, including appropriate material selection

Tufts University School of Dentistry, Postgraduate Prosthodontics Division, 1 Kneeland Street, Boston, MA 02111, USA
E-mail address: Roya.Zandparsa@tufts.edu

Dent Clin N Am 58 (2014) 113–134
http://dx.doi.org/10.1016/j.cden.2013.09.011
0011-8532/14/$ – see front matter © 2014 Elsevier Inc. All rights reserved.

and design; an understanding and evaluation of the biological interaction at the interface between the implant and the tissue; careful and controlled surgical techniques; collaboration between various specialties to optimize patient selection; selection of appropriate implant design, size, and surface; and long-term follow-up care.[1,3]

There have been 3 basic designs of dental implants. The endosseous implant was preceded by the subperiosteal and transosteal implants. The most successful and frequently used implant design is the endosseous type. Dental implants have been made from many different materials, such as platinum, silver, steel, cobalt alloys, titanium and alloy, acrylic, carbon, sapphire, alumina, tantalum, niobium, zirconia, and calcium phosphate compounds.[4–8] An implant is placed in a surgically prepared osteotomy, submerged and integrated within the bone of the mandible or maxilla. Success of endosseous dental implants depends on the formation of the biologic interface between the bone and the implant, which is formed by the growth of new bone. This interface, osseointegration, represents integration of the new bone along the implant surface.

CERAMICS

Ceramics have been used for manufacture of dental implants based on the properties of biocompatibility and inert behavior.[3] Because bone is composed of a calcium phosphate ceramic, hydroxyapatite, bone replacement using a substance of similar composition, such as synthetic hydroxyapatite, could be presumed to be suitable. Ceramics are mixtures of nonmetals and metals and can be divided into metallic oxides or other compounds. Ceramics have been used in manufacture of dental implants because of their high strength, suitable color, and low thermal and electrical conductivity. Nevertheless, the limitation of this type of material is based on low ductility and brittleness.[7] These properties have led to the development of metallic implants, which may be designed with calcium phosphate coatings.[1,2]

Metallic oxides (eg, Al_2O_3, ZrO_2, TiO_2) have been used for root form, endosteal plate form, and pin-type dental implants. Calcium phosphate ($CaPO_4$), also known as calcium phosphate ceramics, has been used in dental reconstructive surgery, endosteal implants, and subperiosteal implants as a coating for stronger implant materials.[7,9]

Zirconia Implants

The first ceramic implant placed in United States and Germany was used as a medical joint substitute in the 1970s.[9] Various zirconia dental implant systems are available commercially as well as the use of zirconia particles comprising a coating material. Many studies have shown enhanced implant osseointegration in titanium implant surfaces coated with zirconia and that zirconia implants are capable of contributing to similar bone-implant contact to that of titanium implants.[10–12]

Yttria stabilized zirconia (Y-TZP) is currently considered an attractive and advantageous endosseous dental implant material because it presents enhanced biocompatibility, improved mechanical properties, high radiopacity, and easy handling during abutment preparation.[13] Zirconia ceramic is well tolerated by bone and soft tissues and possesses mechanical stability.[14] Because the difference in bone-to-implant attachment strength between bioinert ceramics and stainless steel is not significant, the affinity of bone to bioinert ceramics has almost the same capacity as metal alloys.[14] This fact was confirmed in another in vivo study, in which no differences in soft tissue health were seen in peri-implant mucosa adjacent to zirconia and titanium abutment surfaces.[15] From the available data, osseointegration of Y-TZP implants might be comparable with that of titanium implants.[16]

Regarding the impact of the design (1 piece vs 2 piece) on the biomechanical behavior of Y-TZP implants using chewing simulation testing conditions, a prototype 2-piece zirconia implant revealed low fracture resistance at the level of the implant head and therefore questionable clinical performance, whereas 1-piece zirconia implants seem to be clinically applicable. Moreover, it preparation of 1-piece zirconia implant to accept a crown had a statistically significant negative influence on the implant fracture strength.[14] Pirker and Kocher placed an immediate zirconia implant in the maxillary first premolar region and evaluated the clinical outcome of this implant. After a 2-year follow-up, a stable implant and unchanged peri-implant marginal bone level was observed.[17] Lambrich and Iglhaut[18] compared the survival rates for zirconia (Z-systems) and titanium dental implants. Zirconia implants had a comparable survival rate with titanium as long as there was a high primary stability and load-free healing, ideally under complete tooth-supported protective stents. Kohal and colleagues[19] found that yttrium-partially stabilized zirconia (YPSZ) implants had a similar stress distribution to commercially pure Ti implants and presented a pattern of low, well-distributed stress along the implant-to-bone interface. Kohal and colleagues[20] evaluated the cyclic loading and preparation on the fracture strength of a zirconia dental implant system and observed that preparation as well as cyclic loading can decrease the fracture strength resistance of zirconia implants.

Zirconia Implant Abutments

All-ceramic implant abutments made from aluminum oxide ceramic material (glass infiltrated or densely sintered alumina) were first introduced as an esthetic alternative to titanium in the mid-1990s. The alumina abutments presented pleasing optical properties, adequate fracture strength for the anterior regions, and excellent 5-year prognosis. Implant manufacturers are also producing abutments made from zirconia. Besides strength considerations, Y-TZP implant abutments offer enhanced biocompatibility, metal-like radiopacity for better radiographic evaluation, and ultimately reduced bacterial adhesion, plaque accumulation, and inflammation risk. Moreover, Y-TZP abutments may promote soft tissue integration, whereas favorable peri-implant soft tissues may be clinically achieved adjacent to zirconia or alumina-zirconia abutments and zirconia healing caps.[2] Zirconia abutments are successors to the densely sintered high-purity alumina (Al_2O_3) abutments. Zirconia abutments are radiopaque and show significantly higher resistance to fracturing.[21]

Zirconia abutments are available in prefabricated or customized forms and can be prepared in the dental laboratory either by the technician or by using computer-aided design/computer-aided manufacturing (CAM) techniques. The radiopaque esthetic abutment has good biocompatibility and is designed to engage the implant directly. They offer sufficient stability to support implant-retained reconstructions, especially in the incisor and premolar locations. They are indicated in areas with limited gingival tissue height and also minimize the gray color transmitted through the peri-implant tissues associated with metal components.[17,22]

COMPUTER-AIDED NAVIGATION IN DENTAL IMPLANTOLOGY

Computer-assisted navigation systems are widespread in neurosurgery; orthopedics; and ear, nose, and throat surgery.[23–26] In oral and maxillofacial surgery, navigation technology is applied with particular success in arthroscopy of the temporomandibular joint; in the surgical treatment of posttraumatic deformities of the zygomatic bone; in orthognathic surgery; and for distractions, osteotomies, tumor surgery, punctures, biopsies, and removal of foreign bodies.[23]

At present, a trend in the use of computer-assisted navigation in dental implantology can be observed. Navigation systems are developed for research purposes and for use by commercial companies that provide hardware and software to position dental implants. A substantial advantage of navigation is precise preoperative planning, which is optimized by taking into consideration prosthetic and functional aspects. This advantage is of crucial importance to avoid an unfavorable mechanical load, which can lead to peri-implant bone loss and thus an early loss of implants.[23–27] Furthermore, navigation systems improve intraoperative safety, because damage to critical anatomic structures such as nerves or neighboring teeth can be avoided. The accuracy attainable with computer-aided navigation systems has been examined in several studies and found to be sufficient.[23–29]

The work flow consists of getting all vital information from the patient's anatomy using a computed tomography (CT) scan or a cone-beam scan. The converted scan data result in three-dimensional representations of the patient's anatomy and provide vital information needed to plan the implant placement. The treatment planning results in creation of a customized drill guide that links the computer-assisted planning to the surgery and helps the surgeon to place the implants more accurately. The computer-aided surgical guide indicates the angle, position, and depth of the implants in the preoperative plan and can be placed on the bone or on the mucosa to guide the drill in the planned position during the surgery (**Fig. 1**).[30]

At present, three-dimensional CT and cone-beam CT (CBCT) systems allow a more reliable treatment planning than when only two-dimensional data were available, and allow the virtual implant planning driven by restorative considerations and the successive fabrication of surgical guides by means of CAM or rapid prototyping techniques. The developments in computer-aided planning by means of the use of three-dimensional virtual models have modified the interventional possibilities in implant

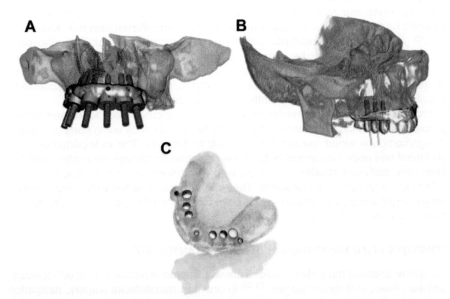

Fig. 1. Navigator system for CT-guided dental implant surgery. (*A*) The three-dimensional image is calculated and implants are planned. (*B*) The relation of the implants to the bone and the planned restoration. (*C*) The SurgiGuide with drill guide. (*Courtesy of* Materialise Dental Inc, Available at: http://www.materialisedental.com.)

dentistry. Multiple appointments are required, beginning with the initial diagnosis, impressions to fabricate the diagnostic casts, the diagnostic waxing, and fabrication of the radiographic template.[31]

CBCT RADIOLOGICAL SYSTEM

CT is routinely used in the diagnosis and treatment planning of dental and maxillofacial structures, with particular reference to dental implant surgery.[32–34] Special application software allows attainment of two-dimensional images perpendicular to the dental arch and panoramic views of the dental arch as well as three-dimensional views. However, the cost and complexity of these machines, along with the problems related to the high dose absorbed by the patient, limit the use of this modality.

There is a new type of CT machine devoted to the imaging of dental and maxillofacial structures and based on the cone-beam technique (CBCT). The CBCT technique has been used in radiotherapy, using fluoroscopic systems or modified simulators in order to obtain cross sections of the patient in the geometric conditions of the treatment.[35–40] The CBCT technique has also been used in vascular imaging and in microtomography of small specimens for biomedical and industrial applications. The technique seems to be promising because of the inherent efficiency in volumetric acquisition and high efficiency in radiograph use. Moreover, it permits manufacture of less costly CT machines. In principle, the CBCT technique allows faster data acquisition than traditional CT. Overall advantages of the CBCT technique are a lower radiation dose, a shorter acquisition time, and reduced costs. Disadvantages of CBCT include the scattered radiation, the limited dynamic range of the x-ray area detectors, the truncated-view artifact, and artifacts caused by beam hardening. These drawbacks need to be considered because they may influence image quality and bone segmentation accuracy.[41–44]

A large number of different computer-assisted guided implant systems are available today in clinical practice. Differing levels and quantity of evidence were noted to be available, revealing a high mean implant survival rate of 96.6% after only 12 months of observation in different clinical indications. In addition, the mean percentage of intraoperative complications and unexpected events was 4.6%.[45]

The accuracy of these systems depends on all cumulative and interactive errors involved. There is not yet evidence to suggest that computer-assisted surgery is superior to conventional procedures in terms of safety, outcomes, morbidity, or efficiency.

LASER SYSTEMS IN DENTISTRY

In recent years, various laser systems have gained importance in dentistry as alternative methods for tooth preparation as well as for soft tissue management.[46]

The use of laser beam for caries removal allows the preservation of the natural shape of decayed cavities without the need for preventive extension of prepared cavities.[46]

In operative dentistry, some laser wavelengths have the ability to produce a melting of dentinal surfaces by heat generation, which is potentially helpful in the treatment of dental hypersensitivity.[46]

The high potential of disinfection of laser beams can be helpful for the eradication of infected oral areas and for the treatment of viral tumors. Laser surgery induces a different process for oral soft tissue healing. The advantages of using the laser beam in oral surgeries are the reduction of inflammation and postoperative discomfort, appreciated quality of healed tissues, disinfection potential, and induction of fibrin production in lased tissues.[46]

The use of some wavelengths of laser beams is also beneficial in oral prosthetic surgery. The nonsuturing of the wounds on patients having removable prostheses such as complete dentures after the ablation by laser beam of tumors or any gingival hyperplasia allows the preservation and, in some cases, increase of vestibular length that is beneficial for the stability and retention of dentures. Laser beams can also be helpful in oral esthetic applications. The removal of gingival pigmentation (eg, melanin or metallic tattoo) by laser beams can be performed in a bloodless surgical field, and it also reduces postoperative discomfort. The use of laser beam seems to be the best alternative for the treatment of mucositis, which is a common side effect of chemotherapy and radiotherapy in patients with cancer.[46]

Laser in Restorative Dentistry

Alternative technologies for cavity preparation, such as erbium yttrium aluminum garnet (Er:YAG) laser, have been studied to reduce the inherent stresses, to minimize the removal of sound tooth structure, and to provide a surface that is more suitable for adhesive restorative materials.[47]

When laser light reaches a tissue, it can be absorbed, reflected, scattered, or transmitted to the surrounding tissues. Absorption by water molecules plays a significant role in thermal reactions.[48] Laser energy is absorbed selectively by water molecules and hydrous organic components of biological tissues in Er:YAG laser irradiation. Erbium, chromium yttrium scandium gallium garnet (Er,Cr:YSGG) laser is more highly absorbed by OH ions than water molecules and is expected to have a performance similar to that of the Er:YAG laser.[47] In both erbium lasers, absorption into water and hydrous organic components occurs quickly, before the absorption into inorganic components (ie, the cause of heat accumulation)[47–49] takes place. Therefore these two laser systems have been shown to remove enamel and dentin as safely as conventional diamond burs.[49–52]

Veneer removal

Veneer removal is generally performed with a rotary instrument. With the introduction of pulsed lasers into dentistry, there may be a beneficial application of such lasers for removing veneers. The Er:YAG laser energy is transmitted through the veneer, and the transmitted amount depends on the veneer thickness and composition. The veneer resin cement absorbs the transmitted energy, which results in an ablation of the cement. When enough cement is ablated through the veneer it slides off the tooth surface.[53]

Laser in Soft Tissue Procedures

Many studies have shown that the use of laser in intraoral soft tissues may result in increased coagulation, a dry surgical field, and better visualization. Laser increases tissue surface sterilization, which reduces bacteremia, and decreases swelling, edema, and scarring. Gingival depigmentation using laser ablation has been recognized as an effective, pleasant, and reliable technique. Finkbeiner in 1994 suggested the usefulness of argon laser in soft tissue welding and soldering compared with conventional tissue closure methods. At present, lasers are used for frenectomy, free gingival graft procedures, crown lengthening, operculectomy, and many other procedures.[54]

NANOTECHNOLOGY IN DENTISTRY

Nanotechnology is engineering of molecularly precise structures. These techniques use molecular machines that are typically equal to or less than 0.1 μm. The prefix nano means 10 to the minus ninth power (10^{-9}), or 1 billionth. The nanoscale is about a 1000 times smaller than micro, which is about 1/80,000 of the diameter of a human hair. It is expected that nanotechnology will be developed at several levels: materials, devices, and systems. At present, the nanomaterials level is the most advanced both in scientific knowledge and in commercial applications. To understand nanodentistry requires a background in nanotechnology and nanomedicine. Nanotechnology aims to manipulate and control particles to create novel structures with unique properties and promises advances in medicine and dentistry. The growing interest in the future of medical applications of nanotechnology is leading to the emergence of a new field called nanomedicine. With nanodentistry, it is possible to maintain comprehensive oral health care by involving the use of nanomaterials, biotechnology, and ultimately dental nanorobotics. Nanorobots induce oral analgesia, desensitize teeth, manipulate the tissue to realign and straighten irregular sets of teeth, and improve durability of teeth. They also can be used for preventive, restorative, and curative procedures.[55,56]

Major Tooth Repair

Many techniques have been proposed for tooth repair using tissue engineering procedures, with the goal of replacing the tooth and all the mineral and cellular components.[57,58]

Nanorobotic Dentifrice (Dentifrobots)

Development of dentifrobotics could lead to recognition and destruction of the pathogens that cause tooth caries. They will be delivered by either mouthwash or toothpaste and could be used to fight plaque formation, halitosis, and possibly calculus.[57,59]

Dentin Hypersensitivity

Many patients have dentinal hypersensitivity. A goal of dental nanorobotics is to target the exposed dentinal tubules and to relieve sensitivity.[57,59]

Orthodontic Nanorobots

Challenges in realignment of natural teeth occur as well as in the timing of tooth movement. Use of orthodontic nanorobotics could affect the timing of tooth movement.[57,59]

Tooth Durability and Appearance

Tooth durability, appearance, and biocompatibility may be improved by replacing enamel layers with covalently bonded artificial materials such as sapphire or diamond, which are 100 times harder than natural enamel or contemporary ceramic veneers. Like enamel, sapphire is susceptible to acid corrosion, but sapphire can be manufactured in virtually any color, offering cosmetic alternatives. Pure sapphire and diamond are brittle and prone to fracture if sufficient shear forces are imposed, but they can be made more fracture resistant as part of the nanostructure of composite materials that possibly include embedded carbon nanotubes.[57,59–62]

Nanocomposites are a new restorative nanomaterial that increases tooth durability. The manufacture of nanocomposites can use nonagglomerated discrete nanoparticles that are homogeneously distributed in resins or coatings to produce nanocomposites. The nanofiller includes an aluminosilicate powder with a mean particle size of about 80 nm and a 1:4 ratio of alumina to silica. The nanofiller has a refractive index of 1.508; it has superior hardness, modulus of elasticity, translucency, esthetic appeal, excellent color density, high polish, and 50% reduction in filling shrinkage. They are superior to conventional composites and blend with a natural tooth structure much better.[59,63–65]

Strength alone does not explain the relationship of filler to wear resistance. Occlusal wear occurs by several different mechanisms but mostly caused by abrasive particles of approximately 0.1-mm diameter that exist within food and that are suspected to be silica.[66]

The matrices all composites are subjected to wear. Manufacturers suggest a microprotection process in the design of the composite materials so that the filler covers and protects the matrix from contacting abrasive food particles. This phenomenon has been seen in some of the available dental composites such as microfills, microhybrids, and now in nanohybrids. Nanocomposites could become the composites of choice in the near future.[63]

Nanofillers are not all the same. A variety of nanofillers have already been shown. 3M uses sol-gel technology to produce tiny nanospheres called nanomers, which can be agglomerated into nanoclusters, and either the spheres or clusters can become filler particles for composite formulations.[67]

3M ESPE Filtek Supreme[68] uses primarily nanoclusters in combination with submicrometer fillers to produce a hybrid. Pentron has had excellent success using polyhedral oligomeric silsesquioxane (POSS) technology borrowed from hybrid plastics.[69] Molecular-sized silicate cages are produced from silane and functionalized for coreaction with matrix monomers. This technology has great potential that is still being explored. Other nanoscale fillers have been designed using tantalum nanoparticles (**Fig. 2**A, B).[70,71]

Implants

Current trends in clinical dental implant therapy include use of endosseous implant surfaces embellished with nanoscale topography. Nanoscale modification of titanium endosseous implant surfaces can alter cellular and tissue responses to benefit dental implant therapy. Three nanostructured implant coatings are in use: diamond, which possess improved hardness, toughness, and low friction; hydroxyapatite, which possesses increased osteoblast adhesion proliferation and mineralization; and graded metalloceramics, which have the ability to overcome adhesion problems (see **Fig. 2**C).[72]

Nanoimpression

Impression material is available with nanotechnology application. Nanofillers are integrated in the vinylpolysiloxanes, producing a unique siloxane impression material. This material has better flow, improved hydrophilic properties, better model pouring, and enhanced detail precision.[59,64]

Nanoanesthesia

One of the most common procedures in dentistry is the injection of local anesthesia, which can involve long procedures, patient discomfort, and many associated complications. To induce oral anesthesia in the era of nanodentistry, a colloidal suspension containing millions of active analgesic micrometer-sized dental robots will be instilled on the patient's gingiva. After contacting the surface of the tooth or mucosa, the ambulating nanorobots reach the pulp via the gingival sulcus, lamina propria, and dentinal tubules. Once installed in the pulp, the analgesic dental robots may be directed by the dentist to shut down all sensitivity in any tooth that requires treatment. After completion of the oral procedure, the dentist directs the nanorobots to restore all sensation, to relinquish control of nerve traffic, and to egress from the tooth by the same pathways that were used for ingress.[57,59]

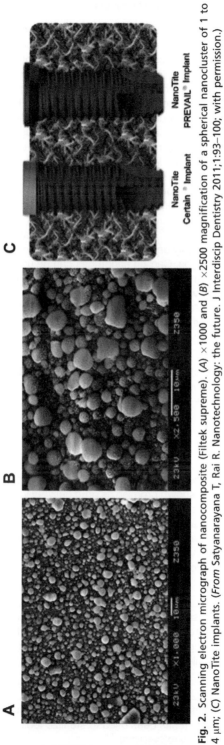

Fig. 2. Scanning electron micrograph of nanocomposite (Filtek supreme). (*A*) ×1000 and (*B*) ×2500 magnification of a spherical nanocluster of 1 to 4 μm; (*C*) NanoTite implants. (*From* Satyanarayana T, Rai R. Nanotechnology: the future. J Interdiscip Dentistry 2011;1:93–100; with permission.)

DETECTION AND TREATMENT OF ORAL CANCER

Nanoparticles play a key role in developing new methods for detecting cancer. Detection of cancer in an early stage is a critical step in improving cancer treatment. The various nanoparticles used are cantilever, nanopore, nanotubes, and quantum dot. As cancer cells secrete their molecular products, the antibodies coated on the cantilever fingers selectively bind to these secreted proteins. The physical properties of the cantilever change in real time and provide information about the presence and also the concentration of different molecular expressions. A simple device for studying single molecule interactions, called a nanomechanical force gauge, has been developed, which consists of nanocantilevers fabricated from single-crystal silicon, an etched nanometer reading scale, and a light microscope to read cantilever deflection along reading scale.[72]

Another nanodevice is nanopore. Improved methods of reading genetic code will help researchers in detecting errors in genes that may contribute to cancer. Nanopores contain tiny holes that allow DNA to pass through 1 strand at a time, making DNA sequencing more efficient.[73] Nanotube carbon rods about half the diameter of a molecule of DNA will not only detect the presence of altered genes but also pinpoint the location of those changes. Carbon nanotubes can be used as sensors for cancer drugs and other DNA-damaging agents inside living cells. Carbon nanotubes fluoresce near infrared light, whereas human tissue does not. The interaction between DNA and the DNA disrupter changes the intensity or wavelength of the fluorescent light emitted by nanotubes.[72]

Quantum Dots

These are tiny crystals that glow when they are stimulated by ultraviolet light. When injected into the body, they drift until encountering cancerous tissue. The cells then attach to a coating on the glowing dots. The light particles show doctors where the disease has spread.[72]

Treatment of Oral Cancer

A single dendrimer can carry a molecule that recognizes cancer cells, a therapeutic agent to kill those cells, and a molecule that recognizes the signal of cell death. Dendrimer nanoparticles have shown promise as drug delivery vehicles capable of targeting tumors with large doses of anticancer drugs. Nanoshells have a core of silica and a metallic outer layer. By manipulating the thickness of the layer, scientist can design beads to absorb near-infrared light, creating an intense heat that is lethal to cancer cells. The physical selectivity to cancer lesion sites occurs through a phenomenon called enhanced permeation retention.[72]

Decay-resistant Teeth

Researchers at the Clarkson Advanced Materials Center have found a way to use nanotechnology to help protect almost any teeth or surface from caries. This protection is achieved by polishing teeth with silica that is made from nanoparticles. This material is 90,000 times smaller than a grain of sand.[72,73]

Surface Disinfectant

EcoTrue is a surface disinfectant that safely kills 100% of human immunodeficiency viruses and other particles. It has been used to sterilize tools and incisions to prevent postoperative infections (EnviroSystems).[72]

Nanotechnology could have a profound effect on dentistry. Once nanomechanics are available, programmable and controllable microscale robots comprising nanoscale parts fabricated to nanometer precision will allow dentists and doctors to perform curative and reconstructive procedures at the cellular and molecular levels. Before that, they the safety norms must be fulfilled. The current materials available from nanotechnology through green nanotechnology have fulfilled the safety norms, and have improved qualities compared with the previous technologies.[74]

TISSUE ENGINEERING

In the last decade, there has been a substantial and growing awareness of a new field of applied biologic research called tissue engineering, which builds on the interface between materials science and biocompatibility, and integrates cells, natural or synthetic scaffolds, and specific signals to create new tissues. This field promises to have enormous clinical potential, including in dentistry.

To date, most of the procedures performed in dentistry are limited to the replacement of damaged tissues with biocompatible synthetic materials that may not present chemical, biological, or physical characteristics and behaviors similar to the host tissues. These discrepancies, together with the hostile environment of the oral cavity, result in short-lived successful outcomes and frequent need for retreatment. Tissue engineering is a multidisciplinary field focused on the development of materials and strategies to replace damaged or lost tissues with biologic materials by merging principles, methods, and knowledge of chemistry, physics, engineering, and biology.[75]

The concept underlying tissue engineering was first proposed in the United States in the mid-1980s in order to reduce the donor scarcity for organ transplantation. The classic cell-based tissue engineering approach involves the seeding of biodegradable scaffolds with cells and/or growth factors, and then implanting it in order to induce and conduct tissue growth. The key ingredients for tissue engineering are stem cells, the morphogens or growth factors that regulate their differentiation, and a scaffold of extracellular matrix that constitutes the microenvironment for their growth.[75]

The principal objectives of the current clinical approaches to tissue replacement and reconstruction are to alleviate pain and to restore mechanical stability and function. Current strategies for treatment of lost tissues include the use of autogenous grafts, allografts, and synthetic materials (alloplasts). Although all of these treatment approaches have had successes and have been major advances in medicine, each of them has limitations.[76]

Strategies to Engineer Tissue

Strategies used to engineer tissue can be categorized into 3 major classes: conductive, inductive, and cell transplantation approaches (**Fig. 3**).[77]

Conductive approaches use biomaterials in a passive manner to facilitate the growth or regenerative capacity of existing tissue; for example, the use of barrier membranes in guided tissue regeneration and osseointegration of dental implant.[77]

Inductive approaches involve activating cells in close proximity to the defect site with specific biological signals. The origins of this mechanism are rooted in the discovery of bone morphogenetic proteins (BMPs). These proteins are now available in recombinant forms and are produced on a large scale by biotechnology companies. BMPs have been used in many clinical trials and are promising as a means of therapy and supplementation in the regeneration and repair of bone in a variety of situations, including nonhealing fractures and periodontal disease.[77]

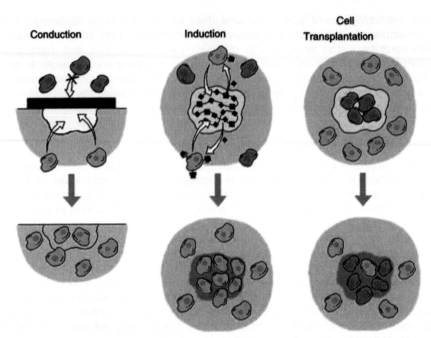

Fig. 3. Tissue engineering strategies. Three different tissue engineering approaches: conductive, inductive, and cell transplantation. (*From* Alsberg E, Hill E, Mooney DJ. Craniofacial tissue engineering. Crit Rev Oral Biol Med 2001;12(1):64–75; with permission.)

Cell transplantation approaches involve direct transplantation of cells grown in the laboratory. The cell transplantation strategy reflects the multidisciplinary nature of tissue engineering, because it requires the clinician or surgeon, the bioengineer, and the cell biologist.[77]

A common feature to all three of the tissue engineering strategies is that they typically involve the use of polymeric materials. In conductive approaches, the polymer is used primarily as a barrier membrane for the exclusion of specific cells that may disturb the regenerative process. Inductive approaches typically use a carrier or vehicle for the delivery of proteins (eg, BMP) or the DNA (gene) that encodes the protein.[77]

FOUNDATIONS OF TISSUE ENGINEERING

The 3 tissue engineering fundamental elements are cells, scaffold, and cell signaling.

Cells

Stem cells are clonogenic cells capable of self-renewal and capable of generating differentiated progenies. These cells are responsible for normal tissue renewal as well as for healing and regeneration after injuries.

Scaffolds

Scaffolds are temporary frameworks used to provide a three-dimensional microenvironment in which cells can proliferate, differentiate, and generate the desired tissue. The design of the ideal scaffold for each tissue to be formed is a challenging task. Scaffolds are usually made from ceramics, natural or synthetic polymers, or composites of these materials. The choice of scaffold material depends on the desired outcome, thus physical as well as chemical characteristics must be considered.[75]

Several fabrication technologies have been applied to process biodegradable and bioresorbable materials into three-dimensional polymeric scaffolds of high porosity and surface area.[78–80]

The scaffold degradation is fundamental to achieve success in tissue engineering therapies. It should ideally reabsorb once it has served its purpose of providing a template for tissue regeneration. The degradation must occur at a rate compatible with the new tissue formation.[75]

Cell Signaling

Cell signaling is part of a complex system of communication that governs cell activities and organizes their interactions. The surface of scaffolding materials is important in tissue engineering because the surface can directly affect cellular response and ultimately the tissue regeneration. An ideal tissue engineering scaffold should mimic extracellular matrix (ECM) and positively interact with cells, including enhanced cell adhesion, growth, migration, and differentiated function. Although a variety of synthetic biodegradable polymers have been used as tissue engineering scaffolding materials, they often lack biological recognition.[81,82]

TISSUES OF SIGNIFICANCE TO THE ORAL-MAXILLOFACIAL COMPLEX

The effect that tissue engineering may have in dentistry stems from its widespread application to many different types of tissues related to the oral cavity, including bone, cartilage, skin and oral mucosa, dentin and dental pulp, and salivary glands.[75,83]

Bone

Tissue engineering will likely have its most significant impact in dentistry via bone tissue engineering and regeneration.[75,83]

Cartilage

The limited capacity of cartilaginous tissue to regenerate and the lack of inductive molecules have focused interest among researchers and manufacturers in developing cell transplantation approaches to engineer cartilage. Transplantation of cells without a carrier is now used clinically to repair small articular cartilaginous defects. Investigators have also shown in animal models that new cartilaginous tissue with precisely defined sizes and shapes relevant to maxillofacial reconstruction (eg, nasal septum, temporomandibular joint) can be engineered using appropriate biodegradable scaffolds for transplanting the cells.[84–86]

Skin and Oral Mucosa

The most successful application of tissue engineering to date is the development of skin equivalents. Skin with both dermal and epidermal components is grown in the laboratory using a combination of cells and various polymer carriers, and engineered skin products were the first tissue-engineered products approved by the US Food and Drug Administration for clinical use. A similar approach has also been developed for the replacement of oral mucosa.[79,80]

Various gene-delivery methods are available to administer growth factors to periodontal defects, offering great flexibility for tissue engineering.[77]

To date, the regeneration of small to moderate-sized periodontal defects using engineered cell-scaffold constructs is technically feasible, and some of the current concepts may represent alternatives for selected clinical scenarios. However, the predictable reconstruction of the normal structure and functionality of a tooth-supporting apparatus remains challenging.[75]

Dentin and Dental Pulp

The production of dentin and dental pulp has also been achieved in animal and laboratory studies using tissue engineering strategies. There is now evidence suggesting that even if the odontoblasts (cells that produce dentin) are lost because of caries, it may be possible to induce formation of new cells from pulp tissue using certain BMPs. These new odontoblasts can synthesize new dentin. Tissue engineering of dental pulp may also be possible using cultured fibroblasts and synthetic polymer matrices.[81,82,87]

Restorative dentistry is trying to develop techniques and materials to regenerate the dentin-pulp complex in a biological manner.[88] Tissue engineering-based approaches have the potential to do this. The regeneration of the dentin-pulp complex with stem cells might be clinically achievable. However, this may not be applicable to all clinical scenarios (ie, old teeth with small pulp chambers and root canals and with closed apices).[89]

Salivary Glands

The most challenging goal of tissue engineering is replacement of complete organs, and significant progress has been made in efforts to engineer salivary gland function. One method of treating salivary gland functional deficiencies makes use of an inductive gene therapy approach. The aim in this approach is to make existing nonsecretory ductal epithelial cells (following irradiation therapy) into secretory cells capable of fluid movement. Success in animal models has been shown. Another method to restore salivary gland function uses cell transplantation. The development of an artificial salivary gland substitute composed of polymer tube lined by epithelial cells has been initiated. This simple device could engraft into the buccal mucosa of patients whose salivary gland tissue has lost function or been destroyed, and would have the physiologic capacity to deliver an aqueous fluid to the mouth via the buccal mucosa. These new approaches could be effective for treating conditions associated with lost salivary gland function, including dysphagia, dysgeusia, rampant caries, and mucosal infections.[90–92]

USE OF STEM CELLS FOR TEETH REGENERATION

Nonbiological approaches have been broadly used for restoring loss of teeth for centuries. Materials such as gold, sapphire, and stainless steel were all used as teeth replacements throughout the generations. However, these devices all induce foreign body reactions and run the risk of rejection by the immune system, and thus biocompatibility is a requirement for the next generation of tooth replacements.[93]

Regenerative medicine offers opportunities to replace or restore tissues of the body after disease and trauma. Biomimetic restorations for partial teeth structures, such as dentin and periodontal ligament (PDL), have also been in development for several years.[93,94]

Use of stem cells, either of embryonic or postnatal derivation, for tissue engineering is attractive because it offers greater scope for using cell fate to try to mimic physiologic tissue architecture.[95] Although tooth development is a complex process governed by redundant and reiterative signaling with temporal and spatial protein expression patterns, efforts have been undertaken by including morphogens such as BMP, and delivery of platelet-derived growth factor gene therapy vectors, which has resulted in partial dental tissue regeneration.[93]

STEM CELL CLASSIFICATION

Stem cells are cells that have the ability to divide for indefinite periods in culture, and to give rise to specialized cells. The cells may be classified according to their origin as embryonic stem cells, embryonic germ stem cells, or adult stem cells. As the name implies, embryonic stem cells come from embryos that have developed from eggs that have been fertilized in vitro. These embryos, used with the consent of the donors, were leftovers from in vitro fertilization clinics. Separated from the other parts of the early developing embryo, primitive cells can be grown in a culture medium to become embryonic stem cells. These cells are not derived from eggs fertilized within the body.[96]

Embryonic germ cells are similar to embryonic stem cells except that they are collected from the fetus later in development. The cells come from a region known as the gonadal ridge, which later develops into the sex organs. Because the cells are farther along the development process, they are limited in their ability to give rise to organs of the body.[96] Adult stem cells originate in a mature organism and help maintain and repair the tissues in which they are found. These stem cells are responsible for replacing blood and tissues on a regular basis. One advantage of using adult stem cells is that samples of tissues, or even patients' own cells, can be used for implantation, avoiding problems of rejection. Furthermore, the use of adult cells does not involve the ethical issues that accompany embryonic research.[96]

Dental Stem Cells

Several populations of cells with stem cell properties have been isolated from different parts of the tooth. These include cells from the pulp of both exfoliated (children's) and adult teeth, from the PDL that links the tooth root with the bone, from the tips of developing roots, and from the tissue (dental follicle) that surrounds the unerupted tooth.[97]

The first stem cells isolated from adult human dental pulp were termed dental pulp stem cells (DPSCs) and were isolated from permanent third molars. In addition, in vivo transplantation into immune-compromised mice showed the ability of DPSCs to generate functional dental tissue in the form of complexes similar to dentine/pulp. Further characterization revealed that DPSCs were also capable of differentiating into other mesenchymal cell derivatives in vitro, such as odontoblasts, adipoctyes, chondrocytes, and osteoblasts. DPSCs differentiate into functionally active neurons, and implanted DPSCs induce endogenous axon guidance, suggesting their potential as cellular therapy for neuronal disorders.[97]

Stem cells from human exfoliated deciduous teeth (SHED) have become an attractive alternative for dental tissue engineering. The use of SHED might bring several advantages for tissue engineering compared with the use of stem cells from adult human teeth:

- SHEDS were reported to have higher proliferation rate and increase cell population doublings compared with stem cells from permanent teeth. This property might facilitate the expansion of these cells in vitro before replantation.[95]
- SHED cells are retrieved from a tissue that is disposable and readily accessible in young patients.[95]

Commercial banking of these cells is becoming widespread to enable them to be used once the child becomes an adult. Limited studies have shown that frozen

SHED cells maintain their properties after cryopreservation for 2 years, but one caveat is that the effects of long-term storage (>10 years) have not yet been assessed. Because children naturally lose 20 deciduous teeth, there are multiple opportunities to bank these cells (unlike cord blood, for example).[95]

PDL Stem Cells

The PDL is a fibrous connective tissue that contains specialized cells located between the bonelike cementum and the inner wall of the alveolar bone socket, which acts as a shock absorber during mastication. The PDL has long been recognized to contain a population of progenitor cells. Several recent studies identified a population of stem cells from human PDL that were capable of differentiating along mesenchymal cell lineages to produce cementoblastlike cells, adipocytes, and connective tissue rich in collagen I in vitro and in vivo. These cells form cementumlike tissue when transplanted into severe combined immunodeficiency mice. They also show the capacity to form collagen fibers, highlighting their potential for PDL regeneration.[97]

Tooth Regeneration

Tissue engineering approaches have proved to be useful for dental tissue and whole-tooth regeneration strategies. Based on preclinical cell and gene therapy strategies used for soft tissue organs, reports of the emerging use of tissue engineering strategies for dentin, pulp, and cementum as an alternative to commonly used root canal and crown therapies are becoming more numerous.[98]

Because bioengineered tooth crown formation requires the interactions of both dental epithelial cell progenitors and mesenchymal cell progenitors (as in natural tooth formation), the ability to bioengineer a tooth of specified size and shape depends on the ability to first identify, and then guide, the interactions of both types of cells.[98]

Stem Cell Therapies

Dental caries is one of the most prevalent diseases in the world. In the United States, more than 50% of children, 85% of adults aged more than 18 years, and more than 50% of the elderly aged more than 75 years have caries lesions.[99]

Researchers have been able to grow human DPSCs in the laboratory to create both soft tissues and mineralized dentin. The problem has been that the ameloblasts die off by a process of apoptosis during tooth development. However, it has been possible to establish ameloblast cell lines from rodents. The next milestone for scientists is to refine the technology to use DPSCs and ameloblasts as part of tissue engineering to synthesize bioengineered replacement tooth substance with a controllable structure and morphology. Once this has been accomplished, it is expected that bioengineered tooth filling materials will quickly become commercially available. Bioengineered filling materials will be attached to existing tooth structure that is not in contact with the systemic immune system; therefore, the risk of these materials creating immune-rejection reactions is very low.[99]

In the future, the pulp tissue may be regenerated using stem cell therapy. The tissue engineering of the dental pulp is less complex than the tissue engineering of a whole tooth, because it is protected inside the tooth, which contributes to the success of stem cell therapy as part of endodontic treatment.[99]

Whole-tooth Regeneration

The ultimate goal in dentistry is to have a method to replace lost teeth biologically; a cell-based implant rather than a metal one. The minimum requirement for a biological replacement is to form the essential components required for a functional tooth,

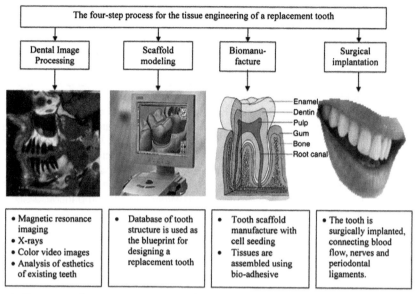

The four-step process for the tissue engineering of a replacement tooth

Dental Image Processing	Scaffold modeling	Biomanu-facture	Surgical implantation

Enamel
Dentin
Pulp
Gum
Bone
Root canal

• Magnetic resonance imaging • X-rays • Color video images • Analysis of esthetics of existing teeth	• Database of tooth structure is used as the blueprint for designing a replacement tooth	• Tooth scaffold manufacture with cell seeding • Tissues are assembled using bio-adhesive	• The tooth is surgically implanted, connecting blood flow, nerves and periodontal ligaments.

Fig. 4. The process for tissue engineering of a replacement tooth. (*Data from* Garcia-Godoy F, Murray PE. Status and potential commercial impact of stem cell-based treatments on dental and craniofacial regeneration. Stem Cells Dev 2006;15(6):881–7.)

including roots, PDL, and nerve and blood supplies. The visible part of the tooth, the crown, is less important because, although essential for function, synthetic tooth crowns function well, and can be perfectly matched for size, shape, and color. Therefore, the challenge for biological tooth replacement is to form a biological root (**Fig. 4**).[94,97,100]

REFERENCES

1. Zandparsa R. Dental biomaterials. Chapter 17. In: Kutz M, editor. Biomedical engineering and design handbook, vols. 1–2, 2nd edition. New york: McGraw-Hill; 2009. p. 397–420.
2. Ferracane JL. Materials in dentistry: principles and applications. 2nd edition. Philadelphia: Lippincott Williams & Wilkins; 2001.
3. Phillips RW, Keith Moore B. Elements of dental materials. 5th edition. Philadelphia: WB Saunders; 1995. p. 274–8.
4. AQB Research Group. The basics. 1st edition. Basics and clinical practice of AQB implants, vol. 1. Tokyo: ADVANCE; 2008. p. 1–4.
5. Albrektsson T, Wennerberg A. The impact of oral implants – past and future, 1966-2042. J Can Dent Assoc 2005;71(5):327.
6. Norton M. The history of dental implants. Available at: http://www.touchbriefings.com/pdf/2262/norton.pdf. Accessed November 12, 2012.
7. Lemons J, Misch-Dietsh F. Biomaterials for dental implants. In: Misch CE, editor. Contemporary implant dentistry. 3rd edition. Mosby; 2008. p. 511–42.
8. Smith DC. Dental implants: materials and design considerations. Int J Prosthodont 1993;6(2):106–17.
9. Koch FP, Weng D, Kramer S, et al. Osseointegration of one-piece zirconia implants compared with a titanium implant of identical design: a histomorphometric study in the dog. Clin Oral Implants Res 2010;21(3):350–6.

10. Özkurt Z, Kazazoglu E. Zirconia dental implants: a literature review. J Oral Implantol 2011;37(3):367–76.
11. Sollazzo V, Pezzetti F, Scarano A, et al. Zirconium oxide coating improves implant osseointegration in vivo. Dent Mater 2008;24:357–61.
12. Möller B, Terheyden H, Acil Y, et al. A comparison of biocompatibility and osseointegration of ceramic and titanium implants: an in vivo and in vitro study. Int J Oral Maxillofac Surg 2012;41(5):638–45.
13. Bormann KH, Gellrich NC, Kniha H, et al. Biomechanical evaluation of a microstructured zirconia implant by a removal torque comparison with a standard Ti-SLA implant. Clin Oral Implants Res 2012;23:1210–6.
14. Koutayas SO, Vagkopoulou T, Pelekanos S, et al. Zirconia in dentistry: part 2. Evidence-based clinical breakthrough. Eur J Esthet Dent 2009;4:348–80, 2–34.
15. Van Brakel R, Meijer GJ, Verhoeven JW, et al. Soft tissue response to zirconia and titanium implant abutments: an in vivo within-subject comparison. J Clin Periodontol 2012;39:995–1001.
16. Wenz HJ, Bartsch J, Wolfart S, et al. Osseointegration and clinical success of zirconia dental implants: a systematic review. Int J Prosthodont 2008;21(1): 27–36.
17. Ozkurt Z, Kazazoglu E. Clinical success of zirconia in dental applications. J Prosthodont 2010;19:64–8.
18. Lambrich M, Iglhaut G. Comparison of the survival rates for zirconia and titanium implants. J Dental Implantology 2008;24(3):182–91.
19. Kohal RJ, Papavasiliou G, Kamposiora P, et al. Three-dimensional computerized stress analysis of commercially pure titanium and yttrium-partially stabilized zirconia implants. Int J Prosthodont 2002;15(2):189–94.
20. Kohal RJ, Wolkewitz M, Tsakona A. The effects of cyclic loading and preparation on the fracture strength of zirconium-dioxide implants: an in vitro investigation. Clin Oral Implants Res 2011;22(8):808–14.
21. Guess PC, Strub JR. Zirconia in fixed implant prosthodontics. Clin Implant Dent Relat Res 2012;14(5):633–45.
22. Swain MV. Unstable cracking (chipping) of veneering porcelain on all-ceramic dental crowns and fixed partial dentures. Acta Biomater 2009;5:1668–77.
23. Ewers R, Schicho K, Truppe M, et al. Computer-aided navigation in dental implantology: 7 years of clinical experience. J Oral Maxillofac Surg 2004;62: 329–34.
24. Kelly PJ. State of the art and future directions of minimally invasive stereotactic neurosurgery. Cancer Control 1995;2:287.
25. Freysinger W, Gunkel AR, Pototschnig C, et al. New developments in 3D endonasal and frontobasal endoscopic sinus surgery. Paris: Kugler Publications; 1995.
26. Thumfart WF, Freysinger W, Gunkel AR. 3D image-guided surgery on the example of the 5,300-year-old Innsbruck iceman. Acta Otolaryngol 1997; 117:131.
27. Hobkirk JA, Havthoulas TK. The influence of mandibular deformation, implant numbers, and loading position on detected forces in abutments supporting fixed implant superstructures. J Prosthet Dent 1998;80:169.
28. Birkfellner W, Solar P, Gahleitner A, et al. In-vitro assessment of a registration protocol for image guided implant dentistry. Clin Oral Implants Res 2001;12:69.
29. Wagner A, Wanschitz F, Birkfellner W, et al. Computer-aided placement of endosseous oral implants in patients after ablative tumour surgery: assessment of accuracy. Clin Oral Implants Res 2003;14:340.

30. SurgiGuide system. Available at: www.SimPlant@materialise.com.
31. Avrampou M. Virtual implant planning in the edentulous maxilla: criteria for decision making of prosthesis design. Clin Oral Implants Res 2012;24(Suppl A100):152–9.
32. Weinberg LA. CT scan as radiologic database for optimum implant orientation. J Prosthet Dent 1993;69:381.
33. Sethi A. Precise site location for implants using CT scans: a technical note. Int J Oral Maxillofac Implants 1993;8:433.
34. Falk A, Gielen S, Heuser L. CT data acquisition as a basis for modern diagnosis and therapy in maxillofacial surgery. Int J Oral Maxillofac Surg 1995;24:69.
35. Baily NA, Keller RA, Jacowatz CW, et al. The capability of fluoroscopic systems for the production of computerized axial tomograms. Invest Radiol 1976;11:434.
36. Harrison RM, Farmer FT. The determination of anatomical cross sections using a radiotherapy simulator. Br J Radiol 1978;51(606):448–53.
37. Arnot RN, Willetts RJ, Batten JR, et al. Investigations using an X-ray image intensifier and a TV camera for imaging transverse sections in humans. Br J Radiol 1984;57(673):47.
38. Cho PS, Johnson RH, Griffin TW. Cone-beam CT for radiotherapy applications. Phys Med Biol 1995;40:1863.
39. Saint-Félix D, Trousset Y, Picard C, et al. In vivo evaluation of a new system for 3D computerized angiography. Phys Med Biol 1994;39:583.
40. Machin K, Webb S. Cone-beam X-ray microtomography of small specimens. Phys Med Biol 1994;39:1639.
41. Lehr JL. Truncated-view artifacts: clinical importance on CT. AJR Am J Roentgenol 1983;141(1):183.
42. Mozzo P, Procacci C, Tacconi A, et al. A new volumetric CT machine for dental imaging based on the cone-beam technique: preliminary results. Eur Radiol 1998;8:1558–64.
43. Schulze D, Heiland M, Thurmann H, et al. Radiation exposure during midfacial imaging using 4- and 16-slice computed tomography, cone beam computed tomography systems and conventional radiography. Dentomaxillofac Radiol 2004; 33:83–6.
44. Brooks RA, DiChiro G. Beam hardening in reconstructive tomography. Phys Med Biol 1976;21:390–8.
45. Jung RE, Schneider D, Ganeles J, et al. Computer technology applications in surgical implant dentistry: a systematic review. Int J Oral Maxillofac Implants 2009;24(Suppl):92–109.
46. Nammour S. Laser dentistry, current advantages, and limits. Photomed Laser Surg 2012;30(1):1–4.
47. Raucci-Neto W, Pécora JD. Thermal effects and morphological aspects of human dentin surface irradiated with different frequencies of Er:YAG laser. Microsc Res Tech 2012;75(10):1370–5.
48. Kimura Y, Yu DG, Fujita A, et al. Effects of erbium, chromium:YSGG laser irradiation on canine mandibular bone. J Periodontol 2001;72:1178–82.
49. Sasaki KM, Aoki A, Masuno H, et al. Compositional analysis of root cementum and dentin after Er:YAG laser irradiation compared with CO_2 lased and intact roots using Fourier transformed infrared spectroscopy. J Periodont Res 2002; 37:50–9.
50. Aoki A, Ishikawa I, Yamada T, et al. Comparison between Er:YAG laser and conventional technique for root caries treatment in vitro. J Dent Res 1998;77: 1404–14.

51. Rizoiu I, Kohanghadosh F, Kimmel AI, et al. Pulpal thermal responses to an erbium, chromium:YSGG pulsed laser hydrokinetic system. Oral Surg Oral Med Oral Pathol Oral Radiol Endod 1998;86(2):220–3.
52. Kilinc E, Roshkind DM, Antonson SA, et al. Thermal safety of Er:YAG and Er, Cr:YSGG lasers in hard tissue removal. Photomed Laser Surg 2009;27(4): 565–70.
53. Morford CK, Buu NC, Rechmann BM, et al. Er:YAG laser debonding of porcelain veneers. Lasers Surg Med 2011;43(10):965–74.
54. Elavarasu S, Naveen D, Thangavelu A. Lasers in periodontics. J Pharm Bioallied Sci 2012;4(Suppl 2):S260–3.
55. Feynman R. There's plenty of room at the bottom. Science 1991;254:1300–1.
56. Feynman RP. There's plenty of room at the bottom. Eng Sci 1960;23:22–36.
57. Frietas RA. Nanodentistry. J Am Dent Assoc 2000;131:1559–69.
58. Somerman MJ, Ouyang HJ, Berry JE, et al. Evolution of periodontal regeneration: from the roots' point of view. J Periodont Res 1999;34(7):420–4.
59. Saravanakumar R, Vijaylakshmi R. Nanotechnology in dentistry. Indian J Dent Res 2006;17(2):62–5.
60. Fartash B, Tangerud T, Silness J, et al. Rehabilitation of mandibular edentulism by single crystal sapphire implants and overdentures: 3–12 year results in 86 patients—a dual center international study. Clin Oral Implants Res 1996;7(3):220–9.
61. Reifman EM. Diamond teeth. In: Crandall BC, editor. Nanotechnology: molecular speculations on global abundance. Cambridge (MA): MIT Press; 1996. p. 81–6.
62. Freitas RA Jr. Nanomedicine. Basic capabilities, vol. 1. Georgetown (TX): Landes Bioscience; 1999. Available at: www.nanomedicine.com. Accessed September 26, 2000.
63. Bayne SC. Dental biomaterials: where are we and where are we going? J Dent Educ 2005;69(5):571–83.
64. Jhaveri HM, Balaji PR. Nanotechnology. The future of dentistry a review. Jr I Prosthetic 2005;5:15–7.
65. Bayne SC, Heymann HO, Swift EJ Jr. Update on dental composite restorations. J Am Dent Assoc 1994;125(6):687–701.
66. Bayne SC, Thompson JY, Taylor DF. Dental materials (Chapter 4). In: Roberson TM, editor. Sturdevant's art and science of operative dentistry. 4th edition. St Louis (MO): Mosby; 2001. p. 135–236.
67. Mitra SB, Wu D, Holmes BN. An application of nanotechnology in advanced dental materials. J Am Dent Assoc 2003;34:1382–90.
68. 3M ESPE. Filtek supreme universal restorative system technical product profile. St Paul (MN); 2002. p. 8.
69. Hybrid plastics. Available at: www.hybridplastics.com/. Accessed October 28, 2004.
70. Chan DC, Titus HW, Chung KY, et al. Radiopacity ofantalum oxide nanoparticle filled resins. Dent Mater 1999;15:219–22.
71. Furman B, Rawls HR, Wellinghoff S, et al. Metal-oxide nanoparticles for the reinforcement of dental restorative resins. Crit Rev Biomed Eng 2000;28:439–43.
72. Satyanarayana T, Rai R. Nanotechnology: the future. J Interdiscip Dentistry 2011;1:93–100.
73. Randooke B. The future of dentistry and dental care –how nanotechnology will change your visit to the dentist. Available at: http://ezinearticles.com. Accessed June 21, 2010.
74. Matthew JE, Julie BZ, Paul TA. Towards green nano: E-factor analysis of several nanomaterial syntheses. J Ind Ecol 2008;12:316–28.

75. Rosaa V, Della Bonaa A, Cavalcanti BN, et al. Tissue engineering: from research to dental clinics. Dent Mater 2012;28(4):341–8.
76. Kaigler D, Mooney D. Tissue engineering's impact on dentistry. J Dent Educ 2011;65(5):456–62.
77. Baum R, Mooney D. The impact of tissue engineering on dentistry. J Am Dent Assoc 2001;131(3):309–18.
78. Naughton G. The advanced tissue sciences story. Sci Am 1999;280:84–5.
79. Mizuno H, Emi N, Abe A, et al. Successful culture and sustainability in vivo of gene-modified human oral mucosa epithelium. Hum Gene Ther 1999;10:825–30.
80. Garlick JA, Fenjves ES. Keratinocyte gene transfer and gene therapy. Crit Rev Oral Biol Med 1996;7:204–21.
81. Lianjia Y, Yuhao G, White F. Bovine bone morphogenetic protein induced dentinogenesis. Clin Orthop Relat Res 1993;295:305–12.
82. Rutherford RB, Wahle J, Tucker M, et al. Induction or reparative formation in monkeys by recombinant human osteogenic protein-1. Arch Oral Biol 1993;38:571–6.
83. Ramseier C, Rasperini G, Batia S, et al. Advanced reconstructive technologies for periodontal tissue repair. Periodontol 2000 2012;59:185–202.
84. Puelacher WC, Mooney DJ, Langer R, et al. Design of nasoseptal cartilage replacements synthesized from biodegradable polymers and chondrocytes. Biomaterials 1993;15:774–8.
85. Puelacher WC, Wisser J, Vacanti CA, et al. Temporomandibular joint disc replacement made by tissue-engineered growth of cartilage. J Oral Maxillofac Surg 1994;52(11):1172–7.
86. Parenteau N. The organogenesis story. Sci Am 1999;280:83–4.
87. Nakashshima M. The induction of reparative dentin in the amputated dental pulp of the dog by bone morphogenetic protein. Arch Oral Biol 1990;35(7):493–7.
88. Mooney DJ, Powell C, Piana J, et al. Engineering dental pulp-like tissue in vitro. Biotechnol Prog 1996;12(6):865–8.
89. Sakai VT, Zhang Z, Dong Z, et al. SHED differentiate into functional odontoblast and endothelium. J Dent Res 2010;89:791–6.
90. Baum BJ, O'Connell BC. In vivo gene transfer to salivary glands. Crit Rev Oral Biol Med 1999;10:276–83.
91. Delporte C, O'Connell BC, He X, et al. Increased fluid secretion following adenovirus mediated transfer of the aquaporin-1 cDNA irradiated rat salivary glands. Proc Natl Acad Sci U S A 1997;94:3268–73.
92. Baum BJ, Wang S, Cukierman E, et al. Re-engineering the functions of a terminally differentiated epithelial cell in vivo. Ann N Y Acad Sci 1999;875:294–300.
93. Yen AH, Sharpe PT. Regeneration of teeth using stem cell-based tissue engineering. Expert Opin Biol Ther 2006;6(1):9–16.
94. Yildirim S, Fu SY, Kim K, et al. Tooth regeneration: a revolution in stomatology and evolution in regenerative medicine. Int J Oral Sci 2011;3:107–16.
95. Mitsiadis TA, Feki A, Papaccio G. Dental pulp stem cells, niches, and notch signaling in tooth injury. Adv Dent Res 2011;23:275.
96. Kelly EB. Stem cells. Westport, CT: Greenwood Publishing Group; 2007. p. 203.
97. Volponi AA, Pang Y, Sharpe PT. Stem cell biological tooth repair and regeneration. Trends Cell Biol 2010;20(12–6):715–22.
98. Duailibi SE, Duailibi MT, Vacanti JP, et al. Prospects for tooth regeneration. Periodontol 2000 2006;41:177–87.

99. Garcia-Godoy F, Murray PE. Status and potential commercial impact of stem cell-based treatments on dental and craniofacial regeneration. Stem Cells Dev 2006;15:881–7.

100. Hu B, Nadiri A, Kuchler-Bopp S, et al. Tissue engineering of tooth crown, root, and periodontium. Tissue Eng 2006;12(8):2069–75.

Digital Imaging and Fabrication

Roya Zandparsa, DDS, MSc, DMD

KEYWORDS

- Digital • Imaging • Fabrication • Bioceramics

KEY POINTS

- Bioceramics have rapidly been adopted in dental restorations for implants, bridges, inlays, onlays, and all-ceramic crowns. The structure of dental bioceramics covers a wide spectrum of glass ceramics, reinforced porcelains, zirconias, aluminas, fiber-reinforced ceramic composites, and multilayered ceramic structures.
- The process of additive manufacturing is ideally suited to dentistry. Models are designed using data from a computed tomography scan or magnetic resonance imaging. The image is downloaded to a computer-aided design (CAD) machine and converted to a standard transformation language (STL) file.
- Since its development in 2001, direct ceramic machining of presintered 3 mol% yttria stabilized tetragonal zirconia ceramics has become increasingly popular in dentistry. The die or wax pattern is scanned, an enlarged restoration is designed by computer software (CAD), and a presintered ceramic blank is milled by computer-aided machining.
- There are wide variety commercially available cements for luting all-ceramic restorations, including zinc phosphate cements, conventional and resin-modified glass ionomer cements, resin cements, and self-adhesive resin cements. However, resin cements possess some advantages compared with the other classes of materials, because they have lower solubility and better aesthetic characteristics.

HISTORY OF DENTAL MATERIALS

Gold was one of the first dental materials known; its use has been traced to circa 500 BC. Its durability and lack of corrosion make it one of the best restorative materials available.

The first dental porcelain, which was used for making complete dentures and individual teeth, was introduced at the end of 1700s. One of the major benefits of ceramic as a dental restorative material was the resemblance to natural dentition.

Since the nineteenth century, other dental materials like high-copper amalgam, polymers including composite resins, elastic impression materials, base metal alloys, orthodontic wires, bonding agents, glass ionomer, and polycarboxylate cements were also developed, which enhanced treatment possibilities. Every year new versions of

Tufts University School of Dentistry, Postgraduate Prosthodontics Division, 1 Kneeland Street, Boston, MA 02111, USA
E-mail address: roya.zandparsa@tufts.edu

Dent Clin N Am 58 (2014) 135–158
http://dx.doi.org/10.1016/j.cden.2013.09.012
0011-8532/14/$ – see front matter © 2014 Elsevier Inc. All rights reserved.

dental materials with better properties are developed and introduced to practitioners. Among them are all-ceramic restorations, better quality composite resin and bonding agents, flowable composites and sealants, resin-modified glass ionomers and resin cements, and more accurate impression materials.[1-4]

The science of dental materials studies the composition and properties of materials and the way they interact with the environment. The selection of materials for any application can thus be undertaken with confidence and sound judgment. Dentists spend much of their professional careers handling materials. The success or failures of many treatments depend on the correct selection of materials and their manipulation. Dental biomaterials are the natural tissues or synthetic products that are used to restore or replace decayed, damaged, fractured, or missing teeth. The major synthetic dental material groups are metals, ceramics, and polymers, including composite structures (**Table 1**).[1,5]

CERAMICS

Teeth are complex organs of the human body and consist of several component tissues, both hard and soft. The tooth is subject to many damaging influences. Restorative dentistry is concerned with repairing damaged teeth and their supporting structures. Aesthetics are of paramount concern, and the only medical material that in any way provides a durable and satisfactory solution to the aesthetic repair of teeth is ceramic.[6]

Historic Perspectives: Ceramics as Restorative Materials

Although routine use of ceramics in restorative dentistry is a recent phenomenon, the desire for a durable and aesthetic material is ancient. Most cultures through the centuries have acknowledged teeth as an integral facial structure for health, youth, beauty, and dignity. Teeth have routinely been designated with an equally powerful, if occasionally perverse, role in cultures in which dentitions were purposely mutilated as inspired by vanity, fashion, and mystical and religious beliefs. Therefore, it has been almost universal that unexpected loss of tooth structure, and particularly missing anterior teeth, creates physical and functional problems and often psychological and social disturbances as well. During the eighteenth century, artificial teeth were made of human teeth, animal teeth carved to the size and shape of human teeth, ivory, bone, or mineral (porcelain). John Greenwood carved teeth from hippopotamus ivory for at least one of the 4 sets of complete dentures he fabricated for George Washington.[1,7,8]

Mineral teeth or porcelain dentures accelerated an end to the practice of transplanting freshly extracted human teeth and supplanted the use of animal products. Feldspathic dental porcelains were adapted from European triaxial white ware

Table 1		
Three basic materials used in dentistry, with some of their applications		
Metals	Alloys	Components of dentures, orthodontic wires, cast restorations
Ceramics	Crystalline ceramics Glasses Inorganic salts	Al_2O_3, SiO_2 Dental porcelain Gypsum product, dental cements
Polymers	Rigid Elastomers	Denture bases, direct filling Impression materials

formulations (clay-quartz-feldspar), nearly coincident with their development. After decades of effort, Europeans mastered the manufacture of fine translucent porcelains, comparable with porcelains of the Chinese, by the 1720s. The use of feldspar to replace lime (calcium oxide) as a flux, and high firing temperatures, were critical developments in fine European porcelain.[9] Around 1774, the first successful porcelain dentures were made at the Guerhard porcelain factory by Nicholas Dubois de Chemant.[1,7,8]

In 1808, Giuseppangelo Fonzi formed individual porcelain teeth that contained embedded platinum pins, which provided a major advance in prosthetic dentistry. In 1723, Pierre Fauchard described the enameling of metal denture bases. Fauchard was credited with recognizing the potential of porcelain enamels and initiating research with porcelains to imitate color of teeth and gingival tissues.[1,7,10]

Classification of Dental Ceramics

Ceramics are classified into 3 main composition categories:

- Predominantly glass, which has a regular pattern of atoms known as an amorphous structure. They are the best at mimicking the optical properties of enamel and dentin and therefore are highly aesthetic. The glass in this category is mainly made up of a mined mineral called feldspar and is based on silica and alumina. Glasses composed of feldspar are resistant to crystallization during firing, have long firing ranges, and are biocompatible.[11–14]
- Particle-filled glass, in which filler particles like Lucite are added to the glass matrix to improve its mechanical properties and to control optical effects such as opalescence, color, and opacity. Another advantage of adding leucite as a filler to ceramics is that its index of refraction is close to feldspathic and maintain translucency. It also etches at a faster rate than the base glass and creates selective etching. This property allows the resin cements to attach and form a good micromechanical bond. Dispersion strengthening is when the fillers are added and uniformly dispersed throughout the glass, creating an increase in strength. Leucite filler allows this phenomenon to occur. All of these advantages help strengthen the material without compromising the aesthetics.[11–14]
- Polycrystalline ceramics contain no glass, the matrix is aluminum oxide or zirconium oxide, and the fillers are not particles but modifying atoms called dopants. These dopants are packed into regular crystalline arrays that are more difficult to crack than the irregular networks found in glasses. In general, polycrystalline ceramics are therefore stronger than glass-based ceramics.[11–14]

Dental Computer-aided Design/Computer-aided Manufacturing Technology

Bioceramics have rapidly been adopted in dental restorations for implants, bridges, inlays, onlays, and all-ceramic crowns.[15] The structures of dental bioceramics cover a wide spectrum of glass ceramics, reinforced porcelains, zirconias, aluminas, fiber-reinforced ceramic composites, and multilayered ceramic structures.[15,16] Bioceramics in dental restorations are essentially oxide-based glass-ceramic systems and other traditional ceramic materials. The materials cover mica-containing glass ceramics, feldspar-containing porcelains, leucite-containing porcelains, glass-infiltrated alumina, and yttria-stabilized tetragonal zirconia.[7,15] With increasing interest in improving the aesthetic quality of restorations, a wide variety of ceramic structures and their composites have also been developed, including the ceramic whisker-reinforced composites[17,18] and the damage-resistant brittle-coating bilayer or trilayer structures.[15,19] Over the past 25 years, computer-aided design (CAD) and computer-aided manufacturing (CAM) have become increasingly popular parts of dentistry. Dental CAD/CAM technology has been used to replace the laborious and time-consuming conventional lost-wax technique for efficient fabrication of restorations. This technology enables dentists to produce complex shapes of ceramic prostheses under the computer-controlled manufacturing conditions directly from the simply shaped blocks of materials within 1 hour.[20] However, dental CAD/CAM systems use abrasive machining processes in which machining damage is potentially induced, resulting in the reduction of the strength of ceramic prostheses and the need for final finishing in oral conditions using a dental handpiece and diamond burs. It is expected that a ceramic restoration should have a high longevity. However, wear and fatigue damage are often observed to cause the failures of bioceramic prostheses. With the CAD/CAM systems, restorations can be produced quicker, which eliminates the need for temporary restorations. Moreover, with CAD/CAM, it is possible to make prostheses with consistent quality.[20]

At present, there are 2 major CAD/CAM systems, one for machinable bioceramics, the other for materials that are difficult to machine. In the first system, the computer-assisted milling process can be used to machine the machinable ceramics directly from their blanks (**Fig. 1**).[21] In the second system, the milling process is first conducted from the presintered blanks of the difficult-to-machine ceramics, and then the sintering is followed to harden the ceramic prostheses, compensating for shrinkage during sintering in a special high-temperature furnace.[15] In the CAD of prostheses, there are 2 digital image-generation systems for data acquisition. The three-dimensional (3D), noncontact, optical/laser scanning systems are most widely applied in dentistry.[15,20–22]

The quality and the speed of intraoral imaging of the CAD/CAM process still need improvement.[23]

CAD/CAM Components

There are 3 main sequences to CAD/CAD systems. The first sequence is to capture or record the intraoral condition to the computer. This sequence involves the use of a scanner or intraoral camera. Once the data have been recorded to the computer, a software program (CAD) is used to complete the custom design of the final desired restoration, which may involve a full contour design of the restoration or just the internal coping or substructure of the final restoration. The final sequence requires a milling device to fabricate the restoration from the design data in the

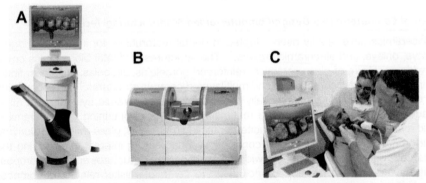

Fig. 1. (*A*) CEREC AC with Omnicam, (*B*) milling unit, and (*C*) data acquisition in CEREC system using Omnicam. (*Courtesy of* Sirona Dental Systems, Available at: www.sirona.com)

CAD program. At present, the most common technique is a wet grinding subtractive milling process during which a preformed block of material is shaped by cutting instruments.[24,25]

Results with in-office milling machines seem to be as good as those from laboratory milling machines. A systematic review of 16 articles that comprised 1957 restorations found no significant differences in 5-year survival rates between chairside CEREC (Chairside Economical Restoration of Esthetic Ceramics) restorations (90.2%–93.8%) and Celay laboratory restorations (82.1%).[26]

Scanner
There are 2 different scanning possibilities:

- Optical scanner. This scanner uses the collection of 3D structures, for which the source of light and the receptor unit are in a definite angle in their relationship to one another. Through this angle the computer can calculate a 3D data set from the image on the receptor unit. Either white light projections or a laser beam can serve as a source of illumination.
- Mechanical scanner. In this scanner variant, the master cast is read mechanically line by line by means of a ruby ball and the 3D structure measured. The Procera Scanner from Nobel Biocare is one of the mechanical scanners in dentistry. This type of scanner is distinguished by a high scanning accuracy, whereby the diameter of the ruby ball is set to the smallest grinder in the milling system, with the result that all data collected by the system can also be milled. The drawbacks of this data measurement technique are in the highly complicated mechanics, which make the apparatus expensive with long processing times compared with optical systems.[27,28]

Design software
Special software is provided by the manufacturers for the design of various kinds of dental restorations. With such software, crown and fixed partial denture (FPD) frameworks can be constructed. Some systems also offer the opportunity to design full anatomic crowns, partial crowns, inlays, inlay retained FPDs, as well as adhesive FPDs and telescopic primary crowns. The software of CAD/CAM systems presently available on the market is being continuously improved. The latest construction possibilities are continuously available to the user by means of updates. The data for the construction can be stored in various data formats. The basis is often standard transformation language (STL) data. However, many manufacturers use their own specific data formats, with the result that data for the construction programs are not compatible with each other.[27]

CAD/CAM Development in Dentistry

The development of CAD/CAM is based around the data acquisition, data processing, and digital fabrication processes.[29,30]

Digital data acquisition methods
The oral information for the patient can be directly extracted from a patient's mouth or indirectly by means of a stone model generated through making an impression. The data acquisition techniques were originally developed for reverse engineering and intensively used in manufacturing industries. Their strengths were gradually recognized and these techniques are also applied in the medical field. The acquisition systems are divided into 2 basic categories: contact and noncontact digitizers.[29,30]

The digital data acquired through various techniques and instruments are converted into a standard format so that the data can be processed using the capabilities of a CAD/CAM system.[29]

This process is exemplified by the recent introduction of intraoral scanners, a number of which are now on the market: Lava COS (chairside oral scanner) from 3M, Trios from 3Shape and iTero from Cadent, and CEREC from Sirona.[31,32]

A further development in the CAD/CAM technologies used in dentistry was the transition from closed to open access systems. Although in the past the digitizing, designing, and manufacturing came as a closed system (eg, CEREC), the technology is increasingly being opened up and the component parts of a CAD/CAM system can be purchased separately, which creates greater flexibility because data can be acquired from a range of sources (intraoral scanner, contact or laser model digitizer, computed tomography, magnetic resonance imaging). Another important consequence of the transition from closed to open systems is that this opens up access to a wider range of manufacturing techniques such that the most appropriate manufacturing processes and associated materials can be selected. Thus, clinicians are no longer constrained by the computer numerically controlled machining technologies that are currently used in most dental CAD/CAM systems.[31,32]

Data processing and remodeling

CAD software is often used to edit and manipulate the point cloud data generated by a digitizer. After the point cloud data are converted into a representation of a surface or solid, the next step involves a digital design process for the dental part.[29]

The shape design of the 3D dental restoration is one of the core elements of successfully fabricating restorations. In these systems the basic models of teeth are available in their own libraries. However, general forms of teeth geometry provided by these CAD/CAM systems can only give raw shapes. There are always some manual alterations and modifications required because every patient is unique and every tooth has its own topological features.[29,33]

Digital fabrication processes

This is the last phase of the dental CAD/CAM process. It involves transforming a CAD model into a physical part that is later postprocessed and polished before being inserted into the patient's mouth.[29]

Industrial 3D printers have existed since the early 1980s, and have been used extensively for rapid prototyping and research purposes. These printers are generally large machines that use proprietary powdered metals, casting media (ie, sand), plastics, or cartridges, and are used for many rapid prototyping uses by universities and commercial companies.[33] Several methods can be used to fabricate the physical parts. These methods can be additive or subtractive.

Subtractive manufacturing Subtractive manufacturing removes material from a raw block to form an object of the desired shape and size, which can be done by conventional machining (eg, milling) and unconventional machining (eg, electrical discharge machining (EDM), laser machining).[29]

CAD/CAM in dentistry is now primarily based around the process of subtractive manufacturing. The technology most people are familiar with is computer numerically controlled machining, which is based on processes in which power-driven machine tools, such as saws, lathes, milling machines, and drill presses, are used with a sharp cutting tool to mechanically cut the material to achieve the desired geometry, with all the steps controlled by a computer program. This method of manufacturing is wasteful because more material is removed than is used in the final product. The main advantage of this type of manufacturing is the ability of the technique to create fine detail such as undercuts, voids, and complex internal geometries. Another limitation of the current dental CAD/CAM systems is that the process does not easily lend itself to mass production, such as crowns and bridges, because only 1 part can be machined at a time.[34]

Additive manufacturing Additive manufacturing describes technologies that can be used anywhere throughout the product life cycle from preproduction (ie, rapid prototyping) to full-scale production (also known as rapid manufacturing) and even for tooling applications or postproduction customization. 3D printing is achieved using additive processes, in which laying down successive layers of material creates an object. The primary advantage of additive construction is its ability to create parts of almost any geometry, and the capability to spatially grade composition and/or microstructure (eg, porosity) to meet specific designs or needs, without requiring a previous mold. Also, this fabrication technology permits internal morphology, shape, distribution, and connectivity to be controlled more precisely. Another benefit from this system is the ability to print with multiple materials at one time as well as to create graded structures.[29,33,35]

Modalities of Rapid Printing

The process of additive manufacturing is ideally suited to dentistry. Models are designed using data from a computed tomography scan or magnetic resonance imaging. The image is downloaded to a CAD machine and converted to an STL file. Various rapid prototyping technologies can be used to produce anatomic models:

- Stereolithography (SLA), which builds models by laser fusing a photopolymer layer by layer. SLA is now routinely used to produce surgical guides for the placement of dental implants. Its use is gradually being extended to include the manufacture of temporary crowns and bridges and resin models for loss wax casting.[31,36]
- Laminated object manufacturing, which uses a laser to cut and fuse successive layers of bonded sheet material.[31]
- Laser powder forming techniques. Laser-based additive manufacturing, such as selective laser melting (SLM) and selective laser sintering (SLS), is accomplished by directing a high-power laser using mirrors at a substrate consisting of a fine layer of powder. Where the beam hits the powder it creates a melt pool and the powder particles fuse together. Compared with other methods of additive manufacturing, SLS/SLM can produce parts from a wide range of commercially available powder materials, including a wide range of polymers such as polyamide to produce a facial prosthesis, ultrahigh-molecular-weight polyethylene, polycaprolactone to provide functionally graded scaffolds, mixtures of polymers such as polycaprolactone and drugs to act as drug delivery devices, and composites such as mixtures of hydroxyapatite and polyethylene and polyamide to produce customized scaffolds for tissue engineering. A range of metal powders can be used that include steel, titanium, titanium alloys, and Co/Cr alloys.[31,33]
- Solid ground curing, which laser polymerizes successive layers of resin through a stencil.[31]
- Fused deposition modeling, which builds models by depositing layers of molten thermoplastic materials.[31]
- Selective electron beam melting, which is a type of additive manufacturing for producing near net shape metal parts. The technology manufactures parts by

melting metal powder layer by layer with an electron beam in a high vacuum. This technology has already found wide application in orthopedics and maxillofacial surgery for the construction of customized implants.[31,37]

- 3D ink-jet printing, which selectively deposits binding material through a print head to fuse a thin layer of powder to a previously fused layer. In direct ink-jet printing, a ceramic suspension provides the possibility of generating dense green bodies at a high resolution and in complex shapes.[31,37]

With the improvements in the speed, reliability, and accuracy of the hardware, additive manufacturing will compete with traditional manufacturing in creating end-use products. One advantage with additive manufacturing is that it eliminates much of the expensive and highly skilled labor associated with traditional manufacturing. It can also make any number of complex products simultaneously so long as the parts fit within the build envelope of the machine. Thus the production of some 50 dental crown units that would normally take a considerable amount of time using loss wax casting can be done within a day, which has a profound influence on the dental technology community (**Fig. 2**).[31,37]

It is possible to build up dense 3D components of the size and shape of a dental crown out of high-strength zirconia ceramics by this technology. Although the microstructures of the printed and fired samples were not completely free of process-related defects, the obtained density was at 96.9% of the theoretic density required

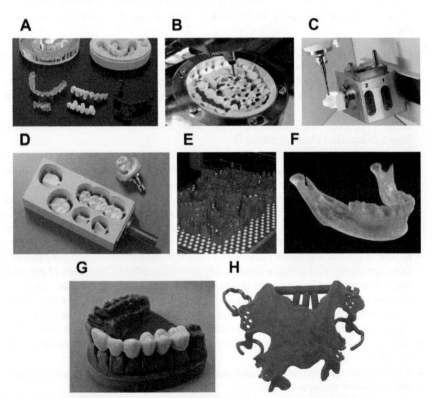

Fig. 2. (*A-D*) CAD/CAM milling (http://www.rolanddga.com/) and (*E-H*) 3D printing (http://envisiontec.com/). (*Courtesy of* [*A-D*] Roland DGA Corporation; and [*E–H*] Envisiontec.)

to provide mechanical properties.[36] The shrinkage caused by drying or sintering can be a critical issue in individually made dental ceramic prostheses.[36]

Two key challenges to successful printing of ceramic crowns by the robocasting technique are the development of suitable materials for printing and the design of printing patterns for assembly of the complex geometry required for a dental restoration.[33]

Solid Free-form Fabrication Concept: Robocasting

Robocasting is a rapid prototyping (RP) that fabricates objects based on layering techniques. Robocasting uses computer-controlled extrusion of colloidal pastes (slurries, gels, or inks) onto a flat substrate without using molds or tooling. Unlike milling, in which blocks are cut back to create a form, robocasting uses a computer-generated scan from computed tomography of a SLA file to create a strategically printed 3D structure.[39]

This process has been used in orthopedics for bone and tissue engineering. Robocasting in the dental setting is a new development with limited information or practice. The advantages of printing versus milling are the ability to make microstructure as needed for the prosthesis without requiring a previous mold; that it allows internal morphology, shape, distribution, and connectivity to be controlled more precisely; and a significant decrease in waste of materials.[38]

To achieve its full potential as a dental restoration production process, robocasting must improve the use of support materials to produce better tolerance for occlusal surfaces. In addition, the digital nature of the layer printing process leads to a stair-stepped surface that may need to be improved for commercial acceptance. The step size is a function of the nozzle diameter used for printing. The issue of support materials/structures seems to be a tractable problem; however, the stair stepping may require some postprocessing (eg, a dip-coating process) before final sintering. Drying issues, such as cracks, sometimes occur (**Fig. 3**).[31,33]

Digital Imaging in Different CAD/CAM Systems

The following are a few of the currently available products for digital impressions in the dental office: CEREC AC (Sirona, Charlotte, NC), E4D Dentist (D4D Technologies, Richardson, TX), iTero (Cadent, Carlstadt, NJ), Lava COS (3M ESPE, St Paul, MN), and 3Shape TRIOS (3Shape, Copenhagen, Denmark). The CEREC and E4D devices can be combined with in-office design and milling, whereas the iTero and Lava COS devices are reserved for image acquisition only. In-office milling allows same-day restorations.[39]

The CEREC system

CEREC, introduced in 1987, was the first dental system to combine digital scanning with a milling unit. The first grinding trials with a simple device on bodies made of feldspathic ceramic (Vita Zahnfabrik, Bad Säckingen, Germany) showed that this material could be removed with a grinding wheel in a few minutes without damaging the rest of the bulk. Then the ceramic block could hold on the block carrier with a spindle and feed it against the grinding wheel, which ground from the full ceramic a new contour with a different distance from the inlay axis at each feed step. This solution proved itself in a prototype implemented in the same year in the CEREC 1 unit (Sirona Dental Systems GmbH, Bensheim, Germany). A CEREC team at Seimens (Munich, Germany) equipped the CEREC 2 with an additional cylinder diamond enabling the form grinding of partial and full crowns. CEREC 3 skipped the wheel and introduced the 2-bur system. The step bur, which was introduced in 2006, reduced the diameter of the

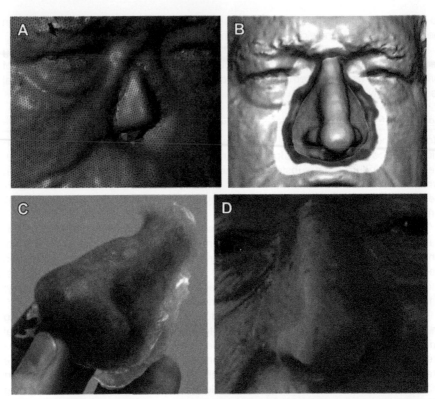

Fig. 3. (*A*) The STL file polygon mesh data of the baseplate and surrounding anatomy. (*B*) The complete digital design with texture. (*C*) Completed prosthesis from the silicone-wrapped direct RP-fabricated pattern. (*D*) Completed prosthesis from the RP-fabricated mold. (*From* Eggbeer D, Bibb R, Evans P, et al. Evaluation of direct and indirect additive manufacture of maxillofacial prostheses. Proc Inst Mech Eng H 2012. Available at: http://pih.sagepub.com/content/early/2012/07/02/0954411912451826; with permission.)

top one-third of the cylindrical bur to a small-diameter tip, enabling high precision form grinding with reasonable bur life.[24,39,40]

In 2009, the newest model known as CEREC AC powered by BlueCam (Sirona, Charlotte, NC) was introduced, which has the ability to take half-arch or full-arch impressions and create crowns, veneers, and bridges. The current acquisition system uses intense blue light from blue light emitting diodes (LEDs). The camera records a series of overlapping single images that the software converts into a 3D virtual model. The camera projects blue light onto the teeth, which reflect it back at a slightly different angle. This method of visualization is referred to as active triangulation.[24,39]

To use the system, the tooth preparation to be scanned is coated with a layer of special titanium dioxide powder, which makes translucent areas of the teeth opaque and permits the camera to register all of the tissues. Several optical impressions are then taken from an occlusal orientation. The shorter wavelength of the LED blue light has been measured to have a higher resolution compared with that of a red laser.[24,39]

After the impression is complete, a 3D rendering of the tooth to be restored appears on the monitor. The dentist is able to mark where the die should begin and end based on this image. The software program then generates a proposed restoration based on comparisons with the surrounding teeth, which can then be altered or fine tuned as needed. After the design is approved, the milling process can begin. A block of ceramic or composite material in the correct color is inserted into the milling unit.[39]

As an alternative, the dentist can obtain a digital impression and send the data to a dental laboratory. The laboratories can then design and mill the restoration using CAD/CAM technology. They can also use the digital image to fabricate a hard resin model based on the data and proceed to fabricate the restoration in the conventional manner.[39]

The E4D dentist system

E4D was introduced by D4D Technologies LLC (Richardson, TX) in early 2008 and it is presently the only other system besides CEREC that permits same-day in-office restorations. The system consists of a cart containing the design center and laser scanner, a separate milling unit, and a job server and router for communication. The scanner, termed the intraoral digitizer, has a shorter vertical profile than that of the CEREC, so the patient is not required to open as wide for posterior scans. The E4D does not require the use of reflected agent powder to enable capture of fine detail on the target site in most cases. Therefore, scanning begins by simply placing the intraoral digitizer directly above the prepared tooth. The scanner must be held a specific distance from the surface being scanned; this is achieved with the help of rubber-tipped boots that extend from the head of the scanner. It is not necessary to scan the opposing arch. Occlusal registration is created with an impression material, trimmed, and then placed on top of the prepared tooth; the scanner captures a combination of the registration material and the neighboring teeth that are not covered by the material. These data are used to design restorations with proper occlusal heights. Once the final restoration is approved, the design center transmits the data to the milling machine. Using blocks of ceramic or composite mounted in the milling machine, and with the aid of rotary diamond instruments that are capable of replacing themselves when worn or damaged, the dentist is able to fabricate the completed restoration.[41]

The Cadent iTero

Cadent introduced iTero in 2007 as the first digital impression system for conventionally manufactured crowns and bridges. Unlike the other systems, which acquire images using triangulation, iTero uses a parallel confocal white light and laser light camera to record a series of single images to create a 3D model. The cadent iTero scanner captures 100,000 points of red laser light and has perfect focus images of more than 300 focal depths of the tooth structure. An advantage of the iTero camera is the ability to scan without the need of any agent powder, resulting in a camera with a larger head than the other systems.[41]

Once the digital impression has been completed the dentist can select from a series of diagnostic tools to evaluate the preparation and complete the impression. The occlusal reduction tool shows in vivid color how much clearance has been created in the preparation for the restoration selected by the dentist. A margin line tool is available to assist in viewing the clearly defined margin. The completed digital impression can be sent through a Health Insurance Portability and Accountability Act (HIPAA)-complaint wireless system to a Cadent facility and the dental laboratory. The model is milled from a property-blended resin and is pinned, trimmed, and articulated based on the digital impression created by the dentist. Cadent uses an industrial 5-axis milling machine to ensure the precision of the milled model and dies.[42]

Lava COS

Lava was created at Brontes Technologies (Lexington, MA) and was acquired by the 3M ESPE (St Paul, MN) in October 2006. The Lava COS system consists of a mobile cart, a touch screen display, and a scanner with a camera at the end. The camera tip of the wand contains 192 lens data system (LDS) and 22 lens systems.

The method used for capturing 3D impressions involves active wave front sampling.

The Lava COS concept of 3D in motion incorporates revolutionary optical design, image processing algorithms, and real-time model reconstruction to capture 3D data in a video sequence and model the data in real time. The scanning wand contains a complex optical system composed of multiple lenses and blue light-emitting diode (LED) cells. The Lava COS is therefore able to capture approximately 20 3D data sets per second or close to 2400 data sets per arch, for an accurate and high-speed scan. After the preparation of the tooth and gingival retraction, the arch is dried and lightly dusted with powder. The Lava COS only requires enough agent powder to allow the scanner to locate reference points, not heavy powdering as with the CEREC. When all the scans have been reviewed for accuracy, the dentist fills out a 1-screen laboratory prescription. The data are wirelessly sent to the laboratory technician, who then uses customized software to digitally cut the die and mark the margin, and also to create an articulated SLA model that a dental laboratory uses to design any type of restoration, such as crowns, inlays, onlays, and bridges, and not just Lava.[39,41]

3M True Definition scanner

The True Definition scanner delivers powerful 3D video-based scanning technology and provides scanning precision, accuracy, and repeatability for taking digital impressions. The technology is contained in a small, ergonomic, lightweight wand the size of a dental headpiece. The system also offers users the 3M connection center, which is built on a secure, cloud-based architecture that provides both trusted and integrated connections to third-party systems, along with the flexibility of open STL file systems. The wand part does not require calibration, and the monitor and computer have been built through a partnership with Hewlett-Packard.[43]

Lava Ultimate Restorative

Lava Ultimate Restorative is a combination of 3M ESPE's Lava COS, Lava Design software, and resin nano ceramic. This combined technology allows clinicians and laboratory technicians to work together as a team to create high-quality restorations. Lava COS provides accuracy in scanning and Lava Design software offers exceptional marginal fit in zirconia and other materials.[44]

3Shape TRIOS

3Shape's Ultrafast Optical Sectioning technology enables dentists to rapidly and easily achieve accurate scans with minimum discomfort for the patient. Unlike most other scanners, 3Shape TRIOS is a no-spray solution.

This technology captures more than 3000 two-dimensional images per second; 100 times faster than conventional video cameras. It combines hundreds or thousands of 3D pictures to create the final 3D digital impression based on real data rather than interpolated artificial surfaces. There is no need to hold the scanner at a specific distance or angle for focus, and dentists can rest the scanner on the teeth for support as they scan. 3Shape TRIOS provides optimized scanning for an extensive range of dental indications including inlays/onlays, crowns (with subgingival preparations), bridges, temporaries, diagnostic wax-ups, veneers, and implant cases.[45]

Influence of Scan Spray Systems on Human Gingival Fibroblasts

Chairside CAD/CAM devices, which can produce ceramic restorations of high durability combined with excellent aesthetic results, usually require opaque surfaces.

Standardized spray systems, which coat the teeth with a titanium dioxide powder to enhance their opacity, represent a necessary and vital part of some systems.

Willershausen and colleagues[46] tested 3 different spray systems (ScanDry, Scan Spray Luer Classic, and CEREC Optispray) to determine their effects on proliferation, viability, and adenylate kinase (ADK) release of human periodontal fibroblasts. Any potential toxic effect would be reflected in the release of ADK after cellular contact of the used materials. The aforementioned results suggest that when scan spray particles are accidentally left in the oral cavity after the spraying process they are not likely to result in increased ADK levels, which showed no harmful effect in vitro.

Dental Materials and CAD/CAM

With the introduction of advanced CAD/CAM technologies, various high-strength ceramic materials were developed and are increasingly used in dentistry.

However yttria-stabilized tetragonal zirconia polycrystalline (Y-TZP) frameworks exhibit unsurpassed mechanical properties, reflected by high survival rates in clinical application. Because of the high reported veneer failure rates with zirconia-based fixed dental prostheses (FDPs), high-strength glass-ceramic systems in monolithic and bilayer applications have regained increased consideration for anterior and posterior restorations.[47,48]

Lithium Disilicate

Lithium disilicate has been indicated for use in thin veneers, minimally invasive inlays and onlays, crowns, implant superstructures, and FPDs. At present there are 2 methods to fabricate a restoration from lithium disilicate glass ceramic. The first method, or the original technique, is the lost-wax/heat-pressing method. A wax pattern is hand made and then the heated ceramic ingot is forced through a heated tube into a mold. More recently, a restoration from lithium disilicate glass-ceramic blocks has been designed and milled from a ceramic block, using CAD/CAM.[12,49]

Lithium disilicate ceramic (IPS Empress II, Ivoclar Vivadent, Schaan, Liechtenstein) using the lost-wax press technique was introduced in 1998 as an enhanced glass-ceramic system for single tooth and anterior 3-unit FDP restorations. Although this all-ceramic system was successful in anterior and posterior crown indications, heterogeneous survival rates ranging from 50% after 2 years to 70% after 5 years were reported for bilayer FDP applications.[50]

In 2001, IPS e.max Press (Ivoclar Vivadent, Schaan, Liechtenstein) was released to the market with significantly improved mechanical and optical properties. Higher translucency and augmented shade variety enabled this lithium-disilicate glass-ceramic material in posterior indication for monolithic full anatomic restoration fabrication with subsequent staining characterization. A promising survival rate of 87.9% after 10 years has been reported for monolithic posterior 3-unit FDP applications.[51]

Silica-based ceramic blocks are offered by several CAD/CAM systems. In addition to monochromatic blocks, various manufacturers now offer blanks with multicolored layers (Vitablocs TriLuxe [Vita], IPS Empress CAD Multi [Ivoclar Vivadent]), for the purpose of full anatomic crowns. Because of their higher stability values, lithium disilicate ceramic blocks are particularly important in this group; they can be used for full anatomic anterior and posterior crowns, for copings in the anterior and posterior region, and for 3-unit FPD frameworks in the anterior region because of their high mechanical stability of 360 MPa. Glass ceramics are particularly well suited to chairside application as a result of their translucent characteristics, similar to that of natural tooth structure; they provide aesthetically pleasing results even without veneering. Lithium disilicate is also biocompatible, provides diminished plaque accumulation, low thermal conductivity, and color stability.[49]

In certain clinical situations, lithium disilicate restorations should not be placed, such as a limited interocclusal distance and in patients with parafunctional habits.[12] Disadvantages of lithium disilicate restorations include the brittleness of the ceramic and their low to moderately high flexural strength and fracture toughness. Because lithium disilicate has these properties, its use and placement should be restricted to low-stress to moderate-stress environments and adequate thickness of the ceramic should be provided to avoid the fracture of the restoration.[52] Another major disadvantage to lithium disilicate is the damaging wear it can cause to the opposing tooth structure. Under certain conditions, the damage can increase, especially when a roughened surface (created through parafunctional habit, premature occlusal contact, and/or inadequate occlusal adjustments) contacts tooth enamel or dentin under high occlusal forces. To decrease this chance of occlusal wear, the clinician should ensure cuspid-guided disclusion.[12]

A dry field and good moisture control from saliva should be maintained during final cementation to ensure a positive outcome when using lithium disilicate restorations.[12] In terms of surface treatment of the ceramic material before final cementation, etch with hydrofluoric acid, application of a silane primer, and using adhesive systems have been recommended and showed improved bond strengths.[53,54]

Infiltration ceramics

These blocks are processed in porous, chalky conditions and then infiltrated with lanthanum glass. They originate from the Vita In-Ceram system (Vita) and are offered in 3 variations:

- Vita In-Ceram Alumina (Al_2O_3): suitable for crown copings in the anterior and posterior regions, and 3-unit FPD frameworks in the anterior region.
- Vita In-Ceram Zirconia (70% Al_2O_3, 30% ZrO_2): suitable for crown copings in the anterior and posterior regions, and 3-unit FPD frameworks in the anterior and posterior regions. Because of its superior masking ability, this ceramic is suitable for discolored abutment teeth.
- VITA In-Ceram Spinell (Mg Al_2O_4): has the highest translucency of all oxide ceramics and is thus recommended for the production of highly aesthetic anterior crown copings, in particular on vital abutment teeth and in young patients.[55]

Oxide high-performance ceramics

At present, aluminum oxide and zirconium oxide are offered as blocks for CAD/CAM technology.

Al_2O_3 This oxide high-performance ceramic is ground in a presintered phase and is then sintered at a temperature of 1520°C in the sintering furnace. Aluminum oxide is indicated in the case of crown copings in the anterior and posterior area, primary crowns, and 3-unit anterior FPD frameworks. The ground frames can be individually stained in several colors with Vita In-Ceram AL Coloring Liquid. Examples of aluminum oxide blocks include In-Ceram AL Block (Vita) and inCoris Al (Sirona), which are available in an ivorylike color.[29]

Yttrium stabilized zirconium oxide (ZrO_2, Y-TZP) Zirconium dioxide is a high-performance oxide ceramic with excellent mechanical characteristics. It has high flexural strength and fracture toughness compared with other dental ceramics, which offers the possibility of using this material as a framework for crowns and FPDs, and, in appropriate indications, for individual implant abutments.[56]

Zirconia

Zirconium minerals were discovered decades ago but are still referred to as jargon, jacinth, and hyacinth. The name zirconium (Zr) comes from the Arabic word zargon (golden in color), which in turn derives from 2 Persian words: zar (gold) and gun (color). The metal dioxide zirconia was discovered by the German chemist Martin Heinrich Klaproth in 1789 and was isolated by the Swedish chemist Jons Jacob Berzelius in 1824.[57,58]

Zirconium dioxide (ZrO_2) Known as zirconia, this is a white crystalline oxide of zirconium. Although pure zirconium oxide does not occur in nature, it is found in the minerals baddeleyite and zircon ($ZrSiO_4$) (**Fig. 4**).[59] Zirconium oxide crystals are arranged in crystalline cells that are categorized in 3 crystallographic phases: (1) the cubic (C) in the form of a straight prism with square sides, (2) the tetragonal (T) in the form of a straight prism with rectangular sides, and (3) the monoclinic (M) in the form of a deformed prism with parallelepiped sides.[59] The cubic phase is stable at more than 2370°C and has moderate mechanical properties; the tetragonal phase is stable between 1170°C and 2370°C and allows a ceramic with improved mechanical properties to be obtained; whereas the monoclinic phase, which is stable at room temperatures up to 1170°C, presents reduced mechanical performance and may contribute to a reduction in the cohesion of the ceramic particles and thus of the density.[59,60]

Stabilized zirconia

This is a mixture of zirconia polymorphs, because insufficient cubic phase–forming oxide (stabilizer) has been added and a cubic plus metastable tetragonal ZrO_2 mixture is obtained. A smaller addition of stabilizer to the pure zirconia brings its structure into a tetragonal phase at a temperature higher than 1000°C and a mixture of cubic phase and monoclinic (or tetragonal) phase at a lower temperature. This partially stabilized zirconia is also called TZP. Several different oxides, such as magnesium oxide (MgO), yttrium oxide (Y_2O_3), calcium oxide (CaO), and cerium oxide (Ce_2O_3), can be added to zirconia to stabilize the tetragonal and/or cubic phases. The addition of stabilizing oxides allows the generation of a multiphase material at room temperature.

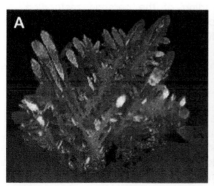
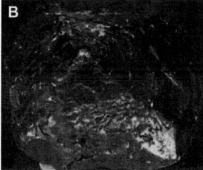

Fig. 4. The minerals (A) baddeleyite (ZrO_2), (B) zircon ($ZrSiO_4$). (Data from Koutayas SO, Vagkopoulou T, Pelekanos S, et al. Zirconia in dentistry: part 1. Discovering the nature of an upcoming bioceramic. Eur J Esthet Dent 2009;4(2):2–23.)

Fully stabilized zirconia is produced when more than 16 mol% CaO (7.9 wt%), 16 mol% MgO (5.86 wt%), or 8 mol% Y_2O_3 (13.75 wt%) is added to ZrO_2, and it has a cubic form. With the addition of smaller amounts of stabilizing oxides, zirconia can also be partially stabilized in a multiphase form, known as partially stabilized zirconia (PSZ). Although a considerable amount of research has been dedicated to magnesia PSZ (Mg-PSZ) for possible biomedical applications, this material has not been successful, mainly because of the presence of porosity, associated with a large grain size (30–60 μm), which can induce wear.[59,61]

Yttrium oxide PSZ Yttrium oxide PSZ is a fully tetragonal fine-grained zirconia ceramic material made of 100% small metastable tetragonal grains (Y-TZP) after the addition of approximately 2 to 3 mol% yttrium oxide (Y_2O_3) as a stabilizing agent. The fraction of the T phase retained at room temperature depends on the processing temperature, the yttrium content, the grain size, and the grade of constraint exerted on them by the matrix. One of the characteristic of the Y-TZP ceramics is the formation of compressive layers on their surface. Surface tetragonal grains are not constrained by the matrix and for that reason can spontaneously transform to monoclinic grains, leading to improved mechanical and wear properties of this material. Y-TZP has been used to manufacture femoral heads in total hip replacement prostheses since the late 1980s but its use in orthopedic surgery has since been reduced by more than 90%, mostly because of a series of failures that occurred in 2001. Y-TZP is available in dentistry for the fabrication of dental crowns and FPDs. The restorations are processed either by soft machining of presintered blanks followed by sintering at high temperature, or by hard machining of fully sintered blocks.[59–61]

Zirconia Properties

Aging
Aging is the mechanical property of degradation in zirconia. Y-TZP ceramics have a low-temperature degradation phenomenon known as aging. Progressive, spontaneous transformation of the tetragonal phase into the monoclinic phase results in the degradation of the mechanical properties of Y-TZP. A slow T-M transformation occurs when Y-TZP is in contact with water or vapor, body fluid, or during steam sterilization, which leads to surface damage.

The strength degradation level varies between TZP ceramics because aging behavior is related to the differences in equilibrium within the microstructural parameters, such as yttrium concentration and distribution, grain size, flaw population, duration of exposure to aging medium, loading of the ceramic restoration, and manufacturing processes.[59,62,63] It is difficult to create aging-free zirconia because the transformation occurring on aging involves a natural return back to the monoclinic equilibrium state.[57]

Effects of aging are reduction in strength, toughness, and density, and an increase in monoclinic phase content.[61,62]

Optical properties
Different grades of zirconium have different levels of translucency. The higher the grade the more translucent the material is. At present, colored zirconia cores are offered by some manufacturers to enhance aesthetic outcomes. Different coloring agents are introduced for a better aesthetic performance of the white shade zirconia frameworks. These frameworks can be further customized in terms of form and aesthetics by veneering with porcelain, through the layering or pressing technique. Coloring of the framework has no influence on the frameworks' flexural strength. Individual characterization of the monochromatic zirconia cores provides aesthetically

comparable results with the common layering techniques and multishade block systems, but no long-term follow-up data on the color stability exist. Zirconia frameworks provide a level of opacity that offers adequate masking of underlying discolored abutments and permits a controlled depth of translucency after veneering.[59]

Polishing
The polishing process produces surface scratches that induce residual stresses in the material. According to the type and the amount of these stresses, polishing may lead to the development of a compressive surface stress layer, which is beneficial for aging resistance. Fine polishing after grinding can remove the compressive layer of the M phase from the surface and reduce the severity and amount of surface defects and flows to a degree at which the internal strength of the material becomes the dominant factor determining its mechanical performance. The flexural strength eventually increases. An in vitro study revealed that, if zirconia is used without veneering material for crowns and FDPs, the surface must be well polished to reduce the wear of the opposing enamel.[57–59]

Sandblasting
Sandblasting zirconia ceramics promotes adhesion of the luting cement to the framework and provides a strengthening technique for Y-TZP at the expense of reduced stability. The lower temperatures and stresses developed by sandblasting compared with grinding induce T-M transformation and allow the maintenance of the resulting M phase. Sandblasting after grinding removes some larger grinding-induced cracks and weakly attached surface grains, and simultaneously produces surface compressive stresses that strengthen the material. Despite the increase in strength values after abrasion with 50-µm aluminum oxide particles, the long-term effect of this induced damage still has to be considered as a potentially weakening factor.[59,64]

FABRICATION OF ZIRCONIA FRAMEWORKS
Soft Machining (Green Machining)

Since its development in 2001, direct ceramic machining of presintered 3Y-TZP has become increasingly popular in dentistry. The die or wax pattern is scanned, an enlarged restoration is designed by computer software (CAD), and a presintered ceramic blank is milled by CAM. The restoration is later sintered at a high temperature. There are several variations of this process, depending on how the scanning is performed and how the large sintering shrinkage of 3Y-TZP is compensated for. Restorations can be colored later, by immersion in solutions of various metal salts (cerium, bismuth, iron, or a combination). The final sintering temperature influences the color obtained. Colored zirconia can also be obtained by adding small amounts of various metal oxides to the starting powder. There are several systems using soft machining of 3Y-TZP for dental restorations, including Cercon (Dentsply International), Lava (3M ESPE), Procera zirconia (Nobel Biocare), yttrium-stabilized zirconium oxide (YZ) cubes for CEREC InLab (Vident), and IPS e.max ZirCAD (Ivoclar Vivadent).[61]

Hard Machining of 3Y-TZP and Mg-PSZ

There are 2 systems available for hard machining of zirconia dental restorations: Denzir (Cadesthetics AB) and DC-Zirkon (DCS Dental AG). The blocks are processed by hot isostatic pressing; they need to be machined using a specially designed milling system. because of the high hardness and low machinability of fully sintered Y-TZP, the milling system has to be particularly robust. Hard machining involves milling the framework directly to the desired dimension out of densely sintered (higher strength and more homogeneous) zirconia blanks.[61,65]

Unlike porcelain, zirconia is free of edge chipping when using any diamond grit size. Yttria-stabilized tetragonal zirconia is less sensitive to machining damage than many other polycrystalline ceramics. Supporters of soft machining claim that hard machining may introduce microcracks in the framework during the milling process. In contrast, hard-machining supporters may claim a superior marginal fit because no shrinkage is involved in their manufacturing process.[65,66]

BONDING TO ZIRCONIA

The longevity of an indirect restoration is closely related to the integrity of the cement at the margin. The best method to promote a durable bond between the ceramic and tooth structure is still unknown, but hydrofluoric acid etching and common silane agents seem not to be effective for zirconia ceramics. There is a wide variety of commercially available cements for luting all-ceramic restorations. These cements include zinc phosphate cements, conventional and resin-modified glass ionomer cements, resin cements, and self-adhesive resin cements. However, resin cements possess some advantages compared with the other materials, because they have lower solubility and better aesthetic characteristics.[67]

Zirconium oxide crowns may be cemented using both conventional and adhesive methods. However, a strong and durable resin bond provides high retention, improves marginal adaptation, prevents microleakage, and increases the fracture resistance of the restored tooth and the restoration.[68,69]

There is some evidence that suggests a better bond to Y-TZP ceramics using resin cements with phosphate ester monomers. The phosphate ester group might chemically bond to metal oxides, such as zirconium dioxide. Other monomers present in resin cements might also have a chemical affinity for metal oxides.[70]

The application of the adhesive phosphate monomer 10-methacryloyloxydecyl dihydrogen phosphate (MDP) or an MDP-containing bonding/silane coupling agent mixture after airborne particle abrasion (110 μm Al_2O_3 at 2.5 bar) and a phosphate-modified resin cement (eg, Panavia 21, Kuraray, Osaka, Japan) may provide a long-term durable resin bond to zirconium oxide ceramic with promising high-tensile bond strengths (39.2 MPa).[71–73] Furthermore, it was shown that the application of a tribochemical silica coating (eg, CoJet, 3M ESPE, Seefeld, Germany) in combination with an MDP-containing bonding/silane coupling agent mixture increased the shear bond strength between zirconium oxide ceramic and phosphate-modified resin cement (Panavia F, Kuraray).[74] The tribochemical silica coating process was also tested with zirconia silanization (prefabricated zirconia posts), which resulted in an increased bond strength.[75] Moreover, a self-curing dental adhesive system containing 4-acryloyloxyethyl trimellitate anhydride/methyl methacrylate-tri-n-butylborane (4-META/MMA-TBB) (eg, Superbond C&B, Sun Medical, Tokyo, Japan) showed high bond strengths regardless of the different surface treatments such as silica coating, airborne particle abrasion, hydrofluoric acid etching, and diamond grinding.[76] The bond strength of bisphenol-A-glycidyl dimethacrylate (Bis-GMA) resin cement (eg, Variolink II, Ivoclar Vivadent, Schaan, Liechtenstein) to the zirconia ceramic can be significantly increased after pretreatment with plasma spraying (hexamethyldisiloxane) or by the use of a low-fusing porcelain layer.[77]

Regardless of surface pretreatments, long-term in vitro water storage and thermocycling can negatively influence the durability of the resin bond strength to zirconia ceramic.[72] Thermocycling induces a higher impact than water storage at a constant temperature.[78] It is essential to avoid contamination of the zirconia bonding surfaces during try-in procedures, either by saliva contact or by a silicone disclosing medium. Air abrasion with 50 mm Al_2O_3 at 2.5 bar for 15 seconds is the most effective cleaning method to regain an optimal bonding surface.[79,80]

Zirconia in Dental Applications

Zirconia crowns

Case selection criteria for zirconia crown restorations (ie, limited interocclusal space, parafunctional habits, malocclusion, short clinical crowns, tooth mobility, tooth inclination) and basic clinical sequence do not differ from other all-ceramic crowns.[63]

Marginal discrepancy of all-ceramic restorations is a vital factor that affects the longevity of dental restorations. Different fabricating systems used in CAD/CAM processing techniques could lead to varied results in terms of the marginal and internal gap width. In addition, span length, framework configuration, and veneering ceramic could affect the fit of zirconia PFDs.[81]

Poor fitting in the axial wall area and occlusal plateau can also reduce the resistance to fracture of all-ceramic restorations.[82]

Because of the inherent opacity of zirconia, the abutment should be adequately prepared to allow enough space for both the substructure and the veneering material. After milling, a 0.5-mm uniform zirconia core should be fabricated for single posterior crowns. Particularly in the anterior region, strength and aesthetic requirements may allow the fabrication of 0.3-mm copings; however, reduction of the coping thickness from 0.5 mm to 0.3 mm can negatively influence the fracture loading capacity (35% decrease) of zirconia single crowns.[63]

Zirconia FPDs

New high-strength core/framework materials have been developed for all-ceramic FPDs, also referred to as FDPs. However, most of these systems are limited with respect to replacement of the anterior and premolar teeth, require large connector dimensions, and may require the use of more technique-sensitive clinical procedures such as adhesive cementation. Posterior 3-unit prostheses represent a new challenge for all-ceramic restorations. There are 2 systems for this type of restoration: a glass-infiltrated alumina/zirconia (In-Ceram Zirconia, Vita Zahnfabrik) and a transformation-toughened polycrystalline zirconia (such as Cercon Zirconia, Dentsply Ceramco, York, PA; Lava, 3M ESPE, St Paul, MN; In-Ceram YZ, Vita Zahnfabrik).[63]

Suarez and colleagues[83] reported a survival rate of 94.5% after 3-year clinical evaluation of In-Ceram Zirconia posterior FPDs. In a different study, the success rate for 33 posterior zirconia FPDs (Cercon) was 97.8%. However, the overall survival rate was 73.9% because of other complications, such as secondary caries and chipping of the veneering ceramic. These two clinical studies reported only 1 fracture of the zirconia-based framework, which suggests a promising future for all-ceramic FPDs (**Fig. 5**).[13]

Zirconia posts

This material has been used for root canal dowels since 1989, for orthodontic brackets since 1994, for implant abutments since 1995, for all-ceramic FPD since 1998, and the first use of zirconia as a dental implant material in humans was reported in 2004. Teeth treated endodontically may require a dowel and core to support the definitive restoration; metal dowel and core systems can produce gray discoloration beneath translucent all-ceramic crowns, limiting the aesthetic potential. Zirconia dowels are biocompatible, radiopaque, and possess high flexural strengths and a modulus of elasticity close to that of dentin, thus reducing the incidence of root fracture. However, this can also be a

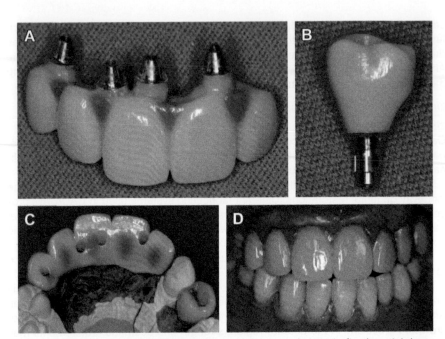

Fig. 5. (*A*) Anterior 5-unit screw-retained implant–supported zirconia fixed partial denture restoration (#6–10). (*B*) Screw-retained implant–supported zirconia crown (left first premolar [#12]). (*C*) Palatal view on the model. (*D*) Frontal view after insertion. Clinical work was performed by Dr R. Zandparsa, Boston, MA.

disadvantage, because it makes the material brittle and therefore it is not recommended for treating patients with bruxism. A stable dowel-core foundation depends on a reliable bond between the core material and the dowel. If composite is used to fabricate the core, then the bond to the zirconia dowel is only mechanical and can only be achieved by roughening the surface using airborne abrasion. For the indirect technique, a castable, zirconia-enriched glass-ceramic material is pressed directly over the prefabricated zirconia dowel. Autopolymerizing or dual-polymerizing composite luting agents are recommended because light units used to polymerize resins cannot penetrate to the apical zone of dowels.[84,85]

Understanding of how all-ceramic restorations perform and fail has improved in recent years. The remaining challenges for future advances present abundant scope for future investigations and innovations.

REFERENCES

1. Zandparsa R. Dental biomaterials. Chapter 17. In: Kutz M, editor. Biomedical engineering and design handbook, vol. 1–2, 2nd edition. McGraw-Hill; 2009. p. 397–420.
2. Ferracane JL. Materials in dentistry: principles and applications. 2nd edition. Philadelphia: Lippincott Williams & Wilkins; 2001.
3. Lygre H. Prosthodontic biomaterials and adverse reactions: a critical review of the clinical and research literature. Acta Odontol Scand 2002;60: 1–9.
4. Szycher M. Szycher's dictionary of biomaterials and medical devices. Lancaster (United Kingdom): Technomic; 1992. p. 21–2.

5. McCabe JF, Walls AW. Applied Dental Materials. Oxford (United Kingdom): Blackwell Science, Blackwell Publishing; 1999. p. 1.

6. Jedynakiewicz NM. Encyclopedia of biomaterials and biomedical engineering. Ceramics in dentistry; School of Dentistry, The University of Liverpool. Liverpool, UK. San Diego, CA: Academic Press; 2006.

7. Kelly RJ, Nishimura I, Campbell SD. Ceramics in dentistry: historical roots and current perspectives. J Prosthet Dent 1996;75:18–32.

8. Ring ME. Dentistry, an illustrated history. New York: HN Abrams; 1985. p. 160–81, 193–211.

9. Kingery WD, Vaudiver PB. Ceramic masterpieces. Art, structure, technology. New York: The Free Press; 1986. p. 7–36.

10. Jones DW. Development of dental ceramics. Dent Clin North Am 1985;29: 621–44.

11. Anusavice K. Philips' science of dental materials. St Louis, MO: Elsevier Science; 2003.

12. Kelly JR, Benetti P. Ceramic materials in dentistry: historical evolution and current practice. Aust Dent J 2011;56(Suppl 1):84–96.

13. Donovan TE. Factors essential for successful all-ceramic restorations. J Am Dent Assoc 2008;139:14S–8S.

14. Robert KJ. Dental ceramics: what is this stuff anyway? J Am Dent Assoc 2008; 139:4S–7S.

15. Yin L, Song XF, Song YL, et al. An overview of in vitro abrasive finishing & CAD/CAM of bioceramics in restorative dentistry. Int J Mach Tool Manufact 2006;46: 1013–26.

16. Kelly JR. Ceramics in restorative and prosthetic dentistry. Mater Sci 1997;27: 443–68.

17. Xu HH, Quinn JB. Whisker-reinforced bioactive composites containing calcium phosphate cement fillers: effects of filler ratio and surface treatments on mechanical properties. J Biomed Mater Res 2001;57:165–74.

18. Xu HH, Schumacher GE, Eichmiller FC, et al. Continuous-fiber preform reinforcement of dental resin composite restorations. Dent Mater 2003;19: 523–30.

19. Lawn BR, Deng Y, Lloyd IK, et al. Materials design of ceramic-based layer structures for crowns. J Dent Res 2002;81(6):433–8.

20. Rekow ED, Erdman AG, Riley DR, et al. CAD/CAM for dental restorations–some of the curious challenges. Biomed Eng 1991;38(4):318–414.

21. CEREC Dental CAD/CAM Systems. Available at: www.sirona.com.

22. M ESPE Lava™ All-Ceramic System, technical product profile, Dental Products, 3M Center, St Paul, MN, USA.

23. Willer J, Rossbach A, Weber HP. Computer-assisted milling of dental restorations using a new CAD/CAM data acquisition system. J Prosthet Dent 1998; 80:346–53.

24. Fasbinder D. Using digital technology to enhance restorative dentistry. Compend Contin Educ Dent 2012;33(9):666–77.

25. Hickel R, Dasch W, Mehl A, et al. CAD/CAM - fillings of the future? Int Dent J 1997;47:247–58.

26. Wittneben JG, Wright RF, Weber HP, et al. A systematic review of the clinical performance of CAD/CAM single-tooth restorations. Int J Prosthodont 2009;22(5): 466–71.

27. Beuer F. Digital dentistry: an overview of recent developments for CAD/CAM generated restorations. Braz Dent J 2008;204(9):505–11.

28. May KB, Russell MM, Razzoog ME, et al. Precision of fit: the Procera AllCeram crown. J Prosthet Dent 1998;80:394.
29. Bártolo P, Bidand B. Bio-materials and prototyping applications in medicine. New York: Springer Science+Business Media, LLC; 2008. p. 125–55, Chapter 8.
30. Ning D, Cheng XS, Liao WH, et al. Deformation design technology of dental restoration model. BioMedical Engineering Informatics 2008;2:793–7.
31. Van Noort R. The future of dental devices is digital. Dent Mater 2012;28:3–12.
32. Miyazaki T, Hotta Y, Kunii J, et al. A review of dental CAD/CAM: current status and future perspectives from 20 years of experience. Dent Mater J 2009; 28(1):44–56.
33. Silva NR, Witek L, Coelho PG, et al. Additive CAD/CAM process for dental prostheses. J Prosthodont 2011;20:93–6.
34. van Roekel NB. Electrical discharge machining in dentistry. Int J Prosthodont 1992;5:114–21.
35. Azari A, Nikzad S. The evolution of rapid prototyping in dentistry: a review. Rapid Prototyping J 2009;15(3):216–25.
36. Ebert1 J, Özkol1 E, Zeichner A. Direct inkjet printing of dental prostheses made of zirconia. J Dent Res 2009;88:673–6.
37. Narayan R, editor. Specialized fabrication processes: rapid prototyping. New York: Biomedical Materials, SpringerScience+BusinessMedia, LLC; 2009. p. 493–523, Chapter 18.
38. Miranda P, Saiz E, Gryn K, et al. Sintering and robocasting of beta-tricalcium phosphate scaffolds for orthopaedic applications. Acta Biomater 2006;2:457–66.
39. Davidowitz D, Kotick P. The use of CAD/CAM in dentistry. Dent Clin North Am 2011;55:559–70.
40. Mormann WH. The evolution of CEREC system. J Am Dent Assoc 2006; 137(Suppl 1):7S–13S.
41. Birnbaum N, Aaronson H, Cohen B. 3D digital scanners: a high-tech approach to more accurate dental impressions. Inside Dentistry 2009;5(4):70–7.
42. Meer W, Andriessen F, Ren Y. Application of intra-oral dental scanners in the digital workflow of implantology. PLoS One 2012;7(8):e43312.
43. 3M True Definition scanner: the future of impressioning technology. Compend Contin Educ Dent 2012;33(9):694.
44. 3MESPE: CAD/CAM guiding dentistry in new direction. Compend Contin Educ Dent 2012;33(7):540.
45. Andersen JB. 3Shape TRIOS next-generation digital impressions, (Brochure) 2011, 1–9. Available at: www.3shapedental.com.
46. Willershausen I, Lehmann KM, Roβ A, et al. Influence of three scan spray systems on human gingival fibroblasts. Quintessence Int 2012;43(6):e67–72.
47. Vult von Steyern P, Carlson P, Nilner K. All-ceramic fixed partial dentures designed according to the DC-Zirkon technique. A 2-year clinical study. J Oral Rehabil 2005;32:180–7.
48. Fasbinder DJ, Dennison JB, Heys D, et al. A clinical evaluation of chairside lithium disilicate CAD/CAM crowns: a two-year report. J Am Dent Assoc 2010; 141(Suppl 2):10S–4S.
49. Tinschert J, Natt G, Mautsch W, et al. Fracture Resistance of lithium disilicate-, alumina-, and zirconia based three-unit fixed partial dentures: a laboratory study. Int J Prosthodont 2001;14:231–8.
50. Valenti M, Valenti A. Retrospective survival analysis of 261lithium disilicate crowns in a private general practice. Quintessence Int 2009;40:573–9.

51. Kern M, Sasse M, Wolfart S. Ten-year outcome of three-unit fixed dental prostheses made from monolithic lithium disilicate ceramic. J Am Dent Assoc 2012;143: 234–40.

52. Ozturk O, Uludag B, Usumez A, et al. The effect of ceramic thickness and number of firings on the color of two all-ceramic systems. J Prosthet Dent 2008;100: 99–106.

53. Sorensen JA, Kang SK, Avera SP. Porcelain composite interface microleakage with various porcelain surface treatments. Dent Mater 1991;7:118–23.

54. Nagai T, Kawamoto Y. Adhesive bonding of a lithium disilicate ceramic material with resin-based luting agents. J Oral Rehabil 2005;32:598–605.

55. Raigrodski AJ, Chiche GJ, Swift EJ Jr. All-ceramic fixed partial dentures, part III: clinical studies. J Esthet Restor Dent 2002;14:313–9.

56. Curtis AR, Wright AJ, Fleming GJ. The influence of surface modification techniques on the performance of a Y-TZP dental ceramic. J Dent 2006;34: 195–206.

57. Chevalier J. What future for zirconia as a biomaterial? Biomaterials 2006;27: 535–43.

58. Mitov G, Heintze SD, Walz S, et al. Wear behavior of dental Y-TZP ceramic against natural enamel after different finishing procedures. Dent Mater 2012; 28(8):909–18.

59. Koutayas SO, Vagkopoulou T, Pelekanos S, et al. Zirconia in dentistry: part 1. Discovering the nature of an upcoming bioceramic. Eur J Esthet Dent 2009; 4(2):2–23.

60. Stawarczyk B, Ozean M, Hallmann L, et al. The effect of zirconia sintering temperature on flexural strength, grain size, and contrast ratio. Clin Oral Investig 2013;17(1):269–74.

61. Denry I, Kelly JR. State of the art of zirconia for dental applications. Dent Mater 2008;24:299–307.

62. Piconi C, Maccauro G. Zirconia as a ceramic biomaterial. Biomaterials 1999;20: 1–25.

63. Koutayas SO, Vagkopoulou T, Pelekanos S, et al. Zirconia in dentistry: part 2. Evidence-based clinical breakthrough. Eur J Esthet Dent 2009;4:348–80, 2–34.

64. Rekow ED, Silva NR, Coelho PG, et al. Performance of dental ceramics: challenges for improvements. J Dent Res 2011;90(8):937–52.

65. Al-Amleh B, Lyons K, Swain M. Clinical trials in zirconia: a systematic review. J Oral Rehabil 2010;37:641–52.

66. Yin L, Jahanmir S, Ives LK. Abrasive machining of porcelain and zirconia with a dental handpiece. Wear 2003;255:975–89.

67. Cavalcanti AN, Foxton RM, Watson TF, et al. Y-TZP ceramics: key concepts for clinical application. Oper Dent 2009;34(3):344–51.

68. Freedman G. Contemporary esthetic dentistry. St Louis, MO: Elsevier, Mosby; 2012. p. 496–508, Chapter 19.

69. Blatz MB, Sadan A, Kern M. Resin-ceramic bonding: a review of the literature. J Prosthet Dent 2003;89(3):268–74.

70. Biscaro L, Bonfiglioli R, Soattin M, et al. An in vivo evaluation of zirconium-oxide based ceramic single crowns, generated with two CAD/CAM systems, in comparison to metal ceramic single crowns. J Prosthodont 2013;22(1):36–41.

71. Wegner SM, Kern M. Long-term resin bond strength to zirconia ceramic. J Adhes Dent 2000;2:139–47.

72. Kern M, Wegner SM. Bonding to zirconia ceramic: adhesion methods and their durability. Dent Mater 1998;14:64–71.
73. Wolfart M, Lehmann F, Wolfart S, et al. Durability of the resin bond strength to zirconia ceramic after using different surface conditioning methods. Dent Mater 2007;23:45–50.
74. Atsu SS, Kilicarslan MA, Kucukesmen HC, et al. Effect of zirconium-oxide ceramic surface treatments on the bond strength to adhesive resin. J Prosthet Dent 2006;95:430–6.
75. Xible AA, de Jesus Tavarez RR, de Araujo Cdos R, et al. Effect of silica coating and silanization on flexural and composite-resin bond strengths of zirconia posts: an in vitro study. J Prosthet Dent 2006;95:224–9.
76. Derand P, Derand T. Bond strength of luting cements to zirconium oxide ceramics. Int J Prosthodont 2000;13:131–5.
77. Derand T, Molin M, Kvam K. Bond strength of composite luting cement to zirconia ceramic surfaces. Dent Mater 2005;21:1158–62.
78. Wegner SM, Gerdes W, Kern M. Effect of different artificial aging conditions on ceramic-composite bond strength. Int J Prosthodont 2002;15:267–72.
79. Yang B, Scharnberg M, Wolfart S, et al. Influence of contamination on bonding to zirconia ceramic. J Biomed Mater Res B Appl Biomater 2007;81:283–90.
80. Quaas AC, Yang B, Kern M, et al. 2.0 bonding to contaminated zirconia ceramic after different cleaning procedures. Dent Mater 2007;23:506–12.
81. Triwatana P, Nagaviroj N, Tulapornchai C. Clinical performance and failures of zirconia-based fixed partial dentures: a review literature. J Adv Prosthodont 2012;4:76–83.
82. Ardekani KT, Ahangari AH, Farahi L. Marginal and internal fit of CAD/CAM and slip cast made and zirconia copings. J Dent Res Dent Clin Dent Prospects 2012;6:42–8.
83. Suárez MJ, Lozano JF, Paz Salido M, et al. Three-year clinical evaluation of In-Ceram zirconia posterior FPDs. Int J Prosthodont 2004;17(1):35–8.
84. Ozkurt Z, Kazazoglu E. Clinical success of zirconia in dental applications. J Prosthodont 2010;19:64–8.
85. Toksavul S, Turkun M, Toman M. Esthetic enhancement of ceramic crowns with zirconia dowels and cores: a clinical report. J Prosthet Dent 2004;92:116–9.

Management of Snoring and Obstructive Sleep Apnea with Mandibular Repositioning Appliances: A Prosthodontic Approach

Reva Malhotra Barewal, DDS, MS[a],*,
Chad Cameron Hagen, MD, DABPN[b]

KEYWORDS

- Sleep apnea • Mandibular advancement • Oral appliances • Snoring
- Practice guidelines • Review

KEY POINTS

- Dentists are becoming increasingly aware of the importance of detection and management of obstructive sleep apnea.
- The anatomic and neuromuscular risk factors in the pathogenesis of obstructive sleep apnea are reviewed with particular emphasis on oral findings.
- Mandibular repositioning appliances hold an important role in the treatment of this condition; however, knowledge of indications and contraindications for treatment, potential areas of oropharyngeal obstruction, appliance design, and treatment steps are vital to ensure maximum treatment success.

INTRODUCTION

The understanding of the complex link between healthy sleep and brain and body function is relatively new. The knowledge base of sleep disorders has exponentially increased over the past 20 years beginning with the publication of the first book on sleep medicine in 1989 titled, *The Principles and Practice of Sleep Medicine*, edited by Kryger and colleagues,[1] recognizing sleep as a specialty in its own right. Dental sleep medicine is also a rapidly emerging discipline that supports sleep specialists, pulmonologists, otolaryngologists, neurologists, and psychiatrists in screening patients for sleep-disordered breathing and providing treatment for many of these patients. The importance of a multidisciplinary approach cannot be understated as the most effective method of treating this condition. New research is showing links

[a] Private Practice, 9300 Southeast 91st Avenue, Suite 403, Portland, OR 97086, USA; [b] Sleep Disorders Program, Oregon Health and Science University, 3181 Southwest Sam Jackson Park Road, Portland, OR 97239, USA
* Corresponding author.
E-mail address: drb@fusiondentalspecialists.com

Dent Clin N Am 58 (2014) 159–180
http://dx.doi.org/10.1016/j.cden.2013.09.010
0011-8532/14/$ – see front matter © 2014 Elsevier Inc. All rights reserved.

between sleep-disordered breathing, nocturnal parafunction, sleep-related movement disorders, and finally, sleep-orofacial pain interactions.[2] A greater awareness of these links would increase skills in providing a more holistic approach to care for patients. Although continuous positive airway pressure (CPAP) remains the first line of treatment for sleep apnea, there is an important role for mandibular advancement devices, which require dentists to have a good understanding of occlusion, temporomandibular disorders (TMD), and removable appliance therapy. In consideration that these areas of learning are already being taught in prosthodontics creates a natural selection for dental sleep medicine in this publication. It is the intention to provide a brief review of sleep apnea and guidelines for the dentist to encourage participation of the dentist in recognition of this condition and understanding of treatment options for their patients.

PREVALENCE/INCIDENCE

Sleep-disordered breathing (SDB) conditions are highly prevalent in society and often undiagnosed. SDB decreases the quality of sleep by breaking its continuity and tends to bring the individual to a state of transient arousal. When these arousals are too frequent or too long, they can cause a multitude of neurocognitive complaints. Compromised airflow can result in oxygen desaturation. Sleep disturbance and oxygen compromise are associated with a variety of consequences (**Box 1**), which can affect the individual and impair their ability to function in society.[3]

Obstructive sleep apnea (OSA) is associated with hypertension, myocardial infarction, coronary artery disease, and arrhythmias.[4] There is also evidence to suggest neurocognitive impairment, excessive daytime sleepiness, fatigue, mood disturbance, structural brain changes, and reduced quality of life.[5–10]

SDB consists of obstructive and nonobstructive breathing disorders during sleep (**Fig. 1**). Obstructive disorders such as upper airway resistance syndrome cause fragmented less efficient sleep and increased work of breathing because of narrowing of the pharynx or narrowness in the nasal airway. There is no oxygen desaturation less than 4%.[11] OSA causes both fragmented sleep and oxygen desaturation. OSA is characterized by repetitive pharyngeal collapse at the level of the soft palate or base of tongue. Obstructive apnea refers to nearly complete cessation of breathing for 10 seconds or more. Obstructive hypopnea refers to partial collapse of the airway resulting in either arousal or oxyhemoglobin desaturation exceeding 3%. Nonobstructive breathing disorders during sleep include central sleep apnea (lack of respiratory drive) and sleep-related hypoventilation or obesity hypoventilation syndrome. Hypoventilation can arise from obesity, chronic obstructive pulmonary disease or asthma,

---

Box 1
Adverse outcomes associated with OSA

Metabolic disturbances: impaired glucose and lipid metabolism, systemic inflammation

Cardiovascular disturbances: hypertension, stroke, congestive heart failure, arterial fibrillation

Excessive daytime sleepiness

Increased risk of motor vehicle accidents

Impaired quality of life

Depression

Cognitive impairment

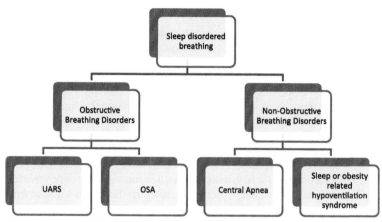

Fig. 1. Classification of SDB. UARS, upper airway resistance syndrome.

neuromuscular disorders, or chest wall defects. Central apnea is more common in patients with a history of stroke, brain injury, heart failure, or opiate use. Oral appliances are contraindicated for both central apnea and hypoventilation.

DEFINITIONS

An apnea-hypopnea index (AHI) is given for the number of apnea events (complete cessation of breathing) and hypopnea events (partial cessation of breathing) per hour of sleep (**Box 2**). This key measure along with the mean and lowest oxyhemoglobin levels during sleep quantifies disease severity.

The prevalence of OSA/hypopnoea syndrome in population-based studies is debatable but estimated to be from 3% to 7% in men and 2% to 5% in women.[12] Specifically, in the middle-age category, the prevalence increases to 9% in women and a remarkable 24% in middle-aged men,[13] although this may vary substantially with geographic, ethnic, and economic factors. Menopause and obesity are significant risk factors for sleep apnea in women.[14] It is likely the prevalence of OSA will continue to increase because one of the main causative factors, obesity, continues to increase dramatically in adults and children in the United States.[15]

Although awareness is increasing among the general public and health professions, OSA remains an underdiagnosed condition in both obese and lean populations and is associated with a range of adverse outcomes. Dentistry offers a key position in the early diagnosis of this condition because of the high frequency of contact intervals and the regular observation of the oropharyngeal structures in the supine position. Communication and partnership with physicians on early identification can reduce the patient's risk of morbidity and mortality associated with OSA.

Box 2
Definitions
Apnea: cessation of breathing for more than 10 seconds
Hypopnea: a reduction in airflow accompanied by arousal or drop in oxygen saturation
AHI: number of apneic and hypopneic events per hour of sleep

DIAGNOSIS

The diagnosis of OSA syndrome typically is formed by a comprehensive sleep history, presence of characteristic clinical features, together with the objective demonstration of SDB.[16]

Screening for OSA can easily be introduced in the dental practice setting. Based on medical history alone, high-risk patients for OSA can be identified (**Box 3**).[17] Self-reported questionnaires given to patients at examination appointments offer incorporation into the routine systemic health evaluation. The most widely used of such questionnaires are the Berlin Questionnaire[18] and the Epworth Sleepiness Score. Emerging questionnaires like the STOP-Bang questionnaire may provide greater clinical utility for identifying the pretest probability of apnea.[19] The STOP-Bang questionnaire is considered positive for high risk of OSA if 3 or more items are positive (**Box 4**). If screening is positive, further questions can be asked pertaining to assessment of risk. It is highly desirable to also interview the bed partner, who can usually provide important additional information based on direct observation of the patient while asleep.[18]

The diagnosis of OSA/hypopnoea syndrome is not based solely on the medical history, self-questionnaires, and detection of clinical features (**Box 5**),[20] but also requires demonstration of abnormal respiratory events with polysomnography (PSG) or home apnea testing. For this reason, if dentists have a suspicion of OSA, it should trigger a comprehensive sleep evaluation by a qualified physician.

OBJECTIVE TESTING

Whether they are home studies or overnight sleep studies, interpretation by a qualified sleep physician is mandatory before a dentist renders treatment. The "gold standard" for the diagnosis of OSA is attended PSG. PSG requires the recording by technical personnel with sleep-related training and the monitoring of the following physiologic signals[20–22]:

- Electroencephalogram
- Electrooculogram
- Nasal pressure
- Oral or oronasal thermistor
- Oxygen saturation
- Respiratory effort
- Electrocardiogram

Box 3
Diagnosis: history taking

Patients at high risk for OSA

    Obesity (body mass index [BMI] >35)

    Congestive heart failure

    Treatment refractory hypertension

    Type 2 diabetes

    Nocturnal dysrhythmias

    Stroke

    Pulmonary hypertension

    High-risk driving populations

Box 4
STOP-Bang questionnaire items

1. Snoring

2. Tiredness

3. Observed apneas

4. Hypertension

5. BMI >35

6. Age >50 years old

7. Neck >40 cm

8. Male gender

- Electromyogram
- Audio, video

The total number of apnea, hypopnea events divided by total sleep time in hours observed on electroencephalogram yields the AHI. Some laboratories will include RERA in the tabulation of AHI, whereas others will add respiratory effort related arousal to the AHI and report a total respiratory disturbance index (RDI = apnea + hypopnea + RERA/total sleep time in hours). A diagnosis based on AHI is shown in **Table 1**. Relevant comorbidity that lowers the threshold for treatment includes insomnia, hypersomnia, fatigue, or other neurocognitive complaints, coronary artery disease, hypertension, history of stroke, myocardial infarction, pulmonary hypertension, heart failure, or arrhythmia.[11]

Box 5
Diagnosis: characteristic symptoms and clinical features

Nocturnal symptoms:

- Snoring

- Witnessed apneas by bed partner

- Nocturnal choking, snorting, or gasping

- Nocturnal reflux

- Bruxism

- Insomnia

- Other nocturnal symptoms: enuresis, nocturia, frequent arousals, diaphoresis, impotence

Daytime symptoms:

- Excessive daytime sleepiness

- Other daytime symptoms: fatigue, memory impairment, personality changes, morning nausea, morning headaches, depression

Physical characteristics/examination:

- Obesity: neck size >17 inches (men), >16 inches (women); BMI >35

- Craniofacial anatomy: retrognathia, micrognathia, tonsillar hypertrophy, macroglossia, inferior displacement of the hyoid bone, narrowing of oropharyngeal airway

- Hypertension: especially drug-resistant hypertension

Table 1 Grading of OSA	
Severity	Grading
Mild OSA	AHI ≥5 and <15 per hour of sleep + symptoms or comorbidity factors
Moderate OSA	AHI ≥15 and <30 events per hour of sleep
Severe OSA	AHI ≥30 events per hour of sleep

Although there has been an increase in need for assessment of patients with possible OSA, the presence of resource limitations for this extensive study has led to a focus of attention on the role of home-based sleep studies. Although there is a clear cost-saving advantage to home-based studies, there are also disadvantages. The raw data is less informative, and the summary reports are thus not as detailed. The AHI denominator is time and can be inflated with home testing if considerable time is spent awake in bed during the test, which can lead to the risk of false negatives. The lack of technician supervision means that dislodged leads are not replaced during the study, and consequently, the likelihood of technically unsatisfactory studies is higher.[20] These home portable monitors should be used in the diagnosis of OSA only in conjunction with a comprehensive sleep evaluation by a sleep physician.[17] These portable monitors should record at a minimum: airflow, respiratory effort, and blood oxygen saturation.[17]

TREATMENT OPTIONS FOR OSA
Treatment

OSA should be treated as a chronic disease requiring long-term, multidisciplinary management. There are medical, dental, behavioral, and surgical treatment options. In many cases there is a primary treatment modality that is supported with adjunctive therapies to manage the condition. The patient performs a vital role in managing his or her own treatment and should be actively involved in understanding the severity of the OSA, their risk factors, and the methods of treatment.[17]

Options for Treatment:
1. Positive airway pressure (PAP)
2. Upper airway surgical procedures
3. Pharmacologic treatment
4. Oral appliances
5. Behavioral modification: weight loss, alcohol avoidance, alteration of sleeping position

PAP was first reported in 1981 and provides pneumatic splinting of the upper airway and still remains the standard treatment of OSA.[23,24] PAP may be delivered in CPAP, bile-vel PAP, or autotitrating PAP modes. Nasal masks are the most frequently used interface but the occurrence of mouth leaks can jeopardize the effectiveness.[25] Oronasal masks (also known as full face masks) allow for nasal and oral breathing, but can worsen apnea if tightening of the interface displaces the mandible and therefore the tongue posteriorly. These oronasal masks are often preferred by patients with impaired nasal breathing.

PAP has proven to improve symptoms, normalize the risk of traffic and workplace accidents, and reduce the elevated sympathetic activity and risk for cardiovascular morbidities, especially arterial hypertension. Most recently, it has been shown that CPAP normalizes mortality in patients with severe OSA syndrome.[26,27] Although CPAP is highly efficacious in terms of reduction of AHI and producing positive outcomes, there has been significant criticism with regards to its expense, and local side effects at the nose or face, or discomfort due to the mask. These side effects have a consequent negative effect on compliance[28] and have led to the search for other options of treatment. Alternative therapies include lifestyle modification, position restriction to avoid supine sleep, nasally applied exhalation pressure valves, oral appliances, and upper airway surgery.[3] Advances in surgically implanted devices show promise in both animal and human models but are not yet available for routine use.

Oral appliance therapy has emerged as an alternative to CPAP for snoring, and mild to moderate OSA in patients who refuse or fail to adhere to the use of the CPAP device. Although mandibular repositioning appliances (MRAs) seem to be less efficacious than CPAP,[29–33] in instances when both treatments are effective, patients usually prefer oral appliances over CPAP. A summary of treatment indications and objectives with oral appliance therapy established by AASM Practice Parameters[34] are shown in **Table 2**.

Mechanism of Action of Oral Appliances

Oral appliance therapy functions by repositioning the tongue and mandible forward and downwards to reduce airway collapse. The treatment aims to widen the lateral aspects of the upper airways to improve the upper airway patency and reduce snoring and OSA.[35] The upper airway can be defined by 3 regions: the velopharynx (hard palate to tip of uvula), oropharynx (tip of uvula to tip of epiglottis), and hypopharynx (tip of epiglottis to vocal cords). The velopharynx is the most common site of primary pharyngeal collapse in OSA.[36,37] The MRA has a lateral wall widening effect on the velopharyngeal and oropharyngeal space.[38,39]

Results of Clinical Trials on the Efficacy of Oral Appliances

A review of the literature on clinical trials testing the use of oral appliances for the treatment of sleep apnea and snoring indicates inhomogeneity in several variables, such as amount of follow-up, respiratory variables measured, measures of success, presentation of results, and type of oral appliances tested. In addition, timing and type of overnight diagnostic testing before and with the appliance differed.

Treatment success with MRA, defined as an AHI of less than 5, was found in 19% to 75% of the patients and, when success was defined as an AHI of less than 10, the range was 30% to 94%.[40–55] Positive effects on blood pressure, cardiac function, endothelial function, markers of oxidative stress, and simulated driving performance have been reported from MRAs.[43,48,53,56–60] Not only can MRAs reduce AHI and improve physiology of the individual but the patient experiences reduced daytime

Table 2
Treatment indications and objectives with oral appliance therapy

Indications	Objectives
Primary snorers without features of OSA	Reduce snoring to a subjectively acceptable level
Mild to moderate OSA with a preference for oral appliances, demonstrated intolerance to CPAP, poor candidates for CPAP, or failure to comply with behavioral changes	Resolution of clinical signs and symptoms of OSA Normalization of the AHI and oxyhemoglobin saturation levels
Severe OSA with initial trial of nasal CPAP Upper airway surgery may precede oral appliance therapy	Resolution of clinical signs and symptoms of OSA Normalization of the AHI and oxyhemoglobin saturation levels

sleepiness and improved quality of life compared with control treatments.[61] Quality of life may further improve because of sleep improvement of the bed partner.

MRA can be considered in combination with CPAP to reduce pressure and stabilize the position of the mandible and is of particular interest in the aforementioned patients that have worsening of mandible position on a CPAP interface that goes over both the nose and the mouth (full face mask). Anecdotal reports are promising, but to date there is limited scientific evidence to support combined use and this area warrants further investigation.

Types of Oral Appliances

Three broad classes of appliances have emerged, namely MRA, tongue retaining devices (TRD), and soft palate lifters. These appliances are listed in order of popularity with the MRA being vastly more common with most of the quantity and quality of scientific literature being greater as well. MRA cover the upper and lower teeth and hold the mandible in an advanced position with respect to the resting position. TRD produce a suction of the tongue into an anterior bulb, thereby widening the upper airway and advancing the tongue. Because the teeth are not used for anchorage of the device, TRDs are proposed as a treatment option for patients with hypodontia, edentulism, and significant periodontal disease.

MRAs are further subdivided into titratable (2-piece appliance) and nontitratable (1-piece appliance) custom-made appliances, and pre-fabricated appliances. Examples of some oral appliances available on the market today are listed in **Table 3**. An analysis of the comparison studies testing the efficacy of different types of appliances show no clear advantage between custom-made MRAs. However, there is a superior treatment response with MRAs that are custom-made over prefabricated designs. The requirements of an MRA are as follows:

1. Good retention form to 1 or 2 arches
2. Sufficient protrusion of the mandible at an increased vertical dimension
3. Appliances that do not restrict jaw movement laterally or vertically are optimal for temporomandibular joint (TMJ) comfort.

Most MRAs use traditional dental orthodontic appliance design and involve a 1- or 2-piece appliance that is retained by one or both dental arches. Design features can include metallic rod and tube fittings, inter-arch elastic, metal or plastic connectors, or even magnets.[32]

Due to the advantages of the oral appliance (**Box 6**), there has been a strong research effort over the last decade to provide evidence and create protocols for the clinical role of MRA in the treatment of snoring and OSA. A treatment flow chart

Table 3
Examples of oral appliances

Somnomed	Aveo-TSD	Adjustable Soft Palate Lifter
The silencer	Tongue-locking appliance	Silent night
Klearway	Snore guard	Snore EX
NAPA	Silent night	TPE
TAP	TheraSnore	Esmark
Herbst	Snore-no-more	HAP
SNOAR	PM positioner	Tessi
SUAD	TheraSnore	Respire

Box 6
Advantages of oral appliances

1. Nonintrusive

2. Lack of noise

3. Simplicity

4. Reversible treatment modality

5. Smaller and more portable than CPAP devices

6. No need for power source

7. Comfortable: fits inside the mouth

8. Potentially lower cost of treatment (**Fig. 2**)

Adapted from Epstein LJ, Kristo D, Strollo PJ, et al. Clinical guideline for the evaluation, management and long-term care of obstructive sleep apnea adults. J Clin Sleep Med 2009;5(3):263–76.

is proposed in **Box 6** to demonstrate the sequence of steps from diagnosis of SDB to treatment options available.

Patient Selection Criteria for MRA

The presence or absence of OSA must be determined before prescribing any treatment with MRAs. The severity of sleep-related respiratory problems must be established by a medical provider with an interpreted PSG or portable monitor and a referral made to the dentist for an MRA. Initiating treatment before establishing a correct diagnosis puts the patient at risk (**Fig. 2**). A correct diagnosis of type of SDB and verification of the presence or absence of central apnea, hypoventilation syndrome, severe oxygen desaturation, or severity of respiratory events must be known before recommending treatment of any modality. Treatment with MRA is largely restricted to adults because of the limited research available to support effective use in children.[62] There is currently no evidence to support the clinical role for MRA in the treatment of other SDB, including central sleep apnea and hypoventilation syndromes,[62] which require attended monitoring and PAP therapies.

Predicting who will respond to oral appliance therapy is not yet possible.[63] Several studies have compared various parameters to establish criteria of success. It is suggested that milder OSA, supine-dependent OSA, female gender, and nonobesity[61] are variables associated with success with MRAs. These findings are relatively consistent with our extensive experience, suggesting that lean patients with less oxygen compromise, modest soft palate, and good nasal breathing tend to have better outcomes and are more likely to approach the extent of respiratory disturbance index reduction seen with CPAP. If positional apnea is present, adding positional restriction typically improves the extent of response. Patient selection is also based on results of the dental examination. More research is needed on isolating ideal patients for oral appliance therapy.

History Intake

OSA is a medical diagnosis. However, the dentist must make an appraisal of the sleep disorder by reviewing the sleep study, current radiographs, recommendations by the physician, clinical history, and dental examination before approving oral appliance therapy.[17] If MRA therapy is initiated, detailed documentation of the subjective and objective data before treatment provide a baseline on which to base treatment efficacy.

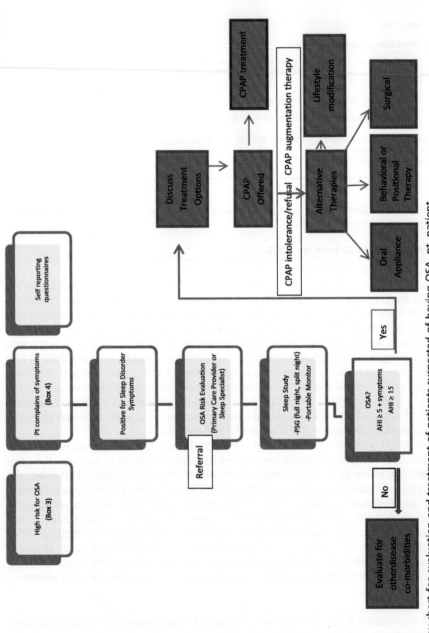

Fig. 2. Flow chart for evaluation and treatment of patients suspected of having OSA. pt, patient.

The clinical history should document the following:
1. Presence and severity of snoring
2. Presence and severity of witnessed apneic events
3. Presence and severity of excessive daytime sleepiness
4. Energy level during day
5. Quality of sleep (provide a scale of 1–10)
6. Quantity of sleep (number of hours of sleep per night)
7. Number of awakenings per night
8. Sleep position: side, back, stomach
9. Presence of other symptoms
   a. Recent weight gain
   b. Bruxism
   c. Morning headache
   d. Gastroesophageal reflux disease
   e. Depression
   f. Impotence
   g. Nasal congestion

Dental Examination

Patients should undergo a thorough dental examination to assess candidacy for an oral appliance. A complete dental history is required, which includes any orthodontic or periodontal treatment rendered. A complete intra-oral examination will provide an assessment of risks to treatment (**Table 4**). This examination should include a caries

Table 4
Relative dental contraindications to oral appliance therapy

Condition	Concern	Risk
Periodontal disease	Status: active or stable Concern: mobility of teeth	Reduced anchorage potential with appliance Increasing degree of mobility, and bite change with MRA Optional use of TRD
Temporomandibular dysfunction	Need to assess degree of TMD	Concern with potential aggravation of TMD and limitation of advancement potential with MRA
Number of remaining teeth	If <6–10 teeth per arch, or uneven distribution	Reduced anchorage
Protrusive capacity of the mandible	If <6 mm	Potential contraindication due to limitation of efficacy of MRA treatment
Bruxism	Patterns of wear	Early damage to appliance from overload or increase in pain with rigid appliance holding them in a fixed position
Occlusion	Number of tooth-to-tooth contacts, horizontal and vertical overjet	Reduced initial contacts will decrease patient awareness of bite change with MRA
Maximum vertical opening	If <25 mm	Inability to seat MRA
Exaggerated gag reflex	Poor adaptation potential	Inability to wear MRA

Table 5
Oral anatomic variables potentially directly or indirectly affecting airway space

Mallampati score		Score of 3 or 4, probability of OSA is 58%–82%
Tonsillar size		
Mandibular tori		Impingement of oral space for the tongue
Macroglossia		Obstructive size effect
Serrations on lateral border of tongue		Indications of tongue size/arch size discrepancy, and possible nocturnal clenching
Steep soft palate drape	 **Residual ridge**	In combination with a large tongue, the soft palate can reduce airway dimension especially in the supine position
Retrognathia and micrognathia		Negative effect on pharyngeal airway dimension

(continued on next page)

Table 5 (continued)		
Loss of vertical dimension of occlusion	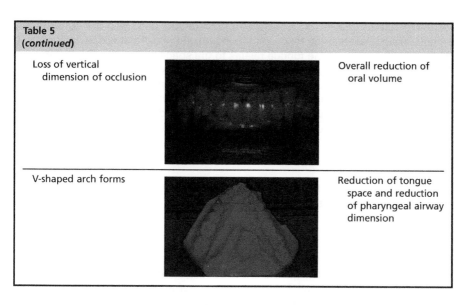	Overall reduction of oral volume
V-shaped arch forms		Reduction of tongue space and reduction of pharyngeal airway dimension

assessment, a periodontal examination, and TMJ evaluation including the muscles of mastication, occlusal analysis, and parafunctional habits. Current dental radiographs should be reviewed for any possible dental pathologic abnormality.[64] Some practitioners obtain a cephalometric radiograph to help prognosticate success with oral appliances[65,66] or monitor for craniofacial change with the appliance use over time. Indications of a successful outcome have been shown to be found with a shorter soft palate and a decreased distance between the hyoid bone and the mandibular plane.[65] Others have found the combination of a narrower SNB (sella, nasion, B point) angle, wider SNA (sella, nasion, A point) angle, shorter soft palate, and narrow oropharynx reflects a more positive outcome with MRAs.[66] More studies are required in this area to formulate more general recommendations.

Other imaging modalities such as computed tomography and magnetic resonance imaging have also demonstrated increases in pharyngeal airway size and volume with mandibular advancement.[67,68] Because increases in the airway size are at least part of the mechanism for the positive effect of MRAs on OSA, pretreatment imaging might provide useful as a predictor of success. The precise utility of magnetic resonance imaging and computed tomography needs to be further verified.

Although predictions of patient response to treatment based on anatomic and physiologic findings are not reliable at this time, understanding the patient's anatomy and possible restrictive effects on the velopharyngeal and oropharyngeal spaces help to understand causes of OSA, help in patient selection for MRA, and guide expectations for treatment. The cause of the smaller sized airway is due to skeletal structures, enlarged soft tissues such as adenoids or tongue, form of soft palate, or obesity.[69,70] Understanding the relationship of the patient's hard and soft tissue to the airway space will help to determine which treatment modality would be most effective in treating this condition. Indicators of oral space limitations are provided in **Table 5**.[28,32,34,65]

PALATO-PHARYNGEAL ASSESSMENT
Mallampati Classification

The American Academy of Sleep Medicine recommends assessing the modified Mallampati score when screening for sleep apnea and should be incorporated into dental practice as well.[17] This assessment is preferably done with the patient in an upright position. Leaving the tongue in the mouth and relaxed provides an important view of how the mass of the tongue relates to the space available within the mouth. Protruding the tongue helps view the extent of tongue length and may improve visualization of tonsillar pillars, length of soft palate, and the posterior oropharynx, further assisted by a tongue blade for some patients (**Fig. 3**). The base of the uvula and the appearance of the soft palates are visualized and scored. A high score (class 3 or 4) is a predictor of sleep apnea.[71,72] **Fig. 4** demonstrates the modified Mallampati classification.

Tonsil Size

Some studies have reported a correlation between tonsil size and AHI,[73] whereas others did not.[74] Tonsil size grading ranges from 0 to 4. **Table 6** defines the grading system.

ADVERSE EVENTS

Side effects and complications are common with oral appliance therapy and can lead to failed treatment adherence. Due to the myriad of appliance designs and lack of standard therapeutic protocol in the use of appliances, there is a wide range of side effects with differing occurrence rates found in the literature.[75–78] Side effects can be grouped into 2 broad categories (**Table 7**)[64]:

1. Minor in severity and temporary: tend to resolve during a short adaptive period of 6 to 8 weeks or are tolerable and do not resolve. Frequency reported from 6% to 86%.[64]
2. Moderate to severe and continuous: these side effects can occur at any stage during treatment and might lead to intolerance and discontinuation of the appliance.

DEGREE OF PROTRUSION

Protrusion of the mandible is required to make the MRA effective[40] unless it is being used as a stabilizing appliance in conjunction with CPAP when the requirement is more reduction of pressure. Determination of the amount of mandibular advancement and vertical opening required to prevent OSA is unclear. Reports of effective degrees of advancement range from 6 to 10 mm, or from 65% to 70% of maximum

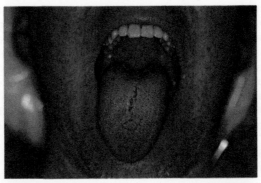

Fig. 3. Protrusion of tongue showing long tongue extension, long soft palate, and lack of visibility of uvula.

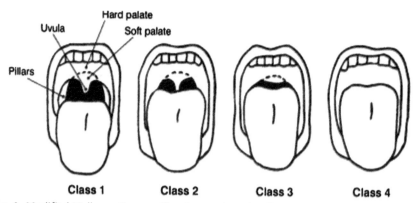

Fig. 4. Modified Mallampati score. Class 1, complete visualization of the soft palate; class 2, complete visualization of the uvula; class 3, visualization of only the base of the uvula; class 4, soft palate is not visible at all. (*Reprinted from* Ginapp T. Ask the clinical instructor. Cath Lab Digest 2012;20(7); with permission.)

protrusive potential.[79] Studies have explored the possibility of a prospective means of determining ideal advancement position using a remotely controlled mandibular positioner test and a temporary oral appliance during the PSG.[80] Further validity testing is required.

The value of a titratable appliance is the opportunity to initiate therapy at a mandibular position that is no more than 50% of maximum protrusion, which although may be below optimal level, would allow for slow advancement thereby reducing negative side effects such as muscular tension or TMD. Patients can remain at this level during an adaptive period of 1 to 8 weeks during which period most if not all of the transient negative side effects resolve.

Titration of an MRA should be slow as well for patient assessment of improvement of OSA symptoms and for the bed partner's assessment of sleep sounds. Rapid advancement could lead to unnecessary side effects and possible rejection of the appliance. In addition, it has been shown that excessive advancement can lead to an increase in airway obstruction.[52,81] Therefore clinicians must make the decision on the initial advancement position based on anatomic and neuromuscular evaluation, periodontal assessment, TMJ assessment, parafunction levels, and severity of OSA, and not on the maximum achievable degree of protrusion (**Fig. 5**). The rate of advancement depends on the patient's pre-existing conditions and the total active titration period could typically last 1 to 4 months. A timeline of events is described in **Fig. 6**.

Table 6 Tonsil size	
Grade	**Definition**
0	Patient had a tonsillectomy
1	Tonsils are in the tonsillar fossa, barely seen behind the anterior pillars
2	Tonsils are visible behind the anterior pillars
3	Tonsils extend three-quarters of the way to the midline
4	Tonsils are completely obstructing the airway

Table 7
Two categories of side effects

Minor and Temporary	Moderate to Severe and Continuous
TMJ pain	TMJ pain
Myofascial pain	Myofascial pain
Tooth pain	Tongue pain (with TRDs)
Salivation	Gagging (mostly with soft palate lifters)
TMJ sounds	Tooth pain
Dry mouth	Gum pain
Gum irritation	Dry mouth
Morning after occlusal changes	Salivation
Bad taste or odor	Tooth movement: decrease in overbite and overjet, mobility of teeth, intrusion, retrusion effects
Loss of crown or restorations	Skeletal changes: change in vertical condylar position, change in arch width

DISCUSSION

The indication for use of MRA is to treat snoring and OSA. MRAs are effective in a substantial number of patients with mild to moderate OSA and to a much lesser degree those with severe OSA. A referral is needed from the physician to the dentist based on clinical history and findings and PSG or home monitoring. Evaluation of the patient by the dentist is necessary to assess possible causes of OSA and possible risk factors in treatment. Response to treatment can be somewhat predicted based on patient preexisting conditions, OSA severity, and protrusive capacity of the mandible. New advances are being made in testing target protrusive positions for the treatment of OSA before fabrication of a permanent MRA (Somnomed MATRx, Frisco, TX, USA) during an overnight sleep study. Also recent publications are demonstrating a link between sleep bruxism and sleep-related micro-arousals. During an overnight polysomnogram, electromyogram patterns related to sleep bruxism are recorded as rhythmic masticatory muscle activity. Dentists, in assessing their patients, must be aware that snoring, with or without apneic or hypopneic events, may be concomitant with sleep bruxism. If sleep bruxism is present, further investigations regarding the presence of a sleep breathing disorder should precede treatment of the dental effects of bruxism.[82]

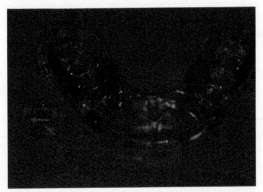

Fig. 5. Breakage of titanium advancement screw in MRA due to significant bruxism.

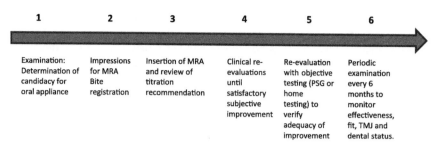

1	2	3	4	5	6
Examination: Determination of candidacy for oral appliance	Impressions for MRA Bite registration	Insertion of MRA and review of titration recommendation	Clinical re-evaluations until satisfactory subjective improvement	Re-evaluation with objective testing (PSG or home testing) to verify adequacy of improvement	Periodic examination every 6 months to monitor effectiveness, fit, TMJ and dental status.

Fig. 6. Time line by visit number.

A multidisciplinary approach with sleep medicine physicians is mandatory to ensure appropriateness of the treatment plan and weigh the risks and benefits of treatment relative to other options. Collaboration with surgeons is also important as adjunctive treatment to improve nasal breathing or reduce collapse at the velopharynx may be necessary for adequate improvement with MRA relative to CPAP. Just as sleep medicine physicians must appreciate the role of MRA therapy and rely on dentists for this much needed treatment, dentists must appreciate the role that CPAP has as the most effective treatment for many patients. Dentists should be aware that most sleep program patients obtain normalization of their sleep and breathing with good tolerability on CPAP. Dentists without adequate training may succumb to the false impression that patients do not succeed with CPAP, which is due to the selection bias of which patients present to clinic for an alternative to CPAP. Surgical interventions, CPAP, and MRA are not equal options for all patients with OSA; rather, each treatment modality has its place in treatment with degree of appropriateness based on a complex combination of factors, including OSA severity, medical comorbidities, craniofacial findings, and patient preference. Dentists and sleep medicine physicians share a duty to assist their patients in obtaining the greatest good independent of which modalities that practitioner can provide. As access to MRA improves, sleep medicine physicians providing CPAP from their office are obligated to refer appropriate cases to a qualified dentist for MRA and not merely place all patients on CPAP. Similarly, dentists have an obligation not to interfere with satisfied patients that are compliant and benefitting from CPAP and to collaborate with sleep medicine physicians on determining an appropriate treatment plan for apnea patients.

Further research aimed at identifying optimum patients for oral appliance therapy will permit more generalizable treatment guidelines and further improve outcomes. Patients with mild forms of apnea, lower body mass index, without significant compromise in nasal airway or at level of the velopharynx seem to have more complete treatment response with oral appliance therapy. Consistent with current guidelines, it is found that many of these mild OSA cases are adequately treated with MRA as their first-line therapy. Normalization of sleep and oxygen saturations is the first goal of apnea treatments. Collaboration with a sleep medicine physician is needed for treatment planning when a patient is electing MRA over CPAP therapy, combining MRA with CPAP therapy, or in cases where the goal of treatment is modified to obtain improvement short of normalization.

Although dental sleep medicine is a relatively new field, major research and clinical advances continue rapidly. Collaborative studies with greater sample sizes, less selection bias, and more control of subjects are needed. Further avenues of research include evaluating how design features affect treatment outcomes and health outcomes; and developing methods for objectively detecting MRA compliance, and predictable single-night titration of MRA to reduce treatment time and improve outcomes.

Because of established training in TMD, removable appliance therapy, and occlusion, prosthodontics is uniquely suited to educating dental students in sleep disorders and oral appliance therapy. Prosthodontists can set a new standard by developing more in-depth dental sleep medicine training within prosthodontic residency programs with access to multidisciplinary teams and to ensuring that dental sleep medicine continues to strive for excellence in the management of sleep apnea with oral appliances.

REFERENCES

1. Kryger MH, Roth T, Dement WC, editors. The principles and practice of sleep medicine. St Louis (MO): WB Saunders; 1989. p. 739.
2. Moldofsky H. Sleep and pain. Sleep Med Rev 2001;5:385–96.
3. Lavigne G, Cistulli P, Smith M. Sleep medicine for dentists: a practical overview. Chicago: Quintessence Publishing; 2009.
4. Redline S, Budhiraja R, Kapur V, et al. The scoring of respiratory events in sleep: reliability and validity. J Clin Sleep Med 2007;3:169–200.
5. Baldwin CM, Griffith KA, Nieto FJ, et al. The association of sleep-disordered breathing and sleep symptoms with quality of life in the Sleep Heart Health Study. Sleep 2001;24:96–105.
6. Beebe DW, Groesz L, Wells C, et al. The neuropsychological effects of obstructive sleep apnea: a meta-analysis of norm-referenced and case-controlled data. Sleep 2003;26:298–307.
7. Joo EY, Tae WS, Lee MJ, et al. Reduced brain gray matter concentration in patients with obstructive sleep apnea syndrome. Sleep 2010;33:235–41.
8. Macey PM, Kumar R, Woo MA, et al. Brain structural changes in obstructive sleep apnea. Sleep 2008;31:967–77.
9. Peppard PE, Szklo-Coxe M, Hla KM, et al. Longitudinal association of sleep-related breathing disorder and depression. Arch Intern Med 2006;166:1709–15.
10. Yang EH, Hla KM, Mchorney CA, et al. Sleep apnea and quality of life. Sleep 2000;23:535–41.
11. American Academy of Sleep Medicine. International classification of sleep disorders. 2nd edition. Diagnostic and coding manual. Westchester (IL): American Academy of Sleep Medicine; 2005.
12. Punjabi NM. The epidemiology of adult obstructive sleep apnea. Proc Am Thorac Soc 2008;5:136–43.
13. Young T, Palta M, Dempsey J, et al. The occurrence of sleep-disordered breathing among middle-aged adults. N Engl J Med 1993;328:1230–5.
14. Bixler EO, Vgontzas AN, Lin HM, et al. Prevalence of sleep disordered breathing in women. Am J Respir Crit Care Med 2001;163:608–13.
15. Young T, Peppard PE, Taheri S. Excess weight and sleep-disordered breathing. J Appl Physiol (1985) 2005;99:1592–9.
16. American Academy of Sleep Medicine Task Force. Sleep-related breathing disorders in adults: recommendations for syndrome definition and measurement techniques in clinical research. Sleep 1999;22:667–89.
17. Epstein LJ, Kristo D, Strollo PJ, et al. Clinical guideline for the evaluation, management and long-term care of obstructive sleep apnea adults. J Clin Sleep Med 2009;5(3):263–76.
18. Netzer NC, Stoohs RA, Netzer CM, et al. Using the Berlin Questionnaire to identify patients at risk for the sleep apnea syndrome. Ann Intern Med 1999;131:485–91.

19. Chung F, Subramanyam R, Liao P, et al. High STOP-Bang score indicates a high probability of obstructive sleep apnoea. Br J Anaesth 2012;108(5):768–75.

20. McNicholas WT. Diagnosis of obstructive sleep apnea in adults. Proc Am Thorac Soc 2008;5(2):154–60.

21. Practice Committee of the American Sleep Disorders Association. Practice parameters for the indications for polysomnography and related procedures. Sleep 1997;20:406–22.

22. Iber C, Ancoli-Israel S, Chesson AL, et al. The AASM manual for the scoring of sleep and associated events: rules, terminology and technical specifications. Westhester (IL): American Academy of Sleep Medicine; 2007.

23. Sullivan CE, Issa FG, Berthon-Jones M, et al. Reversal of obstructive sleep apnea by continuous positive pressure applied through the nares. Lancet 1981;1: 862–5.

24. Elshaug AG, Moss JR, Southcott AM, et al. Redefining success in airway surgery for obstructive sleep apnea: a meta analysis and synthesis of the evidence. Sleep 2007;30(4):461–7.

25. Beecroft J, Zanon S, Lukic D, et al. Oral continuous positive airway pressure for sleep apnea: effectiveness, patient preference, and adherence. Chest 2003; 124:2200–8.

26. Chobanian AV, Bakris GL, Black HR, et al. Seventh report of the Joint National Committee on Prevention, Detection, Evaluation, and Treatment of High Blood Pressure. Hypertension 2003;42:1206–52.

27. Marin JM, Carrizo SJ, Vicente E, et al. Long-term cardiovascular outcomes in men with obstructive sleep apnoea-hypopnoea with or without treatment with continuous positive airway pressure: an observational study. Lancet 2005;365: 1046–53.

28. Giles TL, Lasserson TJ, Smith B, et al. Continuous positive airway pressure for obstructive sleep apnoea in adults. Cochrane Database Syst Rev 2006:CD001106.

29. Ferguson KA, Ono T, Lowe AA, et al. A randomized crossover study of an oral appliance vs nasal continuous positive airway pressure in the treatment of mild-moderate obstructive sleep apnea. Chest 1996;109:1269–75.

30. Ferguson KA, Ono T, al-Majed S, et al. A short-term controlled trial of an adjustable oral appliance for the treatment of mild to moderate obstructive sleep apnoea. Thorax 1997;52:362–8.

31. Randerath WJ, Heise M, Hinz R, et al. An individually adjustable oral appliance vs. continuous positive airway pressure in mild to moderate obstructive sleep apnea syndrome. Chest 2002;122:569–75.

32. Clark GT, Blumenfeld I, Yoffe N, et al. A crossover study comparing the efficacy of CPAP with anterior mandibular positioning devices on patients with obstructive sleep apnoea. Chest 1996;109:1269–75.

33. Engleman HM, McDonald JP, Graham D, et al. Randomized crossover trial of two treatments for sleep apnea/hypopnea syndrome: continuous positive airway pressure and mandibular repositioning splint. Am J Respir Crit Care Med 2002; 166:855–9.

34. Kushida CA, Morgenthaler TI, Littner MR. Practice parameters for the treatment of snoring and obstructive sleep apnea with oral appliances: an update for 2005. Sleep 2006;29:240–3.

35. Kyung SH, Park YC, Pae EK. Obstructive sleep apnea patients with the oral appliance experience pharyngeal size and shape changes in three dimensions. Angle Orthod 2005;75:15–22.

36. Isono S, Tanaka A, Tagaito Y, et al. Pharyngeal patency in response to advancement of the mandible in obese anesthetized persons. Anesthesiology 1997;87: 1055–62.
37. Morrison DL, Launois SH, Isono S, et al. Pharyngeal narrowing and closing pressures in patients with obstructive sleep apnea. Am Rev Respir Dis 1993;148: 606–11.
38. Sutherland K, Deane S, Chan A, et al. Comparative effects of two oral appliances on upper airway structure in obstructive sleep apnea. Sleep 2011;34(4):469–77.
39. Chan AS, Sutherland K, Schwab RJ, et al. The effect of mandibular advancement on upper airway structure in obstructive sleep apnoea. Thorax 2010;65: 726–31.
40. Mehta A, Qian J, Petocz P, et al. A randomized controlled study of a mandibular advancement splint for obstructive sleep apnea. Am J Respir Crit Care Med 2001;163:1457–61.
41. Gotsopoulos H, Chen C, Qian J, et al. Oral appliance therapy improves symptoms in obstructive sleep apnea: a randomized, controlled trial. Am J Respir Crit Care Med 2002;166:743–8.
42. Johnston CD, Gleadhill IC, Cinnamoond MJ, et al. Mandibular advancement appliances and obstructive sleep apnoea: a randomized clinical trial. Eur J Orthod 2002;24:251–62.
43. Barnes M, McEvoy RD, Banks S, et al. Efficacy of positive airway pressure and oral appliance in mild to moderate obstructive sleep apnea. Am J Respir Crit Care Med 2004;170:656–64.
44. Blanco J, Zamarron C, Abeleira P, et al. Prospective evaluation of an oral appliance in the treatment of obstructive sleep apnea syndrome. Sleep Breath 2005; 9:20–5.
45. Naismith SL, Winter VR, Hickie IB, et al. Effect of oral appliance therapy on neurobehavioral functioning in obstructive sleep apnea: a randomized controlled trial. J Clin Sleep Med 2005;1:374–80.
46. Petri N, Svanholt P, Solow B, et al. Mandibular advancement appliance for obstructive sleep apnoea: results of a randomised placebo controlled trial using parallel group design. J Sleep Res 2008;17:221–9.
47. Randerath WJ, Heise M, Hinz R, et al. An individually adjustable oral appliance vs continuous positive airway pressure in mild-to-moderate obstructive sleep apnea syndrome. Chest 2002;122:569–75.
48. Hoekema A, Stegnenga B, Wijkstra PJ, et al. Obstructive sleep apnea therapy. J Dent Res 2008;87:882–7.
49. Gagnadoux F, Fleury B, Vielle B, et al. Titrated mandibular advancement versus positive airway pressure for sleep apnoea. Eur Respir J 2009;34:914–20.
50. Bloch KE, Iseli A, Zhang JN, et al. A randomized controlled crossover trial of two oral appliances for sleep apnea treatment. Am J Respir Crit Care Med 2000;162: 246–51.
51. Pitsis AJ, Darendeliler MA, Gotsopoulos H, et al. Effect of vertical dimension on efficacy of oral appliance therapy in obstructive sleep apnea. Am J Respir Crit Care Med 2002;166:860–4.
52. Tegelberg A, Walker-Engstrom ML, Vestling O, et al. Two different degrees of mandibular advancement with a dental appliance in treatment of patients with mild to moderate obstructive sleep apnea. Acta Odontol Scand 2003;61:356–62.
53. Gauthier L, Laberge L, Beaudry M, et al. Efficacy of two mandibular advancement appliances in the management of snoring and mild-moderate sleep apnea: a cross-over randomized study. Sleep Med 2009;10:329–36.

54. Vanderveken OM, Devolder A, Marklund M, et al. Comparison of a custom-made and a thermoplastic oral appliance for the treatment of mild sleep apnea. Am J Respir Crit Care Med 2008;178:197–202.
55. Aarab G, Lobbezoo F, Hamburger HL, et al. Effects of an oral appliance with different mandibular protrusion positions at a constant vertical dimension on obstructive sleep apnea. Clin Oral Investig 2010;14:339–45.
56. Lam B, Sam K, Mok WY, et al. Randomized study of three non-surgical treatments in mild to moderate obstructive sleep apnoea. Thorax 2007;62:354–9.
57. Gotsopoulos H, Kelly JJ, Cistulli PA. Oral appliance therapy reduces blood pressure in obstructive sleep apnea: a randomized, controlled trial. Sleep 2004;27: 934–41.
58. Coruzzi P, Gualerzi M, Bernkopf E, et al. Autonomic cardiac modulation in obstructive sleep apnea: effect of an oral jaw positioning appliance. Chest 2006;130:1362–8.
59. Itzhaki S, Dorchin H, Clark G, et al. The effects of 1-year treatment with a herbst mandibular advancement splint on obstructive sleep apnea, oxidative stress, and endothelial function. Chest 2007;131:740–9.
60. Trzepizur W, Gagnadoux F, Abraham P, et al. Microvascular endothelial function in obstructive sleep apnea: impact of continuous positive airway pressure and mandibular advancement. Sleep Med 2009;10:746–52.
61. Randerath WJ, Verbraecken J, Anderas S, et al. Non-CPAP therapies in obstructive sleep apnoea. Eur Respir J 2011;37:1000–28.
62. Cistulli P, Gotsopoulos H, Marklund M, et al. Treatment of snoring and obstructive sleep apnea with mandibular repositioning appliances. Sleep Med Rev 2004;8:443–57.
63. Hoffstein V. Review of oral appliances for treatment of sleep-disordered breathing. Sleep Breath 2007;11:1–22.
64. Ferguson KA, Cartwright R, Rogers R, et al. Oral appliances for snoring and obstructive sleep apnea: a review. Sleep 2006;29:244–62.
65. Eveloff SE, Rosenberg CL, Carlisle CC, et al. Efficacy of a Herbst mandibular advancement device in obstructive sleep apnea. Am J Respir Crit Care Med 1994;149:905–9.
66. Mayer G, Meier-Ewert K. Cephalometric predictors for orthopaedic mandibular advancement in obstructive sleep apnoea. Eur J Orthod 1995;17:35–43.
67. Gao XM, Zeng XL, Fu MK, et al. Magnetic resonance imaging of the upper airway in obstructive sleep apnea before and after oral appliance therapy. Chin J Dent Res 1999;2:27–35.
68. Gale DJ, Sawyer RH, Woodcock A, et al. Do oral appliances enlarge the airway in patients with obstructive sleep apnoea? A prospective computerized tomographic study. Eur J Orthod 2000;22:159–68.
69. Vos W, De Backer J, Devolder A, et al. Correlation between severity of sleep apnea and upper airway morphology based on advanced anatomical and functional imaging. J Biomech 2007;40:2207–13.
70. Schwab RJ, Pasirstein M, Pierson R, et al. Identification of upper airway anatomic risk factors for obstructive sleep apnea with volumetric magnetic resonance imaging. Am J Respir Crit Care Med 2003;168:522–30.
71. Nuckton TJ, Glidden DV, Browner WS, et al. Physical examination: Mallampati score as an independent predictor of obstructive sleep apnea. Sleep 2006; 29(7):903–8.
72. Friedman M, Tanyeri H, La Rosa M, et al. Clinical predictors of obstructive sleep apnea. Laryngoscope 1999;109(12):1901–7.

73. Yagi H, Nakata S, Tsuge H, et al. Morphological examination of upper airway in obstructive sleep apnea. Auris Nasus Larynx 2009;36:444–9.

74. Thong JF, Pang KP. Clinical parameters in obstructive sleep apnea: are there any correlations? J Otolaryngol Head Neck Surg 2008;37:894–900.

75. Marklund M, Franklin KA, Persson M. Orthodontic side-effects of mandibular advancement devices during treatment of snoring and sleep apnoea. Eur J Orthod 2001;23:135–44.

76. Pantin CC, Hillman DR, Tennant M. Dental side effects of an oral device to treat snoring and obstructive sleep apnea. Sleep 1999;22:237–40.

77. Fritsch KM, Iseli A, Russi EW, et al. Side effects of mandibular advancement devices for sleep apnea treatment. Am J Respir Crit Care Med 2001;164:813–8.

78. Robertson CJ. Dental and skeletal changes associated with long-term mandibular advancement. Sleep 2001;24:531–7.

79. Charkhandeh S, Topor ZL, Grosse JC, et al. Target protrusive position from mandibular protrusion titration: is it a good estimate of adequate protrusion? Sleep Breath 2012;16:919–31.

80. Dort LC, Hadjuk E, Remmers JE. Mandibular advancement and obstructive sleep apnoea: a method for determining effective mandibular protrusion. Eur Respir J 2006;27:1003–9.

81. Lamont J, Baldwin DR, Hay KD, et al. Effect of two types of mandibular advancement splints on snoring and obstructive sleep apnoea. Eur J Orthod 1998;20:293–7.

82. Lavigne GJ, Khoury S, Abe S, et al. Bruxism physiology and pathology: an overview for clinicians. J Oral Rehabil 2008;35:476–94.

Radiographic Stents
Integrating Treatment Planning and Implant Placement

Ingeborg J. De Kok, DDS, MS[a], Ghadeer Thalji, DDS, PhD[b],
Matthew Bryington, DMD, MS[c], Lyndon F. Cooper, DDS, PhD[a],*

KEYWORDS

- Radiographic stents • Dental implants • Osseointegration • Treatment planning

KEY POINTS

- The use of volumetric imaging is emerging as a valued aid in planning, placement, and restoration of dental implants.
- Any cone beam computed tomography (CBCT) scan intended for these purposes must include a scan prosthesis or integrate an optical scan of a diagnostically waxed cast. When the assembled 3-dimensional model (segmented maxilla, mandible, and prostheses) is visualized, available planning software enables improved planning and enhanced communication.
- The planned treatment can be used to direct computer aided design - computer aided manufacture fabrication of surgical guides that offer 3-dimensional control of implant placement.
- Ongoing development enables clinicians to design and manufacture patient-specific abutments within this 3-dimensional virtual environment to further streamline and improve planning and treatment.
- Clinicians should understand fully the advantages of this technology to appropriately prescribe CBCT scanning for dental implant treatment planning and therapy.

INTRODUCTION

Successful dental implant therapy occurs with the congruent achievement of osseointegration and the location of implants to ideally support the intended restoration. The pivotal point in treatment planning for dental implants occurs when the location of

Financial Disclosures and/or Conflicts of Interest: The authors have nothing to disclose.
[a] Department of Prosthodontics, School of Dentistry, University of North Carolina, 330 Brauer Hall, CB# 7450, Chapel Hill, NC 27599-7450, USA; [b] Department of Prosthodontics, The University of Iowa College of Dentistry, 801 Newton Road, Dental Sciences Building S432, Iowa City, IA 55242, USA; [c] Restorative Dentistry, School of Dentistry, West Virginia University, Post Office Box 9495, Morgantown, WV 26506, USA
* Corresponding author.
E-mail address: Lyndon_Cooper@unc.edu

bone is viewed radiographically in the context of the planned prosthesis. As suggested for any other radiographic diagnostic modality, radiographic planning for dental implant therapy should be used only after a review of the patient's systemic health, imaging history, oral health, and the local oral conditions. It is of further importance to emphasize that the radiological diagnostic and planning procedure for dental implants can only be fully achieved with the use of a well-designed and -constructed radiographic guide. It is the intent of this article to review several methods for construction of radiographic guides and how they may be utilized for the improvement of implant surgery planning and performance.

VOLUMETRIC IMAGING

Cone beam computed tomography (CBCT) has become the prominent method of generating 3-dimensional radiographic images in dentistry. The CBCT scanner produces a cone-shaped radiograph beam that exposes a series of planar images as the focused radiograph beam processes in a circular path around the patient. The computer assembles these multiple images in 3-dimensional volume that can be reoriented to meet the viewing need of the clinician. Although similar in concept to a medical CT scan, the radiation dose is much less, and tailored fields of view offer further dose reduction aligned with the ALARA (as low as (is) reasonably achievable) principles of radiation hygiene and safety.[1] The use of CBCT for dental implant planning has been carefully debated, and several recommendations have been made. For example, the American Dental Association Council on Scientific Affairs recently published an advisory statement on the use of CBCT in dentistry.[2] It is advised that CBCT imaging should be used only after a review of the patient's health and imaging history and the completion of a thorough clinical examination. CBCT imaging should be prescribed only when it is expected that the diagnostic yield will benefit patient care, enhance patient safety, or improve clinical outcomes significantly. There are many situations involving the potential dental implant patient in which these guidelines apply.

The main advantage of CBCT imaging is that a 3-dimensional image of the osseous region of interest may be constructed and viewed in multiple planes. Planning that leads to implant placement results in a reasonable level of accuracy as suggested by a recent systematic review.[3] With regard to osseous architecture, the ability to visualize anatomic landmarks is high.[4] Less clear is the value of CBCT images to accurately estimate or define the density of bone.[5] The quality of the CBCT image may be a limiting factor affecting planning. Although not the objective of this article, it is important to highlight relevant factors that reduce the diagnostic and planning qualities of the CBCT image. An obvious factor is motion-related artifacts that cause blurring. Because the resolution of the machines is typically less than 0.3 to 0.5 mm, even small patient movements create problems. Another factor is the scatter that may be produced from metallic restorations in the mouth, and, unfortunately in CBCT, the streak artifacts occur in all directions. Beam hardening occurs when the beam is attenuated as it passes through dense objects (included dental implants), making the related areas less diagnostic. Noise reduces the ability to resolve features of close radiodensities, and in CBCT imaging, lower power (mA) is one reason for this. The continued development of computational solutions and hardware design suggests progressive improvement in CBCT images for dental implant planning.[6]

Recent guidelines for prescription of CBCT imaging for dental implant treatment planning have been suggested by multiple organizations (**Box 1**).[2,7–9]

Computer-aided implant planning and implant placement have been developed to allow for more efficient preoperative assessment of bone volume and safe implant

---

Box 1
Guidelines for prescription of CBCT imaging for dental implant treatment planning

- Evaluate the morphology of the residual alveolar ridge
- Determine the orientation of the alveolar ridge
- Identify anatomic features that could limit the implant fixture position
- Evaluate pathologic conditions that would restrict the implant fixture placement
- Match imaging findings to the restorative plan
- It should be considered when preoperative cross-sectional imaging is deemed required
- CBCT is desired when there is a need for hard tissue grafting
- It should be used to evaluate hard tissues after augmentation procedures have been performed

---

placement with adequate consideration for a successful implant restoration outcome.[10] Treatment planning by virtual 3-dimensional implant placement is based on both anatomic and prosthetic considerations and criteria.[11] Inclusion of volumetric imaging in this process is the only way to fully appreciate the position of the implant in 3 dimensions. However, without inclusion of the planned tooth or prosthesis position in this 3-dimensional image, such planning is not possible. A central aspect of computer-aided implant planning using radiographic volumetric images is the use of radiographic stents that present the planned tooth or prosthesis position within the radiographic image.

The ideal features of a radiographic stent are listed in **Box 2**.[12] There are many different ways to produce a useful radiographic stent. At least 4 different approaches should be available to clinicians to accommodate the broad array of different clinical circumstances. They include (1) use of an existing prosthesis containing radiopaque markers or fiduciaries (**Fig. 1**), (2) use of a thermoplastic shim incorporating radiopaque markers (**Fig. 2**), (3) use of radiopaque teeth in a mucosa or tooth-supported stent (**Fig. 3**), or (4) fabrication of a radiopaque resin duplicate of a prosthesis or a diagnostic wax-up (**Fig. 4**).

The use of an existing prosthesis as a radiographic stent (and possibly a surgical guide) is simple, direct, and cost-effective. A prerequisite for this is that the position of the tooth or teeth in the existing prosthesis represents the intended position of the future implant-related prosthesis. In such cases, all that is required is the placement of radiopaque markers or fiduciaries onto or within the prosthesis to achieve the scan. Immediately following scanning, the markers may be removed (see **Fig. 1**).

When considering the other 3 approaches, a similar clinical course of action is needed. All 3 procedures require that preliminary study casts are mounted on an

---

Box 2
The ideal features of a radiographic stent

Radiopaque indicator of correct tooth form and position without inducing scatter

Retentive and stable intraorally

Comfortable

Sterilizable, if used as a surgical guide

Compatible with scanner (hardware) platform

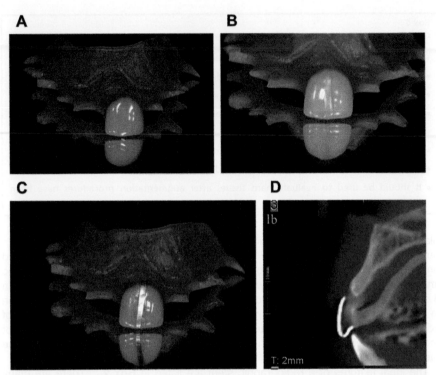

Fig. 1. (*A*) A provisional removable partial denture can be converted to a radiographic guide. Note the absence of clasps that would create artifacts in the CBCT imaging process. (*B*) A line of sticky wax is applied along the midfacial surface of the prosthetic tooth. (*C*) A lead foil strip approximately 0.5 mm wide is applied over the sticky wax. (*D*) The resulting CBCT image revealing the location of the planned prosthesis.

articulator. Next, in all cases, the planned position and form of the proposed prosthesis must be defined by denture tooth arrangement or diagnostic waxing methods. This is true of single-tooth, multiple-tooth (eg, implant-supported fixed dental prosthesis), or full arch restorations.

Use of a thermoplastic shim incorporating radiopaque markers is a relatively inexpensive and rapid method of creating a radiographic stent that embodies the ideal features enumerated previously (see **Fig. 2**). Following the establishment of tooth position (often verified clinically by a wax try-in or temporization), the diagnostically waxed study cast is duplicated in laboratory plaster (or snap stone). The cast is trimmed to display only the alveolar ridge and teeth of the maxilla or mandible to enable rapid trimming of the plastic material. The estimated or desired location of implant(s) is marked on the cast by drawing a line bisecting the intended tooth mesiodistally. Sticky wax is applied to this line, and a 0.5 mm wide strip of lead foil (obtained from radiographic film packets) is applied to this position by rubbing with a warm wax spatula. It is important that the lead foil extend from the midlingual position to the buccal cervical margin of the designated tooth. The cast, now decorated with lead foil strips in the estimated location of implants, is placed onto the vacuformer platform, and a thermoplastic shim is formed directly onto the cast. The heat from the resin typically transfers both the wax and the lead foil to the inner surface of the formed thermoplastic shim. The shim can be trimmed to the height of contour of the majority of teeth, which

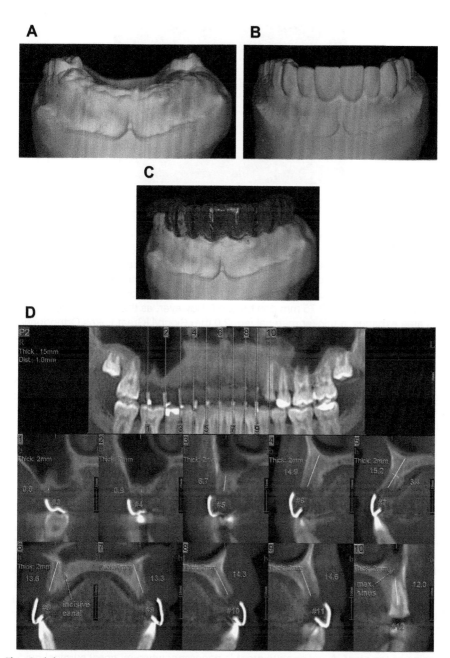

Fig. 2. (*A*) A trauma patient's master cast revealing missing anterior teeth. (*B*) The completed diagnostic waxing is duplicated in dental stone. (*C*) Lead foil strips applied to the stone cast are integrated into a thermoplastic stent. (*D*) The resulting CBCT image revealing the location of the planned prostheses and existing bone.

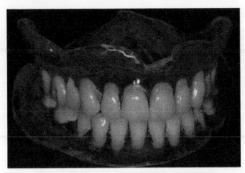

Fig. 3. The incorporation of radiopaque teeth (SR VivoTAC and SR OrthoTAC teeth, Ivoclar Vivadent Inc. Amherst, NY) into a removable prosthesis is another strategy to visualize the prosthetic tooth position in the CBCT image. Note that unless a radiopaque medium is included in the processed resin, only the teeth will be visualized in the radiograph.

enables ease of placement with sufficient stability during scanning and subsequent surgery. It is advantageous to trim the shim to the cervical contour of the planned implant restoration to permit estimation of implant depth. For single-tooth implants, a thin material of 0.5 to 0.75 mm can be used. However, as the extent of the edentulous area expands, a thicker material (eg, 2.0 mm Biocryl [Great Lakes Orthodontics, Tonawanda, NY, USA]) can be used to prevent flexing of the stent intraorally. For distal extension situations, even thicker materials can be used (eg, 3.0 mm Biocryl) to avoid distortion or flexing.

The use of radiopaque teeth to create a surgical guide offers the advantage of displaying the complete 3-dimensional form of the tooth in the CBCT-generated volumetric image (see **Fig. 3**). The process for creating this type of guide again begins with the accurate mounting of diagnostic study casts. Here, the radiopaque teeth are adapted and placed onto the cast to represent the position of the planned implant-related prostheses with acknowledgment of the estimated position of the planned implant(s). There are at 3 three ways of incorporating the radiopaque teeth into the radiographic stent. The first follows the process described herein for the thermoplastic shim and by vacuum forming; the radiopaque teeth are retained within the stent (see **Fig. 4**). It is useful to utilize an acrylic material (eg, 0.75 mm Clear Splint Biocryl). The second way involves the use of composite baseplate material (eg, Triad [Dentsply International, York, PA, USA]) and requires hand forming of the tooth-supported guide using strips of this material adapted to the natural teeth and incorporating the radiopaque teeth within the formed guide. A third method is the processing of the radiopaque teeth into either a removable or complete prosthesis (see **Fig. 3**). When confronted with extensive edentulous regions of an arch or complete edentulous arches, the inclusion of tissue bearing flanges adds to the stability and accuracy of the radiographic stent. When adopting this approach, the processed acrylic resin will be radiolucent unless a radiopaque alternative (eg, Biocryl X) is used in the processing of the stent. A radiopaque stent is necessary when mucosal surgical guides are utilized or when generating a plan by segmentation methods.

For many situations involving partial edentulism and complete edentulism, where the eventual treatment plan will involve an implant-supported partial or complete overdentures, or will result in full arch prosthesis for the edentulous patient, it is often advantageous to complete the waxing of the partial or complete overdenture to verify phonetics, esthetics, and function. In taking full advantage of this strongly recommended diagnostic approach, another way of creating a radiographic template is by means

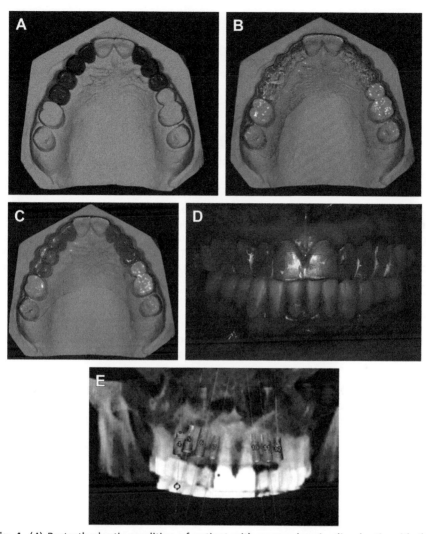

Fig. 4. (*A*) Postorthodontic condition of patient with nonsyndromic oligodontia with the completed diagnostic waxing. (*B*) An acrylic thermoplastic stent was created from a plaster duplicate of the wax up. (*C*) Biocryl X is polymerized within the acrylic thermoplastic stent, creating a radiopaque duplicate of the diagnostic waxing. (*D*) The thermoplastic stent with radiopaque teeth in position, ready for CBCT scanning. The maxillary and mandibular teeth will be separated using cotton rolls. (*E*) The resulting CBCT image revealing the process of implant planning in the derived 3-dimensional model that displays the position of the teeth and existing bone.

of duplicating the partial or complete denture in a radiopaque resin (see **Fig. 5**). Two divergent scanning procedures are possible here. One is an integrated scan that requires the denture to be duplicated in a radiopaque resin (eg, Biocryl X). The radiopaque denture is worn during the CBCT scanning procedure. The duplication of a denture is readily performed in a duplicating flask or by using silicone putty in a clam shell technique (**Fig. 5**). The second approach is the dual scan technique, in which the dentures are scanned by CBCT, and the patient wearing the dentures is scanned

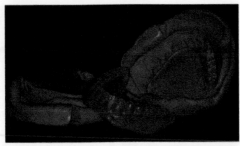

Fig. 5. The duplication of a denture is completed using silicone laboratory putty in a clam shell technique.

by CBCT. Here, the denture must bear radiopaque (and geometrically) identifiable fiduciary markers (4–6) distributed throughout the denture so that the denture may be aligned with the patient following the scanning procedure (**Fig. 6**). Some advantages of the dual scan technique include that the manipulation of the volumetric images is reduced in the process of generating a digital plan and the digital manufacture of a surgical guide.

USING THE GENERATED SCAN DATA

Although it is beyond the scope of this discussion to explore the detailed features of dental implant planning software, the general features of implant planning software include:

1. Acquisition of DICOM (Digital Imaging and Communications in Medicine) data and the generation of a 3-dimensional model
2. Filtering and segmentation of the 3-dimensional data in preparing a cleaned model for evaluation
3. Identification or segmentation of the maxilla and the mandible or regions of interest
4. The 3-dimensional visualization of all data-generated images including soft tissues, bone, teeth, and the scan prosthesis
5. Superimposition of dual scanned or optically scanned data representing the scan prosthesis or diagnostic cast
6. The virtual placement of 3-dimensional implant and abutment models within regions of interest
7. Measurement and evaluation of planned implant position (eg, distances, angles, parallelism) and the design of surgical guides for subsequent digital manufacture

The simplest goal achievable using the generated CBCT data is creation of a 3-dimensional radiographic image representing the patient's osseous structures and the related position of the planned prosthesis. On the computer screen, the clinician is able to establish the geometric relationship between the planned position of the prostheses and the underlying bone. Within the region of space that satisfies this relationship, decisions regarding dental implant dimensions and abutments can be made. This permits evaluation and diagnosis at various levels.

With little additional effort, the superimposition of planned tooth positions can be achieved by segmentation of the scan prostheses or by importation and superimposition of dual scanned prostheses or optically scanned diagnostic casts (**Fig. 7**). Achieving this type of complex virtual model enables detailed planning of implant size and position and abutment size and angulation. It recently was proved possible

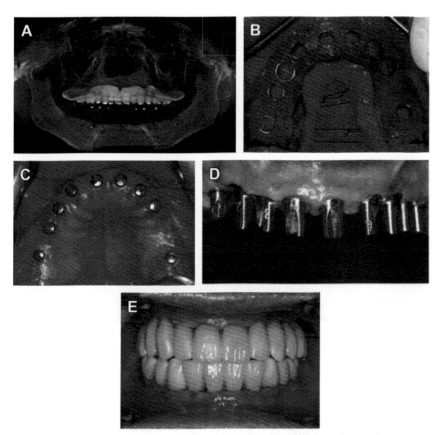

Fig. 6. (*A*) CBCT scan produced using a radiopaque resin (Biocryl-X) duplicate of the patient's maxillary denture. (*B*) Stereolithographic surgical guide produced from the CBCT-derived treatment plan (Simplant 15). (*C*) Resulting implant placement revealed by 1 stage surgery outcome at 4 weeks. (*D*) Position of CAD-CAM abutments (Atlantis) on implants indicates achievement of implant position for FDP construction. (*E*) Final maxillary and mandibular FDPs supported by dental implants placed using surgical guides. (Images courtesy of Dr. Carolina Vera, UNC AstraTech Implant Fellow).

to direct implant abutment design through integrated software when diagnostic casts have been imported (Simplant 16).

An important use of the software is communication. When different treatment concepts are visualized, the clinician is able to share these ideas represented in 3-dimensional models with the patient, with referring specialists, and with supporting laboratory technicians. Remote manufacture centers fabricating surgical guides, frameworks, abutments, and milled crowns have emerged; this communication aspect of planning software is of growing significance to the clinician who must communicate at a distance with treatment team members.

UTILIZING DIGITAL INFORMATION FOR IMPLANT SURGERY

There exist 4 ways to perform dental implant surgery using the information obtained from scanning a patient with a scan prosthesis. Because the scan prosthesis enables estimation or definition of the geometric relationship of the prosthesis and bone, the

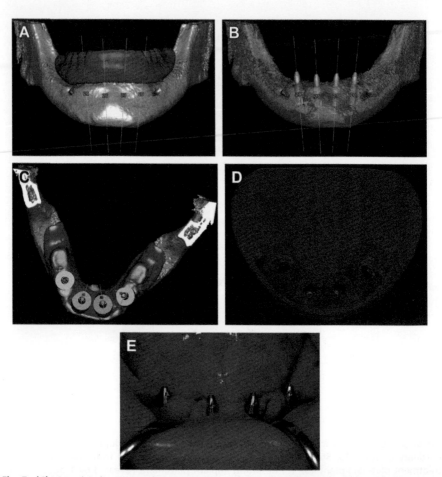

Fig. 7. (*A*) Virtual 3-dimensional reconstruction of the edentulous mandible with the super-imposed scanned prosthesis with planned tooth positions over it, while identifying the location of vital anatomic structures (inferior alveolar nerve). (*B*) Designated dental implant position based on the collected information. (*C*) Designed virtual surgical guide following the developed treatment plan. (*D*) Stereolithographic surgical guide seated on the cast on which surgery was completed prior to the actual patient's surgery. (*E*) Intraoral view of the patient immediately after surgery showing the dental implants in position after using the surgical guide.

trajectory or orientation of the osteotomy can be estimated or defined. Surgery can be performed using free hand-directed placement without a guide, yet with knowledge gained by implant planning in the 3-dimensional digital environment. This might occur in cases in which bone volume is large, and other anatomic structures aid in guiding the surgeon (eg, single-tooth implant placement in a healed alveolar ridge). However, when scan prostheses have been utilized in generating a complete 3-dimensional model, it is almost effortless to convert scan prostheses to surgical guides. This analog surgical guidance can be efficient, and 2 of the more common examples are the simple single tooth implant and implant placement into the parasymphyseal mandible.

The advantages of greater guidance during surgery are seen when implant placement will approximate anatomic structures including the sinuses, the inferior alveolar nerve, and adjacent tooth roots. As well, whenever multiple implants and their precise interimplant orientation are required for prosthesis success, the use of a 3-dimensional model-derived, CAD-CAM generated surgical guide may be used to clinical advantage.

These guides are generated in 2 basic ways. One is exemplified by both the Simplant and Noble Clinician approaches and involves stereolithography to fabricate a resin surgical guide that is supported by bone, mucosa, and/or teeth, and includes metal sleeves to assure accuracy of surgical instrumentation. Contemporary versions of these guides include depth control in the instrumentation systems for true 3-dimensional guidance. The other approach involves creating a surgical guide by CAD-CAM directed drilling of the drill sleeve into either the existing scan prosthesis (as illustrated by SiCAT guides (SICAT GmbH & Co., Bonn, Germany)) or by fabricating a guide for this purpose (Gonyx and CoDiagnostix; Straumann USA LLC, Andover, MA, USA). In both cases, the guides direct the orientation and depth of drills that are positioned using interchangeable metal sleeves.

Navigation differs from surgical guidance and refers to the real-time directional orientation of surgical drilling through global positioning system-mediated techniques. The patient and the 3-dimensional model are linked through hardware and software, and additional software directs the orientation of drilling. Additional information on this related approach to using digital information to direct dental implant placement is available elsewhere.[13–18]

SUMMARY

The use of volumetric imaging is emerging as a valued aid in planning, placement, and restoration of dental implants. Any CBCT scan intended for these purposes must include a scan prosthesis or integrate an optical scan of a diagnostically waxed cast. When the assembled 3-dimensional model (segmented maxilla, mandible, and prostheses) is visualized, available planning software enables improved planning and enhanced communication. The planned treatment can be used to direct CAD-CAM fabrication of surgical guides that offer 3-dimensional control of implant placement. Ongoing development enables clinicians to design and manufacture patient-specific abutments within this 3-dimensional virtual environment to further streamline and improve planning and treatment. Clinicians should understand fully the advantages of this technology to appropriately prescribe CBCT scanning for dental implant treatment planning and therapy.

REFERENCES

1. Eshraghi T, McAllister N, McAllister B. Clinical applications of digital 2-D and 3-D radiography for the periodontist. J Evid Based Dent Pract 2012;12(Suppl 3): 36–45.
2. American Dental Association Council on Scientific Affairs. The use of cone-beam computed tomography in dentistry: an advisory statement from the American Dental Association Council on Scientific Affairs. J Am Dent Assoc 2012;143(8): 899–902.
3. Jung RE, Schneider D, Ganeles J, et al. Computer technology applications in surgical implant dentistry: a systematic review. Int J Oral Maxillofac Implants 2009; 24(Suppl):92–109.

4. Lofthag-Hansen S, Grondahl K, Ekestubbe A. Cone-beam CT for preoperative implant planning in the posterior mandible: visibility of anatomic landmarks. Clin Implant Dent Relat Res 2009;11(3):246–55.
5. Pauwels R, Nackaerts O, Bellaiche N, et al. Variability of dental cone beam CT grey values for density estimations. Br J Radiol 2013;86(1021):20120135.
6. Schulze R, Heil U, Gross D, et al. Artifacts in CBCT: a review. Dentomaxillofac Radiol 2011;40(5):265–73.
7. Tyndall DA, Price JB, Tetradis S, et al. Position statement of the American Academy of Oral and Maxillofacial Radiology on selection criteria for the use of radiology in dental implantology with emphasis on cone beam computed tomography. Oral Surg Oral Med Oral Pathol Oral Radiol 2012;113(6):817–26.
8. Tyndall DA, Brooks SL. Selection criteria for dental implant site imaging: a position paper of the American Academy of Oral and Maxillofacial radiology. Oral Surg Oral Med Oral Pathol Oral Radiol Endod 2000;89(5):630–7.
9. Harris D, Horner K, Grondahl K, et al. E.A.O. guidelines for the use of diagnostic imaging in implant dentistry 2011. A consensus workshop organized by the European Association for Osseointegration at the Medical University of Warsaw. Clin Oral Implants Res 2012;23(11):1243–53.
10. Van Assche N, van Steenberghe D, Guerrero ME, et al. Accuracy of implant placement based on pre-surgical planning of three-dimensional cone-beam images: a pilot study. J Clin Periodontol 2007;34(9):816–21.
11. Vasak C, Kohal RJ, Lettner S, et al. Clinical and radiological evaluation of a template-guided (NobelGuide()) treatment concept. Clin Oral Implants Res 2012. [Epub ahead of print].
12. Floyd P, Palmer P, Palmer R. Radiographic techniques. Br Dent J 1999;187(7): 359–65.
13. Casap N, Tarazi E, Wexler A, et al. Intraoperative computerized navigation for flapless implant surgery and immediate loading in the edentulous mandible. Int J Oral Maxillofac Implants 2005;20(1):92–8.
14. Marchack CB. CAD/CAM-guided implant surgery and fabrication of an immediately loaded prosthesis for a partially edentulous patient. J Prosthet Dent 2007; 97(6):389–94.
15. Hahn J. Single-stage, immediate loading, and flapless surgery. J Oral Implantol 2000;26(3):193–8.
16. Gillot L, Noharet R, Cannas B. Guided surgery and presurgical prosthesis: preliminary results of 33 fully edentulous maxillae treated in accordance with the Nobel-Guide protocol. Clin Implant Dent Relat Res 2010;12(Suppl 1):e104–13.
17. Vercruyssen M, Jacobs R, Van Assche N, et al. The use of CT scan based planning for oral rehabilitation by means of implants and its transfer to the surgical field: a critical review on accuracy. J Oral Rehabil 2008;35(6):454–74.
18. Vasak C, Watzak G, Gahleitner A, et al. Computed tomography-based evaluation of template (NobelGuide)-guided implant positions: a prospective radiological study. Clin Oral Implants Res 2011;22(10):1157–63.

Patient Selection and Treatment Planning for Implant Restorations

Matthew Bryington, DMD, MS[a], Ingeborg J. De Kok, DDS, MS[b],
Ghadeer Thalji, DDS, PhD[c], Lyndon F. Cooper, DDS, PhD[b],*

KEYWORDS

- Implant restorations • Treatment planning • Dental implants

KEY POINTS

- The development of a complete systemic health evaluation with particular emphasis on factors influencing osseointegration is a first step in the evaluation of implant patients.
- An assessment of the overall oral health and ability of patients to maintain ideal oral health is a key step in characterizing potential dental implant patients.
- Without mounted diagnostic casts and simple intraoral and perioral photographs, it is nearly impossible to make the proper assessment of local conditions that impact the delivery of successful dental implant prostheses.
- An important step in the evaluation of implant patients is the radiographic assessment of osseous architecture and quality in relationship to the contours of the planned dental prosthesis.
- Sufficient information to safely and effectively place a dental implant includes the spectrum of diagnostic data that includes the representation of the osseous condition of the intended implant site.

Dental implants have become an indispensible tool for the restoration of missing teeth. Their use has elevated the practice of dentistry by improving both our technical ability to rehabilitate patients and improving general quality of life. To achieve the associated high expectations on a routine basis, diligent attention to details must be observed and addressed from the outset. Of central concern is the attainment of osseointegration and the location of implants to ideally support the intended restoration. The pivotal point in treatment planning for dental implants occurs when the

Financial Disclosures and/or Conflicts of Interest: The authors have nothing to disclose.
[a] Restorative Dentistry, School of Dentistry, West Virginia University, PO Box 9495, Morgantown, WV 26506, USA; [b] Department of Prosthodontics, School of Dentistry, University of North Carolina, 330 Brauer Hall, CB# 7450, Chapel Hill, NC 27599-7450, USA; [c] Department of Prosthodontics, The University of Iowa College of Dentistry, 801 Newton Road, Dental Sciences Building S432, Iowa City, IA 55242, USA
* Corresponding author.
E-mail address: Lyndon_Cooper@unc.edu

Dent Clin N Am 58 (2014) 193–206
http://dx.doi.org/10.1016/j.cden.2013.09.009
0011-8532/14/$ – see front matter © 2014 Elsevier Inc. All rights reserved.

location of bone is viewed radiographically in the context of the planned prosthesis. This diagnostic and planning procedure can only be achieved with the use of a well-designed and constructed radiographic guide (covered in the article by De Kok and colleagues elsewhere in this issue). Notably, the American Dental Association's recommended guidelines for cone beam computed tomography (CBCT) imaging include its use only after a complete clinical evaluation. It is the intent of this report to review the clinical factors that should be considered in the evaluation of dental implant patients.

PATIENT SELECTION

Successful patient selection depends on several key factors concerning the patients' systemic health, the condition of the jaws, and local factors around the proposed implant site. There are few absolute contraindications to implant placement. However, each individual patient presents unique features, and the clinical and radiographic evaluation of individuals accumulates a personal set of risk factors affecting implant outcomes. When selecting patients for implant therapy, it is crucial to obtain a thorough health history to identify conditions that may affect suitability for surgery as well as implant survival (**Box 1**).

One of the most important effectors of implant placement and success is the use of alcohol and tobacco products. Several studies have demonstrated that regular alcohol consumption can cause changes in alveolar bone healing, affecting osseointegration and resulting in greater implant failure.[1,2] The use of tobacco products has been shown to be an even greater detriment not just to the initial placement of implants but to the long-term health and stability. Tobacco use has been shown to increase the chances of initial implant failure by more than 2 times compared with those who do not use tobacco.[2] Smoking negatively impacts healing and damages the delicate tissues around dental implants and has been demonstrated to have a negative effect on several types of bone grafting, limiting the acceptability of potential implant sites. Lastly, the use of tobacco products has been shown to cause complications in fully osseointegrated implants leading to greater chances of long-term implant failure.[3]

In addition to the social habits affecting implant placement, several systemic conditions have been shown to have a negative effect on implant healing and long-term success. The most well-documented condition for affecting implant success is diabetes. Diabetes has been shown to have a wide effect on healing by affecting microvascular health and regeneration as well as cellular responses to trauma.[4] Several studies have demonstrated that this loss of healing potential affects both bone grafting success and implant osseointegration potential, with early failures occurring more frequently compared with nondiabetic patients.[5] It should be noted though that although diabetes should be considered a confounding factor, patients with well-controlled diabetes have been shown to have only slightly worse success rates compared with nondiabetic patients.

Another factor to consider is the presence of osteoporosis. Although it is reasonable to consider that a disease leading to the decalcification of the bones would have an effect on osseointegration, it should not be considered a definitive contraindication because studies have shown that the jaw calcification is only moderately dependent on calcification of the long bones of the body.[6,7] What is of greater concern for the dentist is the pharmacologic agents used to treat osteoporosis, namely, bisphosphonate drugs.[5] Although the risk of bisphosphonate-induced osteonecrosis is a greater risk for those patients receiving intravenous drug therapy, there have been reports of

---

Box 1
Systemic contraindications to implant therapy

Absolute contraindications

   Osteopathies and disorders of bone metabolism

   Renal insufficiency and uremia

   Liver disease

   Hyperthyroidism

   Hypopituitarism

   Connective tissue diseases and specific autoimmune diseases (lupus)

   Leukopoietic and erythropoietic disease (eg, coagulopathies, plasmacytoma)

   High-dosage radiotherapy

Relative somatic conditions

   Osteoporosis

   Aggressive rheumatoid arthritis

   Treated endocrine disorders

   Anticoagulant treatment

   Drug and alcohol abuse

   Low-dosage radiotherapy

Temporary contraindications

   Transient infections

   Systematic therapies affecting wound healing

      Anticoagulant

      Immunosuppressive therapy

      Corticosteroids

      Chemotherapy

Data from Lill W, Solar P. Indications, diagnosis, and recall. In: Watzek G, editor. Endosseous implants: scientific and clinical aspects. Chicago: Quintessence Publishing Co; 1996. p. 153–82.

---

patients developing osteonecrosis while on oral bisphosphonates. Although some estimates place the risk of osteonecrosis at 7.8%, with literature reports ranging from 2.5% to 27.3% for oral bisphosphonates, it is important to advise patients of the potential complications and place implants only after a careful risk-benefit analysis.[8,9]

It is also essential to consider patients with various vascular and heart conditions. Several of our elderly patients can be on various heart medications either for hypertension or anticoagulation therapy. Although neither of these classes of drugs should be used as a contraindication, it is important to note that they can pose complications for the initial implant surgery. Those patients on anticoagulant therapy should be evaluated for their PTT and PT/INR, and drug holidays should be considered only after consultation with their primary care physician and/or cardiologist. With regard to hypertensive patients, careful monitoring of blood pressure should be performed to ensure suitability for dental surgery and to limit the risk of a cardiac incident. *The development of a complete systemic health evaluation with particular emphasis on factors influencing osseointegration is a first step in the evaluation of implant patients.*

Local Factors

When considering the placement of oral implants, it is important to consider the entire oral health of patients. Although it may seem practical to follow a tactical approach of replacing teeth with implants as needed, a more thoughtful strategic approach considered after careful evaluation of the mouth may provide greater restorative options and allow for greater resource management. While implants are not susceptible to oral caries, it is an overall indicator of the patients' oral hygiene and awareness and serves as one indicator of patients' future ability to maintain implant hygiene. In addition, removal of active caries allows for the better planning of dental implants by understanding the restorative viability of the teeth. Failure to do so can result in additional surgery or delayed restorative delivery as other dental matters are addressed.

Also of great concern is periodontitis. Periodontal disease is one of the chief causes of tooth loss. There have been several studies that have demonstrated that periodontal disease increases the likelihood of periimplantitis.[10] Periimplantitis is a serious complication for dental implants that can result in implant failure caused by the loss of bony support around the implant (**Fig. 1**). Although several factors are required to develop periimplantitis, the presence of periodontal oral bacteria can increase the likelihood of its development. In fact, Mombelli and Lang[11] demonstrated a mechanism whereby anaerobic bacterial plaque formations on the implant abutment surface have a negative effect on peri-implant tissues. Most treatments for periimplantitis are palliative in nature and usually only function to arrest the process rather than cure it. Grafting around dental implants to replace the missing bone has been shown to have only limited effectiveness.[12] *An assessment of the overall oral health and ability of patients to maintain ideal oral health is the next step in characterizing potential dental implant patients.*

The local conditions at the intended site of implant placement merit attention only following the general systemic and oral evaluations. Before any radiographic assessment of the intended implant site is performed, important assessments of local conditions should be considered (**Box 2**). More succinctly, the architecture of the implant site, the soft tissue anatomy and health of the local site, and the relative aesthetic impact of the intended site must be fully assessed. Both study casts and intraoral photographs are necessary tools in completing these assessments in an efficient manner that allows rapid clinical data collection and subsequent thoughtful evaluation (**Fig. 2**).

The architecture of the implant site refers to the actual shape and dimension of the intended implant site and the conditions of the teeth, which often frame the site. Although the exact bone volume required to house an implant is not well defined, at

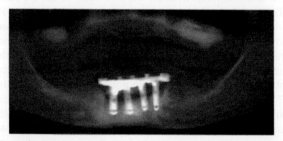

Fig. 1. Panoramic radiograph reveals bone loss reflecting periimplantitis around all 4 mandibular dental endosseous implants that had previously been restored with an implant-supported fixed denture.

Box 2
Local contraindications to implant therapy

Unresolved bone loss attributed to the following:

 Osteomyelitis, osteoradionecrosis, fibrous bone dysplasias

 Apical periodontitis

 Existing residual roots

Unresolvable bone deficiencies

 Vertical bone volume of posterior maxilla or mandible

 Horizontal deficiencies without resolution

Adjacent tooth limitations

 Root proximity

 Aesthetic limitations

Soft tissue and mucosa

 Pathologic conditions

 Deficient attached gingival at proposed implant site

Oral hygiene

 Evidence of unwillingness to perform hygiene

 Local factors that preclude performance of oral hygiene

Data from Lill W, Solar P. Indications, diagnosis, and recall. In: Watzek G, editor. Endosseous implants: scientific and clinical aspects. Chicago: Quintessence Publishing Co; 1996. p. 153–82.

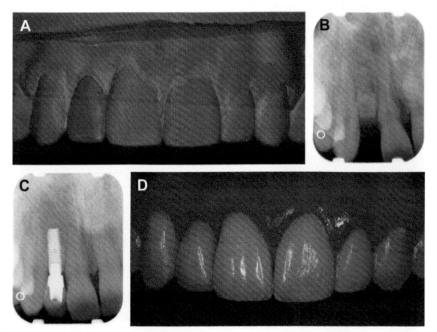

Fig. 2. (*A*) Diagnostic wax-up finished to reproduce ideal contour of the final restoration. (*B*) Preoperative periapical radiograph of the area. (*C*) Postoperative periapical radiograph showing the abutment and definitive crown inserted. (*D*) Frontal view of the completed restoration at time of insertion.

least 1 mm of circumferential bone with 1.5 mm of bone between an implant and the adjacent tooth provides sufficient volume to stabilize the implant. Given that many narrow-diameter implants are approximately 3 mm in diameter, the smallest edentulous space that can be predictably restored is 6 mm by 6 mm (**Fig. 3**). The evaluation of a planned implant site cannot be a simple matter of space measurements because successful planning requires the analysis of soft and hard tissue anatomy, adjacent tooth condition, interdental spatial relationship, and the desired aesthetic outcome.

The soft tissue anatomy of the intended implant site must be well defined. The abundance or lack of keratinized mucosa, the biotype (thickness of the mucosa), and the location of adjacent tooth connective tissue attachments and gingival margins must be defined. This information can be readily assessed in anesthetized patients by bone sounding and periodontal probing (**Fig. 4**). The lack of keratinized mucosa, a thin biotype, and the loss of connective tissue attachment are known risk factors affecting the aesthetic success of dental implants.

The relative aesthetic impact of the intended implant site must be acknowledged. Anterior sites including the first premolar sites may present sufficient osseous dimension for successful implant placement but may, at the same time, be deficient and result in marked aesthetic deficits (**Fig. 5**). When larger prostheses are involved, any local architectural change of the alveolus that leads to marked asymmetry of gingival display or leads to the presentation of large gingival embrasures should be identified. Regarding the maxillary or mandibular fixed prostheses, the location of

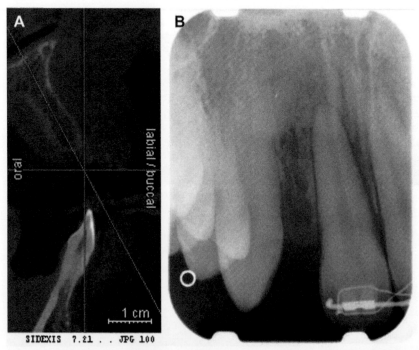

SIDEXIS 7.21 . . JPG 100

Fig. 3. (*A*) Cross-sectional CBCT image of the missing lateral incisor examining the bone available for the planned dental implant surgery. (*B*) Periapical radiograph of a limited restorative space to replace a lateral incisor. Note the existing space between roots, which would indicate the use of a narrow dental implant.

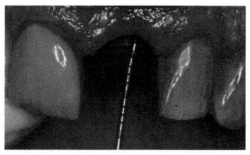

Fig. 4. Preoperative evaluation of the thickness of the mucosa using a periodontal probe.

the prostheses/alveolus finish line must be considered. The potential display of this finish line must be aesthetically managed through treatment planning.

Without mounted diagnostic casts and simple intraoral and perioral photographs, it is nearly impossible to make the proper assessment of local conditions that impact the delivery of successful dental implant prostheses.

Adjacent tooth conditions are also important in the consideration of dental implants. Anterior tooth loss is often attributed to recent or past trauma. The condition of the adjacent teeth must be fully defined. Visual inspection, periodontal probing, and vitality testing should be performed. The near zone connective tissue attachment levels should be measured and defined. The radiographic assessment is discussed later. The color of adjacent teeth and the condition of possible existing restorations should be considered for potential repair or replacement; here, the added value of photography is underscored. The management of the vitality and the appearance of adjacent teeth represent an important part of site development for dental implant therapy.

Another key but often overlooked is that of interdental relationships. It is important to address the dimensions of bound and unbound edentulous spaces both regarding adjacent teeth and between antagonistic teeth. Changes encountered lead to both increased and reduced dimensions. Alveolar ridge resorption following tooth loss is now well characterized. The alveolar process begins to collapse, resulting in less bone both in a vertical occlusal-apical direction and in the horizontal buccolingual direction. Although socket preservation surgery has been proposed as a means to preserve bone height and width, resorption will continue to occur. In posterior regions, this resorption can result in limited available bone before reaching critical structures, such as the maxillary sinus or the inferior alveolar nerve in the mandible. *The third step,*

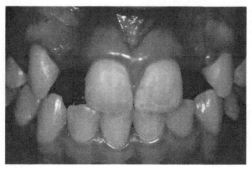

Fig. 5. Frontal view of missing lateral incisors, the edentulous space lacks soft and hard tissues to allow proper esthetics.

the evaluation of local conditions affecting dental implant therapy, is only fully achieved using mounted diagnostic study casts.

At this point in the evaluation of dental implant patients, the role of radiology has yet to be introduced. There are 2 main reasons for this relegated role for radiographs. First, in practical terms, many of the systemic and aesthetic risks affecting implant therapy cannot be readily modified (eg, diabetes or loss of attachment at adjacent teeth), and it is important to define what cannot be modified first. Bone volume, particularly horizontal bone dimension, can be enhanced by a wide number of clinical procedures that are highly successful **(Fig. 6)**.[13] Although bone volume is critical for implant placement, the initial available volume does not eliminate the possibility of eventual implant placement. Second, radiation safety requires that patient exposure be limited according to the principle of being as low as reasonably achievable; this implies that planning radiographs for dental implants be exposed only *after* the diagnostic waxing of the planned prosthesis and development of an illustrative radiographic stent. Based on this logic, the diagnostic process for dental implant therapy is fully revealed. After the stepwise consideration of systemic health, followed by oral health, and the clinical assessment of the intended implant site using mounted diagnostic casts, a proposed restoration is modeled using wax (or digital techniques). The location of the proposed restoration must now be revealed in the exposed radiographic assessment of the intended implant site. That location can be revealed using several radiopaque materials that define the full contour of the restoration. In this way, it is now possible to solve the geometric puzzle of reconciling the position of the restoration with the possible implant position **(Fig. 7)**. *The fourth step in the evaluation of implant patients is the radiographic assessment of osseous architecture and quality in relationship to the contours of the planned dental prosthesis.*

What is the appropriate radiographic imaging technique for dental implants? Although debated, there are guidelines that indicate the volumetric assessment of implant patients using CBCT imaging is of growing importance.[14] Regarding the anterior maxillary aesthetic zone, periapical radiographs remain important because

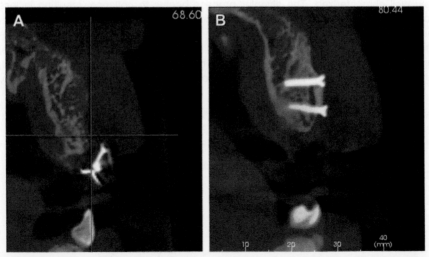

Fig. 6. (A) Cross-sectional CBCT image of the missing tooth showing lack of sufficient bone to place a dental implant. (B) Cross-sectional CBCT image of the area after the bone grafting procedure was completed.

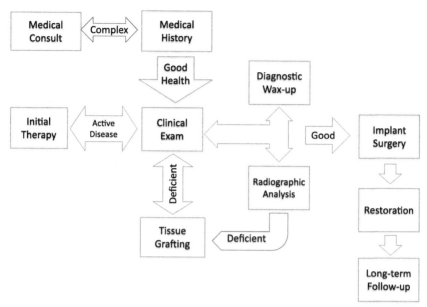

Fig. 7. When evaluating new patients, it is important to begin with an accurate medical history receiving consults as necessary. All patients should then be evaluated clinically for suitability of implant placement as well as treatment of active disease processes, such as caries and periodontal disease. Following the clinical examination, radiographic analysis should be performed with a radiographic stent devised from a diagnostic wax-up. With careful planning, successful implant restoration and follow-up will lead to long-term success.

they assist in evaluation of adjacent tooth connective tissue attachment and bone levels that aid in control of aesthetics. Panoramic radiographs may be sufficient for mandibular overdenture therapy involving 1 or 2 implants in the parasymphyseal mandible when the intended implant location is 5 to 10 mm medial to the inferior alveolar nerve bilaterally. Other implant therapies begin to involve considerations whereby the value of CBCT imaging is easily recognized. *Sufficient information to safely and effectively place a dental implant includes the entire spectrum of diagnostic data that includes the representation of the osseous condition of the intended implant site.*

Implant components, being of fixed and limited vertical dimensions require a defined restorative space represented by the space existing between antagonistic teeth or the tooth and the opposing edentulous ridge. Although initial residual bone measurements can be made from a panoramic radiologic examination, 3-dimensional computed tomography imaging should be considered to ensure that there is adequate space for the implant. In anterior regions, the loss of vertical bone height can result in implants placed lower than the cementoenamel junctions of neighboring teeth, resulting in gingival margin discrepancy (**Fig. 8**). Although a low smile line can sometimes mask this discrepancy, this can be an aesthetic challenge for patients with the proverbial gummy smiles.

In a similar fashion, tooth loss can result in a loss of bone width. The loss of the root causes the collapse of the buccal plate toward the lingual. In the posterior, this may not be a large concern; but in the anterior in particular, this can cause major aesthetic and functional challenges. For maxillary cuspids, this loss of buccal bone results in

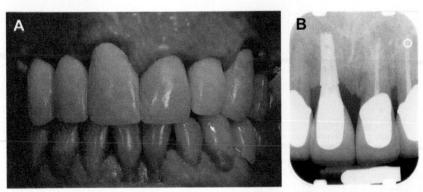

Fig. 8. (*A*) Frontal view of a maxillary central incisor, with an implant-supported crown with compromised aesthetics as a result of deep orientation of the implant caused by prior vertical bone loss. (*B*) Bone height discrepancy between the 2 central incisors can be observed in the periapical radiograph.

obliteration of the canine eminence resulting in teeth that either have higher-than-expected gingival margins or teeth placed more palatally than preferred for the arch form (**Fig. 9**). The situation is equally dire for lateral incisors whereby the horizontal bone loss could compromise a site to the point that an implant is not an aesthetically viable option. Complicating the matter is any adjacent teeth that may be present. On the loss of a tooth, natural tooth crowding may result in further constriction of the proposed implant site. In addition, proximal root convergence particularly in the anterior regions can result in potential sites too limited for conventional implant therapy.

One of the most common errors seen with dental implant therapy is a lack of restorative space for the planned restoration (**Fig. 10**). The amount of space required varies greatly depending on the type of planned restoration. For single-tooth screw-retained restorations, a crown can be directly screwed to the implant with 6 mm of space required from the restorative platform of the implant to the occlusal plane. A single cement-retained crown or fixed dental prosthesis requires approximately 8 mm of space in order to account for the abutment and the prosthesis. An additional 2 mm of distance from the implant/abutment interface is required to allow formation of the biologic width along the abutment. For bar-retained restorations, as much as 16 to 18 mm of space from the implant/abutment interface to the planned occlusal table is needed to provide sufficient space for the abutment, bar, acrylic, and teeth. These

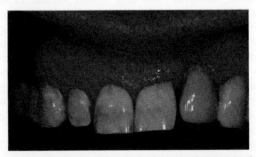

Fig. 9. Frontal view of an implant-supported restoration with poor aesthetics, the result of a poorly placed (unnecessarily superior and facial) dental implant resulting in an unattractive crown replacing tooth number 10.

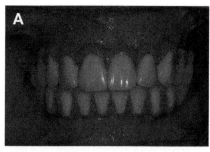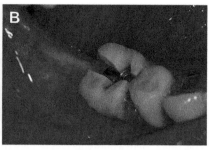

Fig. 10. (*A*) Maxillary and mandibular implant-supported fixed dentures were completed. It can be observed that the lack of restorative dimension (occlusogingivally) of the mandibular prosthesis has limited the amount of resin surrounding the metal framework and prosthetic teeth. (*B*) Fracture of the prosthetic tooth and resin can be appreciated, most probably as a result of the reduced height of the prosthesis.

prosthesis-specific dimensional requirements underscore the need to evaluate mounted study casts when assuring there is sufficient occlusogingival restorative space.

These details affecting implant success may be daunting, but it is important to realize that the complexity of implant placement and restoration can be managed by a thorough and methodical treatment planning methodology. All implant treatment plans should begin with accurate and mounted study models. For single-tooth cases, the models should be mounted in maximal intercuspation, whereas larger rehabilitations may require careful mounting in centric relation. Mounted study models allow for accurate and easy measurements of the residual alveolar ridges and interproximal spaces. In addition, mounted models allow for far greater evaluation of available interocclusal space than can be achieved during the clinical examination.

For patients receiving anterior implant retained restorations, a smile analysis may be required to help achieve optimal aesthetics. A smile analysis is most easily performed using diagnostic intraoral photographs of the anterior tooth display. A smile analysis is performed by a careful assessment of pink, white, and black components of the smile. *Pink aesthetics* refers to an analysis of the shape of gingival tissues around the gingival margins and at edentulous spaces. *White aesthetics* refers to the analysis of the tooth shape, position, and angulation of the clinical crowns within the arch of the aesthetic zone. Lastly, *black* or *dark aesthetics* refers to the embrasure spaces around teeth, which help to frame the aesthetic zone and define the overall tooth shape (**Fig. 11**). Further details planning with a focus on dental implant esthetics are summarized by Cooper[15] (2008). In conjunction with the information obtained by the diagnostic waxing, a smile analysis can determine if an anterior restoration will require additional dental procedures to improve the final aesthetics. Examples of this include the need for soft tissue grafting or gingivectomy to improve pink aesthetics, additional restoration of exiting teeth to improve white aesthetics, and adjustment of embrasure spaces to provide an overall pleasing aesthetic form.

The phrase *restoratively driven implant placement* is mentioned throughout the literature and it refers to the determination of implant location and angulation with regard to the proposed restoration. With mounted diagnostic study models, it is possible to perform a diagnostic wax-up to assess if the proposed restoration will interfere with the existing occlusion or prevent an aesthetic restorative outcome.

The diagnostic waxing can also reveal the need for additional hard or soft tissue grafting by demonstrating unappealing gingival aesthetics. For straightforward,

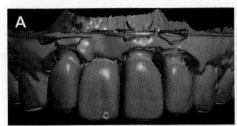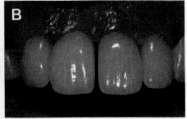

Fig. 11. A diagnostic waxing informs the clinician about potential esthetic limitations and possible goals. Here a diastema was requested and affected the implant position in a mesio-distal direction. (*A*) Virtual design of the definitive prostheses evaluating tooth shape, position, and angulation of the clinical crowns. (*B*) Buccal view of the implant crowns replacing all maxillary incisors.

single-tooth implants, clinicians can use the Rules of Six to determine if they have sufficient restorative space to allow for successful implant restorations. The Rules of Six[16] state that clinicians should attempt to achieve the following:

1. 6 mm of inter-radicular space
2. 6 mm of buccal-lingual osseous dimension
3. 6 mm of minimum implant length
4. 6 mm of interocclusal distance to allow for prosthesis and component construction without functional compromise
5. Less than 6 mm of distance from the bone crest to the interproximal contact point to allow for papilla formation
6. Placement of the implant-abutment interface located 3 mm apical and 2 mm palatal/lingual to the planned gingival zenith.

Following these guidelines allows for implants to be placed with sufficient bone and soft tissue support to provide for aesthetic, stable, and successful implant treatment.

For patients receiving FDP therapy, the Rules of Six are effective guidelines for short spans in the anterior region. For larger spans or those planned in the posterior segment, it is important to consider occlusal forces in relation to implant placement. For posterior bridges, it is necessary to consider the implant placement to allow for occlusal forces to be directed through the body of the implant. Careful implant positioning allows for force distribution through the supporting bone while reducing forces on the restorative screw, lowering the risks of screw fracture and providing for greater prosthetic success. Although this may result in minor aesthetic compromises in posterior cases, the benefits of improved implant and prosthetic survival are worth it.

With regard to implant treatment planning for completely edentulous patients, the Rules of 10 function as an excellent starting point. Similar to the Rules of Six, the Rules of 10 allow for the planning of implants with enough restorative space to provide for successful implants and a full-arch implant-retained prosthesis.[17] The first Rule of 10 is that the inferior/superior dimension of the mandible must be greater than or equal to 10 mm. Although longer implants may seem attractive, there is little evidence to support that longer implants result in great implant success, particularly when placed in the parasymphyseal mandible. In a 5-year prospective study, Gallucci and colleagues[18] demonstrated a 100% implant survival rate while using 4 to 6 implants of 8 to 16 mm in length to support implant supported fixed dentures, showing that the implant length was not a key factor in restorative success. The second rule is that the interocclusal/restorative space from the crest of the ridge to the occlusal plane

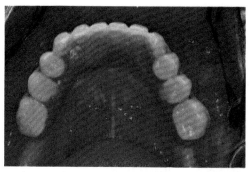

Fig. 12. Occlusal view of an implant-supported fixed denture showing effective cantilever and anteroposterior spread.

must be equal to or greater than 10 mm, which provides acceptable restorative space for uncompromised strength and aesthetic rehabilitation. Various restorative materials, such as acrylics, may need a greater bulk of material to imbue strength; this will require additional restorative space as necessary. Ten millimeters represents the mimimal restorative dimension for creating an implant supported fixed denture or overdenture; ideally, at least 15 mm is advised. Lastly, the anterior-posterior distribution of implants must be at least 10 mm when using an implant-supported fixed prosthesis. When the anatomy of the mandible is considered, the parasymphyseal mandible is bound by the right and left inferior alveolar nerve. Placing implants as far posterior as possible without impinging the inferior alveolar nerve typically results in the distal implant in the first premolar space. This placement typically results in at least the required 10-mm anteroposterior spread. Considering that the average premolar is approximately 6 mm in width and the average first molar is approximately 10 mm, the cantilever required posterior to the most posterior implant is 16 mm. This measurement approximates the recommended anterior-posterior cantilever ratio of 1.5:1.0 the A-P spread (**Fig. 12**). By following the Rules of 10, it is possible to provide an implant-retained fixed restoration, which is of sufficient bulk and size to resist typical function and provide both esthetics and comfort. It must be recognized that these rules represent minimal dimensions for treatment. Again 10 mm of occlusogingival dimension is restrictive, and striving for greater dimension (often by way of alveolectomy) is recommended.

When considering patient selection and implant treatment planning, there are several factors that must be considered when using implant therapy. Beyond the simple idea of replacing a missing tooth with an implant, a careful analysis of patients' oral and systemic health, the amount of residual supporting tissues, and the planned restoration must all factor into the planning of dental implants. Much of this information can only be accurately obtained by careful and diagnostic photographs and models followed by diagnostic wax-up of the planned prosthesis. Using the Rules of Six and the Rules of 10, it is possible to plan for implant restorations that have sufficient restorative space to not only provide an aesthetic outcome but also provide for prosthetic longevity leading to great restorative success.

REFERENCES

1. Heitz-Mayfield LJ. Peri-implant diseases: diagnosis and risk indicators. J Clin Periodontol 2008;35(Suppl 8):292–304.

2. Baig MR, Rajan M. Effects of smoking on the outcome of implant treatment: a literature review. Indian J Dent Res 2007;18(4):190–5.
3. Strietzel FP, Reichart PA, Kale A, et al. Smoking interferes with the prognosis of dental implant treatment: a systematic review and meta-analysis. J Clin Periodontol 2007;34(6):523–44.
4. Fiorellini JP, Nevins ML. Dental implant considerations in the diabetic patient. Periodontol 2000 2000;23:73–7.
5. Bornstein MM, Cionca N, Mombelli A. Systemic conditions and treatments as risks for implant therapy. Int J Oral Maxillofac Implants 2009;24(Suppl):12–27.
6. Jacobs R, Ghyselen J, Koninckx P, et al. Long-term bone mass evaluation of mandible and lumbar spine in a group of women receiving hormone replacement therapy. Eur J Oral Sci 1996;104(1):10–6.
7. Otomo-Corgel J. Osteoporosis and osteopenia: implications for periodontal and implant therapy. Periodontol 2000 2012;59(1):111–39.
8. Otto S, Abu-Id MH, Fedele S, et al. Osteoporosis and bisphosphonates-related osteonecrosis of the jaw: not just a sporadic coincidence–a multi-centre study. J Craniomaxillofac Surg 2011;39(4):272–7.
9. Di Fede O, Fusco V, Matranga D, et al. Osteonecrosis of the jaws in patients assuming oral bisphosphonates for osteoporosis: a retrospective multi-hospital-based study of 87 Italian cases. Eur J Intern Med 2013. [Epub ahead of print].
10. Van der Weijden GA, van Bemmel KM, Renvert S. Implant therapy in partially edentulous, periodontally compromised patients: a review. J Clin Periodontol 2005;32(5):506–11.
11. Mombelli A, Lang NP. The diagnosis and treatment of peri-implantitis. Periodontol 2000 1998;17:63–76.
12. Romanos GE, Weitz D. Therapy of peri-implant diseases. Where is the evidence? J Evid Based Dent Pract 2012;12(Suppl 3):204–8.
13. Chiapasco M, Casentini P, Zaniboni M. Bone augmentation procedures in implant dentistry. Int J Oral Maxillofac Implants 2009;24(Suppl):237–59.
14. Harris D, Horner K, Grondahl K, et al. E.A.O. guidelines for the use of diagnostic imaging in implant dentistry 2011. A consensus workshop organized by the European Association for Osseointegration at the Medical University of Warsaw. Clin Oral Implants Res 2012;23(11):1243–53.
15. Cooper LF. Objective criteria: guiding and evaluating dental implant esthetics. J Esthet Restor Dent 2008;20(3):195–205.
16. Cooper LF, Pin-Harry OC. "Rules of Six"–diagnostic and therapeutic guidelines for single-tooth implant success. Compend Contin Educ Dent 2013;34(2):94–8, 100–1; quiz 102, 117.
17. Cooper LF, Limmer BM, Gates WD. "Rules of 10"–guidelines for successful planning and treatment of mandibular edentulism using dental implants. Compend Contin Educ Dent 2012;33(5):328–34; quiz 335–6.
18. Gallucci GO, Doughtie CB, Hwang JW, et al. Five-year results of fixed implant-supported rehabilitations with distal cantilevers for the edentulous mandible. Clin Oral Implants Res 2009;20(6):601–7.

Prosthodontic Management of Implant Therapy

Ghadeer Thalji, DDS, PhD[a], Matthew Bryington, DMD, MS[b],
Ingeborg J. De Kok, DDS, MS[c], Lyndon F. Cooper, DDS, PhD[c],*

KEYWORDS

- Implant prosthesis • Endosseous implant • Computer-aided design • Abutments

KEY POINTS

- When considering implant prosthodontic treatment for rehabilitation of the partially or fully edentulous patient, the clinician has several choices to choose from including, but not limited to:
  - Use of fixed or removable prostheses
  - Use of individual attachments or bars for retention of removable overdentures
  - Use of screw-retained or cement-retained prostheses
  - Use of stock versus custom abutments
  - Different restorative and abutment materials
- Implant-supported restorations can be screw-retained, cement-retained, or a combination of both, whereby a metal superstructure is screwed to the implants and crowns are individually cemented to the metal frame. Each treatment modality has advantages and disadvantages.
- Survival of zirconia abutments may be influenced by:
  - Manufacturing methods, and clinical and laboratory handling
  - The abutment wall thickness; a minimum wall thickness of 0.5 mm has been recommended
  - Implant-abutment connection
  - Aging of materials (low-temperature degradation)
  - Implant location

Continued

Financial Disclosures and/or Conflicts of Interest: The authors have nothing to disclose.
[a] Department of Prosthodontics, The University of Iowa College of Dentistry, 801 Newton Road, Dental Sciences Building S432, Iowa City, IA 55242, USA; [b] Restorative Dentistry, School of Dentistry, West Virginia University, PO Box 9495, Morgantown, WV 26506, USA; [c] Department of Prosthodontics, School of Dentistry, University of North Carolina, 330 Brauer Hall, CB# 7450, Chapel Hill, NC 27599-7450, USA
* Corresponding author.
E-mail address: Lyndon_Cooper@unc.edu

Dent Clin N Am 58 (2014) 207–225
http://dx.doi.org/10.1016/j.cden.2013.09.007
0011-8532/14/$ – see front matter © 2014 Elsevier Inc. All rights reserved.

Continued

- The use of computer-aided design/computer-assisted manufacture technologies for the manufacture of implant superstructures has proved to be advantageous in the quality of materials, precision of the milled superstructures, and passive fit.
- Maintenance and recall evaluations are an essential component of implant therapy. The longevity of implant restorations is limited by their biological and prosthetic maintenance requirements.

INTRODUCTION

Current tooth-replacement strategies typically consider the alloplastic-integrated replacement of missing teeth using endosseous dental implants as a primary choice among available modes of therapy.[1–6] Implants may help preserve adjacent teeth from long-term biological complications. Clinical data indicate that abutment teeth of fixed or removable prostheses are at increased risk for caries, pulp injury, or even tooth loss as a result of these complications.[7–9] The use of implants improves the stability and retention of removable prostheses.[10] Of importance, the prescription of dental implants provides an alternative for patients who desire a fixed prosthesis or are psychologically unable to accept a removable prosthesis.[11]

Despite the favorable long-term outcomes achieved with prosthetic rehabilitations with implants, biological and technical complications are frequent.[12] Systematic reviews of the survival and complications of implants and associated prostheses identified 6 categories of complications: surgical complications, implant loss, bone loss, peri-implant soft-tissue complications, mechanical complications, and aesthetic/phonetic complications.[13] Such complications are affected by many factors, including the operator's skills and judgments in treatment planning, prosthesis design, materials, patient-specific factors, and local and systemic conditions and habits such as bruxism, smoking, presence of periodontal disease, and maintenance. Prosthetically driven treatment planning for implant placement that is properly communicated to the surgeon is critical to ensure adequate restorative space for the various prosthetic designs, appropriate implant angulation, and minimizing cantilevers. Ultimately, long-term success of the fabricated prosthesis also relies on the patient's commitment to proper hygiene measures and recall appointments to ensure good-quality maintenance of restorations.

When considering implant prosthodontic treatment for rehabilitation of the partially or fully edentulous patient, the clinician has several choices including, but not limited to:

- Use of fixed or removable prostheses
- Use of individual attachments or bars for retention of removable overdentures
- Use of screw-retained or cement-retained prostheses
- Use of stock versus custom abutments
- Different restorative and abutment materials

A consensus statement suggested the 2-implant–supported overdenture as the minimum standard of care for the edentulous mandible (**Fig. 1**).[10] In addition, maxillary removable overdentures may be considered as a satisfactory treatment option for patients with complaints about the retention and stability of their dentures.[14,15] A main advantage of this treatment modality is hygiene access, in addition to providing proper lip support for patients with insufficient alveolar bone volume. Maxillary and

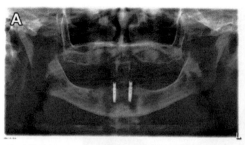
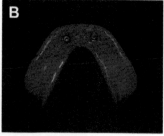

Fig. 1. (A) Panoramic radiograph of 2 implants placed in the mandibular symphysis area used to retain a mandibular overdenture. (B) An occlusal view of the intaglio surface of an implant-retained overdenture with 2 locator attachments.

mandibular removable overdentures are typically fabricated with acrylic resin prosthetic teeth processed on a rigid acrylic resin base that may be reinforced with a metal frame, often used for the maxillary overdentures with a horseshoe-shaped design (**Fig. 2**).[16] The use of metal reinforcement is advisable, owing to the frequent base fracture that may be encountered because of the reduced bulk of acrylic resin in accommodating the attachment systems.[17] Overdentures can be retained either by bar-and-clip attachments or by nonsplinted magnets, locators, ball-and-clip attachments, or cone-shaped telescopic copings. Maintenance demands vary with the different prosthetic designs and attachments used.

The prosthodontic literature is controversial regarding the choice of splinted/unsplinted implants when used to retain maxillary overdentures. Unsplinted implant prostheses are less costly, provide easier access for cleaning, are less technique sensitive, and require less prosthetic space within the prostheses. An essential component for the use of either solitary attachments or bars is the restorative space required, which should be integrated in the treatment-planning phase to ensure the fabrication of durable restorations. The minimum vertical distance requirement from the implant platform to the incisal edges, as suggested by Phillips and Wong,[18] is 13 to 14 mm when bars are used. By contrast, solitary attachments require only 10 to 11 mm (**Fig. 3**). Implant angulation, however, plays a critical factor in the retention of solitary anchors,[19] and surgeons should place implants in these cases with focused concern for parallelism.

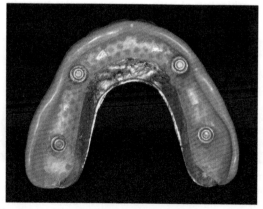

Fig. 2. A maxillary implant-retained overdenture that is reinforced with a metal framework.

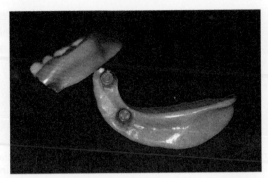

Fig. 3. A mandibular implant-retained overdenture at the site of the locator housing was fractured as a result of insufficient restorative space.

When implant angulation is compromised, the use of either splinted designs involving bars or fabrication of custom anchors may be required. In a systematic review assessing differences between splinted and unsplinted oral implants for implant-retained overdentures. Stoumpis and Kohal[20] reported no differences in implant survival rates or peri-implant outcome between splinted and unsplinted designs, although the bar-supported overdentures have been shown to need less prosthetic maintenance. The observed greater peri-implant mucosal inflammation beneath bar-retained overdentures indicates another important, yet manageable issue when bars are required.

The use of fixed prostheses for maxillary and mandibular complete and partial edentulism is documented in several systematic reviews and many prospective cohort investigations. The general observation of high implant survival (>90% at 5 years) is applicable to the range of applications, but reflects the careful nature of clinical investigations and the training of the investigators.[12,21,22] When patients desire fixed prosthetic reconstruction to replace missing teeth, implants may be used. Guidelines that define the number of implants, the nature of the components, and the nature of the prosthetic construction remain incomplete and in flux.[23]

CEMENT-RETAINED AND SCREW-RETAINED PROSTHESES

Implant-supported restorations can be screw-retained (see **Fig. 4**), cement-retained (see **Fig. 5**), or a combination of both, whereby a metal superstructure is screwed

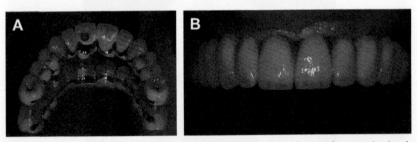

Fig. 4. Full-arch maxillary complete denture screw-retained metal ceramic implant-supported fixed partial denture (FDP) #3-14. (*A*) Occlusal view of screw-retained implant-supported FDP demonstrating absence of unaesthetic access holes. (*B*) Frontal view of screw-retained implant-supported FDP.

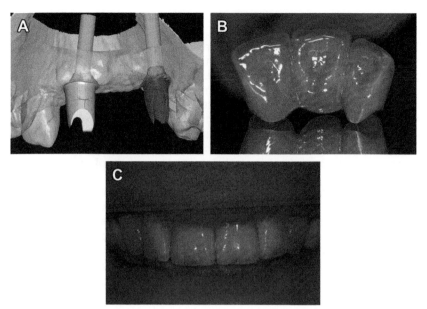

Fig. 5. Cement-retained zirconia implant-supported FDP #8-10. (*A*) A computer-aided design (CAD) of customized abutments for implant-supported FDP #8-10, allowing for proper parallelism and depth of margin placement. (*B*) A zirconia cement-retained implant-supported FDP #8-10. (*C*) Frontal view of smile with implant-supported FDP #8-10 cemented.

to the implants and crowns are individually cemented to the metal frame. Each treatment modality has advantages and disadvantages.

The use of screw-retained restorations provides clinicians with the accessibility of retrieving these restorations if needed for repairs, hygiene, and abutment-screw tightening.[24] If implants are improperly positioned, screw-access holes may compromise aesthetics and occlusion because of the wear of restorative materials used to cover the screw-access channel.[25] A possible complication of screw-retained prostheses is porcelain fracture at the screw-access channel resulting from unsupported porcelain.[26] Ultimately, proactive planning and involvement of the restorative dentist in determining implant positions initially through the diagnostic wax-up phase, and digital planning with the use of cone-beam computed tomography, has become a critical factor in determining the feasibility of this restorative choice and its long-term success.

Cement-retained restorations may offer aesthetic advantages when access holes are visible facially and occlusally (see **Fig. 5**). These restorations may be simpler to fabricate, and provide easier insertion in posterior areas of the mouth for patients with limited jaw openings. In addition, for an implant-supported fixed-denture prosthesis (FDP), the potential for achieving a passive fit is higher with cement-retained restorations.[27,28] Elements that are important for the retention of the cement-retained restorations are essentially the same as those for natural teeth; including taper of axial walls, surface area, height of the abutment, roughness of the surface, and type of cement.[29] Most abutments are manufactured to approximately a 6° taper, which has been considered optimal for crown preparation.[30,31] The minimum abutment height for use of cement-retained restorations with predictable retention was documented as 5 mm.[32] Direct screw fixation at the implant level may be advisable in these instances when the interocclusal space is as little as 4 mm (limited interarch space) (**Fig. 6**).

The main drawbacks of cement-retained restorations are difficult retrievability and retention of excess cement, especially when the restoration margins are placed subgingivally or the implants are deeply placed. Diligence in cement removal at time of cementation is critical. The presence of cement residue can be detrimental to peri-implant health (**Fig. 7**). Residue can cause peri-implant inflammation associated with swelling, soreness, deeper probing depths, bleeding and/or exudation on probing, with radiographic evidence of peri-implant bone loss, and may eventually result in implant loss.[33] A prospective endoscopic clinical study showed that excess cement was associated with signs of peri-implant disease in the majority of cases investigated (81%).[34]

Agar and colleagues[35] demonstrated that when the restorative margins of the abutments are placed 1.5 to 3 mm subgingival, the likelihood of leaving excess cement occurs. Use of screw-retained restorations or custom abutments for cement restorations with higher margins may be used to avoid cement-related complications in situations where implants are deeply placed.

Several techniques have been proposed to help clinicians in eliminating the presence of cement in the peri-implant sulcus, including:

- Using plastic scalers[35,36]
- Reducing the amount of cement placed in the restorations

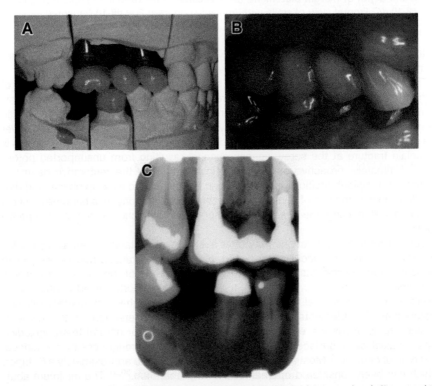

Fig. 6. Screw-retained implant-supported FDP #3-5 with limited interocclusal distance. (*A*) Mounted master cast. (*B*) Clinical photograph. (*C*) Bitewing radiograph.

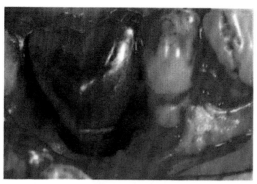

Fig. 7. A clinical photograph demonstrating bone loss around implant #30 caused by excess residual cement not removed at the time of cementation.

- Seating the restoration after placing the cement on the fitting surface on the abutment analog before cementing the restoration intraorally[37]
- Creating a lingual vent hole in the implant-supported crowns[38]
- Using an internal abutment space as a means of decreasing the extrusion of excess cement[39]

Radiographic examination should only be a supplementary method for detection of excess cement. Radiographic density of many implant restorative cements is poor and depends on the thickness of the extruded cement, and radiographic examination cannot be trusted to detect residues of excess cement, especially when present on the facial or lingual aspects of the implant.[40]

Consensus statements from the third consensus conference of the European Association for Osseointegration concluded that both types of reconstructions influenced the clinical outcomes, but none of the fixation methods was clearly advantageous.[23] Cemented and screw-retained single-unit reconstructions had similar survival rates for their supporting implants, whereas cemented multiunit reconstructions had lower survival rates than the screw-retained multiunit reconstructions for their supporting implants. It is important to consider, however, that screw-retained single-unit and multiunit reconstructions tended to have lower reconstruction survival rates. Cemented reconstructions more frequently exhibited serious biological complications (bone loss >2 mm), which may reflect abutment design, margin location, or cement extrusion. The risk for this complication increased with the span of the reconstruction.[41] Clinicians should weigh the advantages and disadvantages of cement-retained and screw-retained types of restorations, so as to select the most appropriate for a given clinical situation. If feasible, long-span and full-arch FDPs as well as riskier cantilever FDPs may be best treated with the screw-retained option, as the complications of these restorations are more frequent.[42]

SELECTION OF ABUTMENTS

The main principles for selecting the appropriate abutment should be aimed to allow for:

- A proper biological response of the tissues
- Provision of the retention and resistance forms essential for cement-retained restorations

- Mechanical strength adequate enough to tolerate fatigue and loading
- Accurate fit with their mating implants
- Achievement of an adequate aesthetic result using the proper emergence profile and abutment material

Abutments used in cement-retained implant restorations maybe either stock pre-fabricated abutments or customized abutments. Several materials have been used, including metal cast with gold alloys, titanium, alumina, and zirconia. In contrast to stock abutments, customized abutments, either cast or built using computer-aided design/computer-assisted manufacture (CAD/CAM), can be made to approximate natural tooth morphology, thereby increasing the total surface area, improving crown retention, and providing a form that supports peri-implant gingival tissue. Moreover, CAD/CAM abutments have advantages over cast abutments including their reduced cost, elimination of the dimensional inaccuracies associated with the casting process, and elimination of the need for additional reductions in stock zirconia abutments that may compromise their strength.

Available clinical data presume that metal abutments made of titanium represent a 'benchmark' with few technical complications the exception being loosening of the abutment screw.[43] One limitation often encountered with the use of metal abutments is the gray discoloration of the peri-implant mucosa in patients with thin tissue biotype.[44] This phenomenon affects aesthetically sensitive areas, especially for patients with a high smile line. In addition, soft-tissue recession in some patients can yield the gray titanium color, which could lead to aesthetic failure of the reconstruction. Ceramic abutments made of high-strength alumina and, more recently, zirconia were developed in efforts to overcome the graying phenomenon associated with metal abutments.

In a spectrophotometric analysis of the color change of the peri-implant soft tissue with different materials, Bressan and colleagues[45] demonstrated that while the color of the soft tissue around titanium implants differed significantly from the gingival color around natural teeth, no significant differences were present in the color performance of abutments made of gold and zirconium oxide. Ultimately, manufacturers developed titanium abutments with nitride coatings that have a gold-shaded hue. These abutments can best be used as an alternative to ceramic abutments in cases with high aesthetic demands.

Analysis of the data collected from clinical settings using ceramic abutments demonstrated a poor performance for alumina abutments; they exhibited a high failure rate, with fracture in 7% of single-implant cases and 1.9% of implant-supported FDPs.[46,47] Hence, the higher-strength zirconia with a bending strength of 900 MPa (574 MPa for alumina) and fracture toughness of 9 MPa m$^{1/2}$ (3.55 MPa m$^{1/2}$ for alumina)[48] may be considered a better choice when ceramic abutments are to be used.

Survival of zirconia abutments may be influenced by[1]:

- Manufacturing methods, and clinical and laboratory handling
- The abutment-wall thickness; a minimum wall thickness of 0.5 mm has been recommended[2]
- Implant-abutment connection
- Aging of materials (low-temperature degradation)
- Implant location

In internal-connection implants, the zirconia abutments can be connected either internally to the implant as one piece by the abutment itself or via a secondary titanium metallic component (**Fig. 8**). Preliminary in vitro data suggested that superior strength maybe achieved by means of internal connection via a secondary metallic component.[49] However, in vivo data are still lacking.

Most of the current studies involving zirconia abutments are limited to implants in the region of premolar and anterior teeth.[1] A concern exists in the first molar region where the highest forces exist.[50] Limited data are available on zirconia abutments in the posterior regions. Zembic and colleagues[1] evaluated the technical and biological complication rates of customized zirconia and titanium abutments placed in the maxillary and mandibular canine and posterior regions 5 years after crown insertion, and reported no abutment fracture throughout that period. While, the existing data on the performance of ceramic abutments are promising, currently available studies on all-ceramic abutments are limited in their numbers and follow-up period. The use of ceramic abutments may be primarily indicated in the aesthetically demanding anterior region, and special consideration should be given to patients with functional disorders, such as bruxism.

Material properties of abutments can influence their integration with the circumferential soft tissues. Conflicting data on the influence of abutment material on the mucosal barrier have been reported. Although reports using the dog model have shown a negative impact of the gold-alloy abutment in its integration with the connective tissue and marginal bone loss,[51,52] evidence from clinical trials shows no difference between gold-alloy abutments and titanium abutments in terms of peri-implant bone stability.[53] However, the connective tissue interface at both titanium and ZrO_2 abutments appears to be similar.[51] The zirconium oxide abutments were shown to have a reduced susceptibility to bacterial adhesion.[54]

Establishment of a direct connective tissue attachment to the supracrestal implant components can be advantageous, as this would prevent the apical downgrowth of the junctional epithelium and act as a physiologic barrier. Scientific evidence pertaining to histologic and radiologic assessments of abutments treated by controlled laser ablation is showing promising results, with reduced crestal bone loss and direct connective tissue attachment to the abutments.[55–57]

FRAMEWORK AND BAR FABRICATION

Traditionally, fabrication of superstructures for full-arch implant-supported FDPs and bars for overdentures was done using the lost-wax technique, which can be very labor

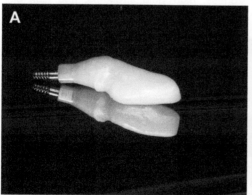 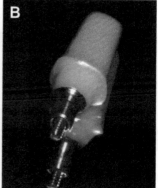

Fig. 8. (*A*) A 1-piece zirconia abutment. (*B*) A zirconia abutment connected to the implant via a secondary metallic piece.

intensive when multiple implants are involved. These techniques often fail to achieve a passive fit.[58–60] Precision of framework fit may be essential for optimal screw mechanics. Several longitudinal clinical studies demonstrated that poorly fitting frameworks could be one of the primary causes of screw loosening or fracture, abutment fractures, and even implant fracture.[61–63] Efforts targeted at improving the adaptation of multiunit fixed restorations included various technical procedures such as soldering, luting and laser welding, spark erosion, and CAD/CAM procedures. The use of CAD/CAM technologies for manufacturing implant superstructures has proven to be advantageous in the quality of materials, precision of the milled superstructures, and passive fit.[3–5] Observations on the clinical outcomes associated with screw-retained fixed-implant prostheses made with laser welding versus frameworks made with milled pure titanium demonstrated significantly more complications in the laser-welded framework group than in the milled framework group.[64] Milled frameworks may be designed, scanned, and milled in a process called copy milling, or can be designed using computer software before milling (**Fig. 9**).

Criteria to be used as design principles essential to the fabrication of implant framework may include adequate access for oral hygiene measures, mechanical strength, and minimal display of metal on the facial and occlusal surfaces.[65]

The long-term performance of implant-supported prostheses may be impaired when access to oral hygiene measures is limited. Hygienic designs for implant frameworks can be achieved readily in mandibular prostheses. However, such designs are often challenging for maxillary implant prostheses regarding the impact on speech and achievement of optimal aesthetics.

The minimum bulk of the framework depends on the material used in each particular case. Several materials have been used in the manufacture of implant frameworks, including:

- Noble metals, in particular type III gold and palladium/silver alloys
- Base-metal alloys
- Titanium and its alloys
- Zirconia

The choice of metal is largely dependent on its casting accuracy, hardness, modulus of elasticity, and handling properties.[65]

Traditionally, noble metals were considered the gold standard for the fabrication of cast frameworks using the lost-wax technique. Although base metals such as chrome-cobalt (Cr-Co) have significant hardness, high yield strengths, and high elastic

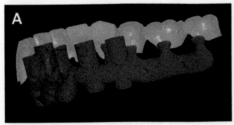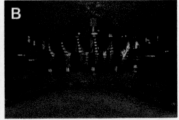

Fig. 9. CAD/computer-assisted manufacture (CAM) mandibular complete denture implant-supported resin-metal FDP. (*A*) Generated CAD of a full-arch implant-supported FDP, based on a diagnostic wax-up. This approach allows proper design for strength and retention. (*B*) Clinical photograph of the CAD/CAM mandibular complete denture implant-supported framework. This framework is fabricated from Co-Cr base metal alloy.

modulus, their use has been limited by the high cost associated with their handling when cast. Recent efforts using the CAD/CAM milling system have facilitated the fabrication of Cr-Co frameworks at a reduced cost. Several investigators suggested that Cr-Co superstructures may well be used as an alternative to gold alloy veneered with ceramic or acrylic resin.[64,66] Milled titanium frameworks possess several advantageous properties including high corrosion resistance, biocompatibility, lower cost, and mechanical strength. Although titanium alloy can be a good material of choice for the fabrication of frameworks for bars in overdentures and for resin-veneered implant-supported complete dentures, its reported performance as a substrate for porcelain veneering is poor. In a 6-year long-term study on metal-ceramic fixed prosthesis with CAD/CAM fabricated substructures, Hey and colleagues[67] reported a success rate of only 58.6%, with porcelain veneer fracture and substructure fracture as causes of failure. Moreover, Ortorp and Jemt[68] documented an overall 10-year cumulative prosthesis survival rate of 88.4% when titanium was used as the superstructure for metal ceramic implant restorations, compared with 100% with the use of conventional metal alloys. This relative failure is largely attributed to the excessive oxidation of the titanium metal during firing of the porcelain veneering.

Implant-supported fixed prostheses can be fabricated with metal frameworks with either acrylic resin and porcelain veneers, or layered and monolithic zirconia superstructures. Porcelain veneering was later introduced as an alternative option to achieve superior aesthetic results, minimal wear, and minimal complications related to resin veneer fracture (**Fig. 10**). A common complication encountered with implant-supported FDPs is the fracture of the veneering material (acrylic, composite, or ceramic). In a systematic review on survival and complication rates of implant-supported FDPs, Pjetursson and colleagues[12] reported higher cumulative 5- and 10-year failure rates for gold-acrylic FDPs (10.7% and 22.6%, respectively) compared with metal ceramic FDPs (5.3% and 6.1%, respectively). A major contributory factor to the high failure rate of gold-acrylic FDPs is the high incidence of veneer fractures.

In certain circumstances a cantilever implant support may be prescribed to provide a simpler rehabilitation procedure, as it may help preclude the need for extra surgical measures such as sinus graft lifts or repositioning of the inferior alveolar nerve. Ultimately, this can circumvent the economic burden of such procedures, and reduce the therapeutic time and potential morbidity that may be associated with such interventions. However, technical complications such as chipping of acrylic resin, screw

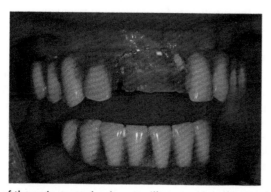

Fig. 10. Chipping of the resin veneering in a maxillary complete denture implant-supported FDP.

loosening, abutment fractures, and framework fractures are not uncommon, especially in cases with inadequate restorative space or anterior-posterior spread. Proper treatment planning, including a prosthodontic diagnostic workup, and consultation between the restoring dentist and the surgeon are imperative in ensuring the appropriate position for implant placement, angulation of the implants, and the need for adjunctive surgical intervention such as alveoloplasty.

SINGLE-IMPLANT RESTORATIONS

Outcomes assessment of single crowns based on the type of reconstruction did not reveal significant differences in the overall survival rates between all-ceramic crowns and metal ceramic crowns. Jung and colleagues,[69] reporting on the survival and complications of single crowns in a systematic assessment of longitudinal studies with a mean follow-up of 5 years, observed common technical complications in both types of reconstruction, with the most common being abutment or screw loosening (8.8%), followed by loss of retention (4.1%) and fracture of the veneering material (3.5%). No differences were observed between porcelain fused to metal crowns and all-ceramic crowns.

MAINTENANCE

Maintenance and recall evaluations are an essential component of implant therapy. The longevity of implant restorations is limited by their biological and prosthetic maintenance requirements.[6] The prosthetic designs of implant restorations should also ensure access for cleaning. It is generally implied that implant patients should be followed up within 6 months of restoration, and at least annually thereafter.[70] Patients should be educated about the importance of proper oral hygiene measures and recall visits.

Recommendations by the American Academy of Periodontology suggest that evaluations of implants at recalls should include[71]:

- Oral hygiene status
- Clinical appearance of peri-implant tissues
- Bleeding on probing and/or presence of exudate
- Pocket probing depths
- Radiographic appearance of peri-implant alveolar bone and its levels related to the implant-abutment junctions
- Stability of the prostheses; screw loosening or cement failure
- Assessment of the prostheses for presence of fractures
- Occlusal assessment
- Denture teeth wear
- Patient comfort and function

Maintenance for implant overdentures may require more postinsertion maintenance than implant-supported fixed prostheses.[72] The highest frequency of complications occurs in the first year.[73] Similarly, reports on complications of implant-supported fixed restorations noted a time-related course, with an increased prevalence of resin fractures at the beginning of the clinical period and progression of severe wear in the later stages of follow-up.[74]

Long-term success of overdenture therapy depends on patients' commitment to periodic maintenance, with the most common requirement being replacement of the matrix portion of the different attachments. The frequency of replacement of the matrices varies with each clinical situation and may be influenced by patient-related factors (eg, parafunctional habits, dietary habits) and implant-related factors (interimplant distance, attachment angulations in relation to the occlusal plane, type of attachment).[6,75] It is recommended that the rubber O-ring is replaced annually or biannually.[76] The prevalence of wear reported for ball abutments with metal clips is lower than with the resilient rubber O-rings[77] or nylon inserts.[78] However, resilient clips may be more advisable, as they produce less wear on their respective patrices.[17] On the other hand, reported maintenance events are very frequent with magnet-attachment systems because of their corrosion and wear.[17] Nissan and colleagues[79] reported that the incorporation technique of the attachment system had some influence on maintenance aftercare, visits with a higher immediate (relief of pressure sores) and long-term (attachment replacement) effect using the indirect technique (laboratory) rather than the direct technique (intraoral chairside). Another issue with implant overdentures is gingival hyperplasia, especially with maxillary prostheses. The incidence of hyperplasia adjacent to a bar was reported to be as high as 64% over a 7-year follow-up period.[80] The mucosal inflammation is often aggravated by patients' continuously wearing their prosthesis (**Fig. 11**). Naert and colleagues[14] reported that although patients were advised to remove their dentures nocturnally, only half complied. Mechanical complications with overdentures are among the most common reported, especially for maxillary prostheses, most often because of the limited restorative space available. Again, surgical planning becomes a critical factor in helping to reduce the incidence of such complications. Prosthetic reinforcement with a cast Cr-Co framework may help to eliminate this complication.[81]

Studies reporting on the technical complications associated with implant-supported FDPs documented fracture of the veneering material (acrylic, ceramic, or composite) as the most common technical complication (**Fig. 12**).[12] In a systematic review, Pjetursson and colleagues[12] reported that 13.5% of the FDPs had minor or major fractures of the veneering material after 5 years. This technical complication was reduced when the analysis was limited to FDPs with ceramic veneering material (7.8%). By contrast, the prevalence rate of this complication when acrylic was used as the veneering material was 20.2%. Other technical complications reported to occur include loss of screw-access hole restoration (5.4%), abutment of occlusal screw loosening (5.3%), fractures of the luting cement (4.7%), fracture of abutments and occlusal screws (1.3%), and fracture of implants and frameworks (0.5%). Long-term

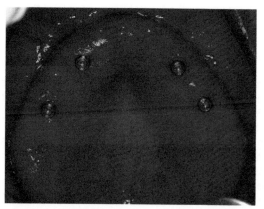

Fig. 11. Erythematous appearance of the maxillary alveolar ridge in a patient who continuously wears her horseshoe-shaped overdenture.

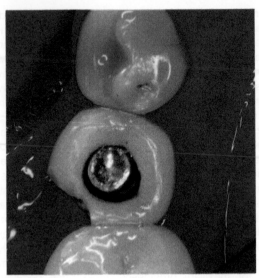

Fig. 12. Occlusal view of a screw-retained implant crown with chipping off the veneering porcelain, a commonly reported technical complication.

studies on implant-supported complete dentures show a longevity-related prevalence of complications, with increased prevalence of resin fractures at the beginning of the clinical period and progression of severe wear in the later stages of follow-up.[74]

REFERENCES

1. Zembic A, Bosch A, Jung RE, et al. Five-year results of a randomized controlled clinical trial comparing zirconia and titanium abutments supporting single-implant crowns in canine and posterior regions. Clin Oral Implants Res 2013; 24(4):384–90.
2. Denry I, Kelly JR. State of the art of zirconia for dental applications. Dent Mater 2008;24(3):299–307.
3. Al-Fadda SA, Zarb GA, Finer Y. A comparison of the accuracy of fit of 2 methods for fabricating implant-prosthodontic frameworks. Int J Prosthodont 2007;20(2): 125–31.
4. Drago C, Saldarriaga RL, Domagala D, et al. Volumetric determination of the amount of misfit in CAD/CAM and cast implant frameworks: a multicenter laboratory study. Int J Oral Maxillofac Implants 2010;25(5):920–9.
5. Ortorp A, Jemt T, Back T, et al. Comparisons of precision of fit between cast and CNC-milled titanium implant frameworks for the edentulous mandible. Int J Prosthodont 2003;16(2):194–200.
6. Payne AG, Solomons YF. The prosthodontic maintenance requirements of mandibular mucosa- and implant-supported overdentures: a review of the literature. Int J Prosthodont 2000;13(3):238–43.
7. Goodacre CJ, Bernal G, Rungcharassaeng K, et al. Clinical complications in fixed prosthodontics. J Prosthet Dent 2003;90(1):31–41.
8. Tan K, Pjetursson BE, Lang NP, et al. A systematic review of the survival and complication rates of fixed partial dentures (FPDs) after an observation period of at least 5 years. Clin Oral Implants Res 2004;15(6):654–66.

9. Vermeulen AH, Keltjens HM, van't Hof MA, et al. Ten-year evaluation of removable partial dentures: survival rates based on retreatment, not wearing and replacement. J Prosthet Dent 1996;76(3):267–72.

10. Feine JS, Carlsson GE, Awad MA, et al. The McGill consensus statement on overdentures. Mandibular two-implant overdentures as first choice standard of care for edentulous patients. Montreal, Quebec, May 24-25, 2002. Int J Oral Maxillofac Implants 2002;17(4):601–2.

11. Albrektsson T, Blomberg S, Branemark A, et al. Edentulousness—an oral handicap. Patient reactions to treatment with jawbone-anchored prostheses. J Oral Rehabil 1987;14(6):503–11.

12. Pjetursson BE, Thoma D, Jung R, et al. A systematic review of the survival and complication rates of implant-supported fixed dental prostheses (FDPs) after a mean observation period of at least 5 years. Clin Oral Implants Res 2012; 23(Suppl 6):22–38.

13. Goodacre CJ, Bernal G, Rungcharassaeng K, et al. Clinical complications with implants and implant prostheses. J Prosthet Dent 2003;90(2):121–32.

14. Naert I, Gizani S, van Steenberghe D. Rigidly splinted implants in the resorbed maxilla to retain a hinging overdenture: a series of clinical reports for up to 4 years. J Prosthet Dent 1998;79(2):156–64.

15. Zembic A, Wismeijer D. Patient-reported outcomes of maxillary implant-supported overdentures compared with conventional dentures. Clin Oral Implants Res 2013. [Epub ahead of print].

16. Bryant SR, MacDonald-Jankowski D, Kim K. Does the type of implant prosthesis affect outcomes for the completely edentulous arch? Int J Oral Maxillofac Implants 2007;22(Suppl):117–39.

17. Osman RB, Payne AG, Ma S. Prosthodontic maintenance of maxillary implant overdentures: a systematic literature review. Int J Prosthodont 2012;25(4): 381–91.

18. Phillips K, Wong KM. Space requirements for implant-retained bar-and-clip overdentures. Compend Contin Educ Dent 2001;22(6):516–8, 520, 522.

19. Gulizio MP, Agar JR, Kelly JR, et al. Effect of implant angulation upon retention of overdenture attachments. J Prosthodont 2005;14(1):3–11.

20. Stoumpis C, Kohal RJ. To splint or not to splint oral implants in the implant-supported overdenture therapy? A systematic literature review. J Oral Rehabil 2011;38(11):857–69.

21. Papaspyridakos P, Mokti M, Chen CJ, et al. Implant and prosthodontic survival rates with implant fixed complete dental prostheses in the edentulous mandible after at least 5 years: a systematic review. Clin Implant Dent Relat Res 2013. [Epub ahead of print].

22. Vouros ID, Kalpidis CD, Horvath A, et al. Systematic assessment of clinical outcomes in bone-level and tissue-level endosseous dental implants. Int J Oral Maxillofac Implants 2012;27(6):1359–74.

23. Gotfredsen K, Wiskott A, Working Group 4. Consensus report—reconstructions on implants. The Third EAO Consensus Conference 2012. Clin Oral Implants Res 2012;23(Suppl 6):238–41.

24. Nissan J, Narobai D, Gross O, et al. Long-term outcome of cemented versus screw-retained implant-supported partial restorations. Int J Oral Maxillofac Implants 2011;26(5):1102–7.

25. Chee W, Felton DA, Johnson PF, et al. Cemented versus screw-retained implant prostheses: which is better? Int J Oral Maxillofac Implants 1999; 14(1):137–41.

26. Hebel KS, Gajjar RC. Cement-retained versus screw-retained implant restorations: achieving optimal occlusion and esthetics in implant dentistry. J Prosthet Dent 1997;77(1):28–35.

27. Michalakis KX, Hirayama H, Garefis PD. Cement-retained versus screw-retained implant restorations: a critical review. Int J Oral Maxillofac Implants 2003;18(5):719–28.

28. Karl M, Taylor TD, Wichmann MG, et al. In vivo stress behavior in cemented and screw-retained five-unit implant FPDs. J Prosthodont 2006;15(1):20–4.

29. Emms M, Tredwin CJ, Setchell DJ, et al. The effects of abutment wall height, platform size, and screw access channel filling method on resistance to dislodgement of cement-retained, implant-supported restorations. J Prosthodont 2007;16(1):3–9.

30. Enkling N, Ueda T, Gholami H, et al. Precision of fit and retention force of cast non-precious-crowns on standard titanium implant-abutment with different design and height. Clin Oral Implants Res 2013. [Epub ahead of print].

31. Wilson AH Jr, Chan DC. The relationship between preparation convergence and retention of extracoronal retainers. J Prosthodont 1994;3(2):74–8.

32. Edward GK, David HC, Laurence C. Factors influencing the retention of cemented gold castings. J Prosthet Dent 1961;11(3):487–502.

33. Gapski R, Neugeboren N, Pomeranz AZ, et al. Endosseous implant failure influenced by crown cementation: a clinical case report. Int J Oral Maxillofac Implants 2008;23(5):943–6.

34. Wilson TG Jr. The positive relationship between excess cement and peri-implant disease: a prospective clinical endoscopic study. J Periodontol 2009;80(9):1388–92.

35. Agar JR, Cameron SM, Hughbanks JC, et al. Cement removal from restorations luted to titanium abutments with simulated subgingival margins. J Prosthet Dent 1997;78(1):43–7.

36. Dmytryk JJ, Fox SC, Moriarty JD. The effects of scaling titanium implant surfaces with metal and plastic instruments on cell attachment. J Periodontol 1990;61(8):491–6.

37. Dumbrigue HB, Abanomi AA, Cheng LL. Techniques to minimize excess luting agent in cement-retained implant restorations. J Prosthet Dent 2002;87(1):112–4.

38. Schwedhelm ER, Lepe X, Aw TC. A crown venting technique for the cementation of implant-supported crowns. J Prosthet Dent 2003;89(1):89–90.

39. Wadhwani C, Pineyro A, Hess T, et al. Effect of implant abutment modification on the extrusion of excess cement at the crown-abutment margin for cement-retained implant restorations. Int J Oral Maxillofac Implants 2011;26(6):1241–6.

40. Pette GA, Ganeles J, Norkin FJ. Radiographic appearance of commonly used cements in implant dentistry. Int J Periodontics Restorative Dent 2013;33(1):61–8.

41. Sailer I, Muhlemann S, Zwahlen M, et al. Cemented and screw-retained implant reconstructions: a systematic review of the survival and complication rates. Clin Oral Implants Res 2012;23(Suppl 6):163–201.

42. Chaar MS, Att W, Strub JR. Prosthetic outcome of cement-retained implant-supported fixed dental restorations: a systematic review. J Oral Rehabil 2011;38(9):697–711.

43. Pjetursson BE, Bragger U, Lang NP, et al. Comparison of survival and complication rates of tooth-supported fixed dental prostheses (FDPs) and implant-supported FDPs and single crowns (SCs). Clin Oral Implants Res 2007;18(Suppl 3):97–113.

44. Jung RE, Sailer I, Hammerle CH, et al. In vitro color changes of soft tissues caused by restorative materials. Int J Periodontics Restorative Dent 2007; 27(3):251–7.
45. Bressan E, Paniz G, Lops D, et al. Influence of abutment material on the gingival color of implant-supported all-ceramic restorations: a prospective multicenter study. Clin Oral Implants Res 2011;22(6):631–7.
46. Andersson B, Taylor A, Lang BR, et al. Alumina ceramic implant abutments used for single-tooth replacement: a prospective 1- to 3-year multicenter study. Int J Prosthodont 2001;14(5):432–8.
47. Andersson B, Scharer P, Simion M, et al. Ceramic implant abutments used for short-span fixed partial dentures: a prospective 2-year multicenter study. Int J Prosthodont 1999;12(4):318–24.
48. Anusavice K. Phillips' science of dental materials. 11th edition. St Louis (MO): Elsevier Health Sciences; 2003.
49. Sailer I, Sailer T, Stawarczyk B, et al. In vitro study of the influence of the type of connection on the fracture load of zirconia abutments with internal and external implant-abutment connections. Int J Oral Maxillofac Implants 2009;24(5):850–8.
50. Ferrario VF, Tartaglia GM, Maglione M, et al. Neuromuscular coordination of masticatory muscles in subjects with two types of implant-supported prostheses. Clin Oral Implants Res 2004;15(2):219–25.
51. Welander M, Abrahamsson I, Berglundh T. The mucosal barrier at implant abutments of different materials. Clin Oral Implants Res 2008;19(7):635–41.
52. Abrahamsson I, Berglundh T, Glantz PO, et al. The mucosal attachment at different abutments. An experimental study in dogs. J Clin Periodontol 1998; 25(9):721–7.
53. Vigolo P, Givani A, Majzoub Z, et al. A 4-year prospective study to assess peri-implant hard and soft tissues adjacent to titanium versus gold-alloy abutments in cemented single implant crowns. J Prosthodont 2006;15(4):250–6.
54. Scarano A, Piattelli M, Caputi S, et al. Bacterial adhesion on commercially pure titanium and zirconium oxide disks: an in vivo human study. J Periodontol 2004; 75(2):292–6.
55. Botos S, Yousef H, Zweig B, et al. The effects of laser microtexturing of the dental implant collar on crestal bone levels and peri-implant health. Int J Oral Maxillofac Implants 2011;26(3):492–8.
56. Nevins M, Kim DM, Jun SH, et al. Histologic evidence of a connective tissue attachment to laser microgrooved abutments: a canine study. Int J Periodontics Restorative Dent 2010;30(3):245–55.
57. Nevins M, Camelo M, Nevins ML, et al. Connective tissue attachment to laser-microgrooved abutments: a human histologic case report. Int J Periodontics Restorative Dent 2012;32(4):385–92.
58. Carr AB, Stewart RB. Full-arch implant framework casting accuracy: preliminary in vitro observation for in vivo testing. J Prosthodont 1993;2(1):2–8.
59. Haselhuhn K, Marotti J, Tortamano P, et al. Assessment of the stress transmitted to dental implants connected to screw-retained bars using different casting techniques. J Oral Implantol 2012. [Epub ahead of print].
60. Mitha T, Owen CP, Howes DG. The three-dimensional casting distortion of five implant-supported frameworks. Int J Prosthodont 2009;22(3):248–50.
61. Jemt T, Book K, Linden B, et al. Failures and complications in 92 consecutively inserted overdentures supported by Branemark implants in severely resorbed edentulous maxillae: a study from prosthetic treatment to first annual check-up. Int J Oral Maxillofac Implants 1992;7(2):162–7.

62. Naert I, Quirynen M, van Steenberghe D, et al. A study of 589 consecutive implants supporting complete fixed prostheses. Part II: prosthetic aspects. J Prosthet Dent 1992;68(6):949–56.

63. Zarb GA, Schmitt A. The longitudinal clinical effectiveness of osseointegrated dental implants: the Toronto study. Part III: problems and complications encountered. J Prosthet Dent 1990;64(2):185–94.

64. Hjalmarsson L, Smedberg JI, Pettersson M, et al. Implant-level prostheses in the edentulous maxilla: a comparison with conventional abutment-level prostheses after 5 years of use. Int J Prosthodont 2011;24(2):158–67.

65. Drago C, Howell K. Concepts for designing and fabricating metal implant frameworks for hybrid implant prostheses. J Prosthodont 2012;21(5):413–24.

66. Teigen K, Jokstad A. Dental implant suprastructures using cobalt-chromium alloy compared with gold alloy framework veneered with ceramic or acrylic resin: a retrospective cohort study up to 18 years. Clin Oral Implants Res 2012;23(7):853–60.

67. Hey J, Beuer F, Bensel T, et al. Metal-ceramic-fixed dental prosthesis with CAD/CAM-fabricated substructures: 6-year clinical results. Clin Oral Investig 2013; 17(5):1447–51.

68. Ortorp A, Jemt T. Laser-welded titanium frameworks supported by implants in the partially edentulous mandible: a 10-year comparative follow-up study. Clin Implant Dent Relat Res 2008;10(3):128–39.

69. Jung RE, Zembic A, Pjetursson BE, et al. Systematic review of the survival rate and the incidence of biological, technical, and aesthetic complications of single crowns on implants reported in longitudinal studies with a mean follow-up of 5 years. Clin Oral Implants Res 2012;23(Suppl 6):2–21.

70. Academy of Osseointegration. 2010 Guidelines of the academy of osseointegration for the provision of dental implants and associated patient care. Int J Oral Maxillofac Implants 2010;25(3):620–7.

71. Parameter on placement and management of the dental implant. American Academy of Periodontology. J Periodontol 2000;71(Suppl 5):870–2.

72. Engquist B, Bergendal T, Kallus T, et al. A retrospective multicenter evaluation of osseointegrated implants supporting overdentures. Int J Oral Maxillofac Implants 1988;3(2):129–34.

73. Walton JN, MacEntee MI. Problems with prostheses on implants: a retrospective study. J Prosthet Dent 1994;71(3):283–8.

74. Jemt T, Johansson J. Implant treatment in the edentulous maxillae: a 15-year follow-up study on 76 consecutive patients provided with fixed prostheses. Clin Implant Dent Relat Res 2006;8(2):61–9.

75. Fromentin O, Lassauzay C, Nader SA, et al. Clinical wear of overdenture ball attachments after 1, 3 and 8 years. Clin Oral Implants Res 2011;22(11):1270–4.

76. Watson RM, Jemt T, Chai J, et al. Prosthodontic treatment, patient response, and the need for maintenance of complete implant-supported overdentures: an appraisal of 5 years of prospective study. Int J Prosthodont 1997;10(4):345–54.

77. Cordioli G, Majzoub Z, Castagna S. Mandibular overdentures anchored to single implants: a five-year prospective study. J Prosthet Dent 1997;78(2):159–65.

78. Kleis WK, Kammerer PW, Hartmann S, et al. A comparison of three different attachment systems for mandibular two-implant overdentures: one-year report. Clin Implant Dent Relat Res 2010;12(3):209–18.

79. Nissan J, Oz-Ari B, Gross O, et al. Long-term prosthetic aftercare of direct vs. indirect attachment incorporation techniques to mandibular implant-supported overdenture. Clin Oral Implants Res 2011;22(6):627–30.

80. Ekfeldt A, Johansson LA, Isaksson S. Implant-supported overdenture therapy: a retrospective study. Int J Prosthodont 1997;10(4):366–74.
81. Smedberg JI, Nilner K, Frykholm A. A six-year follow-up study of maxillary overdentures on osseointegrated implants. Eur J Prosthodont Restor Dent 1999;7(2): 51–6.

Caries Management by Risk Assessment Care Paths for Prosthodontic Patients
Oral Microbial Control and Management

Roy T. Yanase, DDS[a,b], Hamilton H. Le, DMD[c],*

KEYWORDS

- Caries management • Risk assessment • Care paths • Prosthodontic • Patients

KEY POINTS

- Current trends in dental disease management are centered on the identification or presence of disease and the mechanical elimination of the infected structures.
- The development of an oral care path redirects the focus on the identification of the early indicators of disease, before its existence. Once the risks have been identified and diagnosed, then the proper therapies can be selected and prescribed.
- The initial protocol of Featherstone's research centered on the wide spectrum of caries, from white demineralized lesions to severe loss of tooth structure. He emphasized the effects of established preventive measures of xylitol, chlorhexidine, fluorides of increasing strengths, including varnish applications, and diet control.
- Some of the results are noncarious cervical lesions and some are caused by bacteria-induced inflammation, whereas others include bacteria-saturated harmful biofilm, which contributes to the effects on damaged tooth structure, lost supporting periodontium, multiple restorations, and missing teeth.
- The experienced practitioner must meld clinical experience and observation with rapidly evolving, evidence-based scientific dentistry and information on the treatment and prevention of continued disease for the prosthodontic patient after restorations have been completed.
- The incorporation of dental implants, once thought of as a 98% successful procedure, has not allowed for complications of caries and periodontal disease on teeth and implants. Thus, osseoseparation is necessary for justification of continued maintenance.

[a] American Board of Prosthodontics, Advanced Prosthodontic Education, Ostrow School of Dentistry at USC, Los Angeles, CA, USA; [b] Continuing Dental Education, Ostrow School of Dentistry at USC, Los Angeles, CA, USA; [c] California Section, Department of Post Graduate Prosthodontics, American College of Prosthodontists, Tufts University School of Dental Medicine, Boston, MA, USA
* Corresponding author.
E-mail address: hamle216@gmail.com

Dent Clin N Am 58 (2014) 227–245
http://dx.doi.org/10.1016/j.cden.2013.09.013
0011-8532/14/$ – see front matter © 2014 Elsevier Inc. All rights reserved.

INTRODUCTION

Current evidence-based dentistry studies on caries control in children (ref.) have changed the standard of care from the pediatric dental specialty to the medical model of infectious disease. Featherstone and colleagues have a renewed interest in caries management for all patients, beyond the boundaries of pediatric dentistry, from the young to the elderly. The Baby Boomer generation combines a population of health care–dependent and pharmacologically reliant aging individuals. In 2010, the population was estimated to have 40.3 million people 65 years of age and older, and was projected to reach 88.5 million individuals by 2050, a growth of nearly 20%.[1] This paradigm shift has significant implications for the need and demand for general and oral health, and included in this demographic is the prosthodontic patient (**Fig. 1**).

The management of oral and general health becomes more difficult as every decade progresses for these individuals. Hypertension, cholesterol, diabetes, depression, and decreased manual dexterity are among the more common medical conditions that afflict the aging. Caries continues to pose great challenges in prosthetic and restorative dentistry. Pjetursson and colleagues[2] found that natural tooth abutment caries was the second most prevalent complication behind tooth devitalization. Goodacre and colleagues[3] in an 8-year study found that there was a 27% incidence of failure with fixed partial dentures, of which 18% was caused by caries in the abutment teeth.

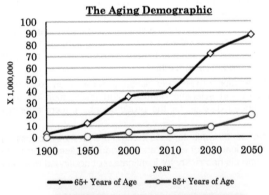

Year	Age 65+	Age 85+
1900	3,100,000	120,000
1950	12,300,000	580,000
2000	35,000,000	4,200,000
2010	40,300,000	5,700,000
2030	72,100,000	8,700,000
2050	88,500,000	19,000,000

Fig. 1. The Aging Demographic. (*Data from* US Administration on Aging/US Census Bureau. Available at: http://www.aoa.gov/Aging_Statistics/Census_Population/Index.aspx.)

Most Common Fixed Partial Denture Complications

The largest obstacle for prosthodontics is not the fabrication of exceptional prosthetics but long-term supportive therapy to balance the risk factors for bacterial management (**Table 1**).

Prevention for the Prosthodontic Practice

For decades, as remains true, the 2 diseases that have accounted most for tooth loss are dental caries and periodontal disease.[4–7] Evidence of tooth decay was recorded as far back as 5000 BC, when a tooth worm was described as the cause of the demineralization of dental enamel. The legend of the worm is also found in the writings of Homer, and as late as the 14th century AD, the surgeon Guy de Chauliac still promoted the belief that worms cause tooth decay.[8] Current clinical studies have shown that caries is associated with increases in the proportions of acidogenic and aciduric (acid-tolerating) bacteria, especially streptococci (such as *Streptococcus mutans* and *Streptococcus sobrinus*) and lactobacilli, which are capable of demineralizing enamel.[9–12]

The role of caries management by risk assessment (CAMBRA) for the primary and secondary dentition identifies the causes of dental disease by assessing the degree of risk that an individual possesses and targeting the cause of caries, periodontal disease, recession, and xerostomia, for the prevention of tooth loss. Identification of these factors, which regulate the natural homeostasis present in plaque during health, but when disrupted drive the enrichment of oral pathogens, is crucial to the management of oral bacteria. Further manipulation of these ecologic influences could help maintain the beneficial microbial composition and normal metabolic activity of plaque biofilms and augment more conventional approaches to control caries (**Table 2**).[13]

A prosthodontic practice is not always exclusively comprehensive and restorative in nature, and often includes patients with removable and fixed appliances, special needs limitations, and developmental deficiencies. Prosthodontics has incorporated predictable dental implants into the established protocols of recent generations of restorative dentists, who previously had mainly concentrated on restoring and reresstoring damaged dentition. The application of ossseointegrated implants in restorative dentistry has contributed to the expanded role of prosthetic reconstruction. Long-term

Table 1
The most common complications in fixed prosthodontics

Cause of Failure	Number of Prostheses or Abutments Studied/Affected	Mean Incidence (%)
Caries	3360/602 abutments	18
	1354/113 prostheses	8
Need for endodontic treatment	2514/276 abutments	11
	13576/88 prostheses	7
Loss of retention	1906/137 prostheses	7
Esthetics	1024/58 prostheses	6
Periodontal disease	1440/62 prostheses	4
Tooth fracture	1602/44 prostheses	3
Prosthesis fracture	1192/24 prostheses	2
Porcelain veneer fracture	768/17 prostheses	2

Data from Goodacre CJ, Bernal G, Rungharasseng K, et al. Clinical complications with implants and implant prostheses. J Prosthet Dent 2003;90(2):121–32; with permission.

Table 2
Risk factors contribute to the increased prevalence of dental caries by affecting the oral environment to favor the conditions suitable for bacterial proliferation

Common Risk Factors	
Medical Conditions	Dietary Habits
Xerostomia	Eating disorders
Sjögren syndrome	Sport drinks
Celiac disease	Soda
Gastroesophageal reflux disease	Citrus fruits and juices
Intravenous bisphosphonates	Energy drinks
Chemotherapy	Pickled foods or vinegar
Diabetes	Candy
Alzheimer disease or dementia	Lifestyle
Sleep apnea	Stress
Prescribed medications	Smoking
Dental Conditions	Alcohol excess
Fixed and removable oral Rehabilitation	Pregnancy
	Substance abuse

research for periodontal prosthetics, at the University of Pennsylvania, established the role of prosthodontics in the retention of the natural dentition with full and partial arch prosthetic restorations. The inclusion of combined interdisciplinary periodontal, endodontic, and prosthetic recall supportive therapy was essential to long-term supportive maintenance for success. Endodontic failure, prosthetic complication, and caries were implicated as major problems if periodontal therapy was successfully maintained.

The principles of informed consent remain a primary legal right for all patients to understand the risks and benefits of treatment options before allowing the removal of teeth that can be treated within their financial responsibilities. Informed patients can demand that every effort to retain as many of their natural teeth for as long as possible be considered an option. The specialty of prosthodontics is a cerebral specialty. As with all specialties, prosthodontics includes the knowledge of all available procedures within that specialty. It is just as important to know how and when to perform a procedure as well as when not to perform a procedure. It is essential to include the patient in a long-term program for supportive maintenance and control of the causes of the most common cause of prosthetic failure, caries.

Caries Initiation

Caries is a result of changes in the environment caused by acid production from the fermentation of dietary carbohydrates, which selects for acidogenic and acid-tolerating species such as mutans streptococci and lactobacilli.

In any ecosystem, homeostasis can break down on occasion because of a substantial change in a parameter that is critical to maintaining ecologic stability at a site.[14]

The formation of the pellicle on the tooth surface is the first and most important step of the bacteria colonization process (Fig. 5.1). The pellicle acts as a protective layer to slow the diffusion of acid as well as being a reservoir for calcium and phosphate. It also acts as an attachment catalyst for early bacterial colonizers, *Streptococcus sobrinus* and *Actinomyces viscosus*.

The polysaccharide surface proteins produced by these bacteria enable cell to pellicle surface adhesion, which in turn attracts the attachment of *S mutans*, and the opportunistic colonization of lactobacilli. These bacteria can rapidly metabolize dietary sugars to acid, creating locally a low pH. These organisms multiply and metabolize optimally at low pH. Under such conditions, they become more competitive, whereas most species associated with enamel health are sensitive to acidic environmental conditions.[13] Carious disease could be prevented not only by targeting the pathogens directly but also by interfering with the key environmental factors driving the deleterious ecologic shifts in the composition of the plaque biofilms.[14]

XEROSTOMIA

The production and presence of saliva are crucial in maintaining the health of the oral soft tissues and providing antimicrobial and pH buffering effects. A normal flow of 1.5 L per day contains calcium and phosphate, bicarbonate, immunoglobins, mucins, and proteins, all of which are essential in contributing to the remineralization of tooth enamel and the neutralization of acids in the oral cavity (**Table 3**). Reduced salivary flow can be a result of damaged salivary glands but is commonly an associated side effect of various medical conditions; uncontrolled diabetes, chemotherapy, head and neck radiation, and autoimmune disorders.

Eighty percent of the most common prescriptions in the United States, more than 500 medications, list xerostomia as a known side effect.[15] More commonly referred to as dry mouth, it is highly correlated with the initiation and progression of dental caries. More than half of all adults take prescription medications and 1 in 5 takes 4 or more medications per day.[16] It is common for individuals to be taking a prescription medication, and when multiple drugs are taken, the effects are compounding, increasing the severity (**Fig. 2**).

pH: Demineralization Versus Remineralization

Carbonated hydroxyapatite (cHAP), a calcium-deficient form of hydroxyapatite (HAP), is the principle mineral in teeth and bones. The substitution of phosphate (PO_4^-), in HAP can take place with various metal ions, most commonly, carbonate (CO_3). The substitution disturbs the crystal lattice of enamel and thus creates cHAP, an acid-soluble substrate more soluble than HAP, which is in turn more soluble than fluorapatite (FAP) (**Table 4**).[17]

HAP demineralization begins at pH 5.5, but under healthy circumstances, when conditions reach these levels, saliva frequently neutralizes the acid attack and restores balance to the oral cavity. The substitution of the hydroxide ions (OH^-) in HAP with fluoride (F^-) anions yields a FAP surface.

Fluoride

The physical characteristics of the fluoride ion (F^-) closely resemble the hydroxide ion (OH^-). This similarity enables the substitution of the hydroxide ion (OH^-), in HAP, by fluoride (F^-) forming FAP, a more resistant structure that resists the demineralization process up to pH 4.5, whereas HAP demineralizes at pH 5.5.[18]

Little agreement exists surrounding effect of fluorides (F^-) on bacterial cell inhibition. Previous studies highlight an F^--induced reduction in acid production contributed by the inhibition of the glycolytic enzyme, enolase, which converts 2-P-glycerate to P-enolpyruvate (PEP). The decreased output of PEP in the presence of F^- results in the inhibition of sugar transport.[19]

Bacterial accumulation of fluoride involves the transport of HF, a process requiring a transmembrane pH difference or pH gradient, which is generated only by metabolically active cells. The uptake of HF into the more alkaline cytoplasm results in the dissociation of HF to H+ and F^- and, if allowed to continue, the accumulation of

Table 3
Eighty percent of the most commonly prescribed medications in the United States list dry mouth as a known side effect. Medications that control blood pressure, diabetes, depression, and even antihistamines for allergies cause drying of the mouth

Commonly Prescribed Medications		
Adrenergic Agonist Agent Ephedrine Phenylpropanolamine Pseudoephedrine (Actifed) α-Adrenergic Receptor Agonist Clonidine (Catapres) Analgesic, Narcotic Levorphanol (Levo-Dromoran) Meperidine (Demerol) Methadone hydrochloride (Dolophine) Morphine sulfate (MS Contin) Oxydodone and acetaminophen (Percocet) Oxycodone and aspirin (Percodan) Pentazocine (Talwin) Proxyphene (Darvon)	Antidepressant, Tricyclic Amitriptyline hydrochloride (Elavil) Amoxapine (Asendin) Clomipramine hydrochloride (Anafranil) Desipramine hydrochloride (Nopramin) Doxepin hydrochloride (Sinequan) Imipramine (Tofranil) Loxapine (Loxitane) Maprotiline hydrochloride (Ludiomil) Nortriptyline (Aventyl, Pamelor) Protriptyline hydrochloride (Vivactil)	Antihypertensive Captopril (Capoten) Clonidine (Catapres) Carvedilol (Coreg) Guanethidine (Ismelin) Prazosin (Minipress) Reserpin (Serpasil) Guanabenz (Wystensin) Antiparkinsonian Amantadine (Symmetrel) Benztropine mesylate (Cogentin) Biperiden (Akineton) Carbidopa with levodopa (Sinemet) Levodopa (Larodopa) Trihexyphidyl (Artane) Antispasmodic
	Anorexiant Phentermine (Adipex, Ionamin, Zantryl) Phendimetrazine (Anorex, Adipost) Mazindol (Mazanor, Sanorex) Fenfluramine (Pondimin, Fen-Phen) Diethylpropion (Tenuate, Ten-Tab) Antianxiety Alprazolam (Xamax) Chlordiazepoxide (Librium) Clorazepate dipotassium (Tranxene) Diazepam (Valium) Halazepam (Paxipam)	

Antiacne
  Isotretinoin (Accutane)
Antiallergic, Inhalation
  Cromolyn sodium (Intal)
Antiarrhythmic
  Propafenone (Rhythmol)
  Disopyramide (Norpace)
Anticholinergic
  Atropine sulfate belladonna and opium
  Bentropine mesylate (Cogentin)
  Diphenoxylate and atropine
  glycopyrrolate (Robinul)
  Hyscyamine sulfate (Donnatal)
  Ipratropium bromide (Atrovent)
  Methascopolamine bromide (Pamine)
  Scopolamine (Transderm-Scop)
  Trimipramine (Surmontil)
Antidiarrheal
  Difenoxin with atropine (Motofen)
  Diphenoxylate with atropine (Lomotil)
  Loperamide (Immodium AD)
Adrenergic Agonist, Bronchodilator
  Albuterol (Proventil, Ventolin)
  Bitoterol (Tomlate)
  Isoproterenol (Bronkometer, Bronkosol)
  Terbutaline (Brethaire, Brethine)
α-Adrenergic Receptor Blocker
  Doxazosin (Cardura)
  Guanabenz (Wystensin)
  Guanadrel sulfate (Hylorel)
  Guanethidine (Ismelin)
  Methyledopa (Aldomet)
  Prazosin (Minipress)
  Reserpine (Serpalan)
  Terazosin (Hytrin)
  Hydroxyzine (Atarax, Vistaril)
  Lorazapam (Ativan)
  Meprobamate (Equanil, Miltown)
  Oxazepam (Serax)
  Prazepam (Centrax)
Anticonvulsant
  Carbamazepine (Tegretol)
  Clonazepam (Klonopin)
  Felbamate (Felbatol)
  Gabapentin (Neurontin)
  Lamotrigine (Lamictal)
Antidepressant, SSRI
  Fluoxetine (Prozac)
  Fluvoxamine (Luvox)
  Paroxetine (Paxil)
  Sertaline (Zoloft)
Antidepressant, Miscellaneous
  Buproprion (Welbutrin)
  Fluoxetine (Prozac)
  Nefazodone (Serzone)
  Phenelzine (Nardil MOA)
  Venlafaxine (Effexor)
  Dicyclomine (Bentyl)
  Flaxovate (Urispas)
  Oxybutynin (Ditropan)
Antitussive
  Guaifenesin and codeine
Bronchodilator
  Albuterol (Proventil, Ventolin)
  Ipratropium (Atrovent)
  Isoproterenol (Isuprel)
Decongestant
  Phenylpropanolamine (Ornade)
  Pseudoephedrine (Sudafed)

Abbreviation: SSRI, selective serotonin reuptake inhibitor.

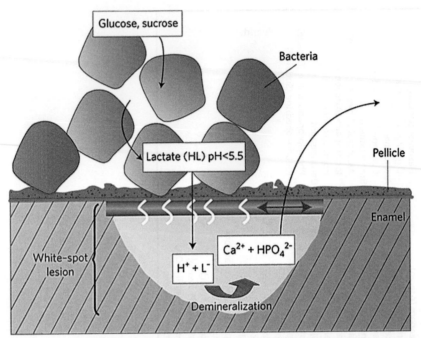

Fig. 2. The combination of fermentable carbohydrates, acidogenic bacteria, and time lead to the slow localized demineralization of tooth enamel. This stage of enamel destruction remains reversible. (*From* Hannig M, Hannig C. Nanomaterials in preventive dentistry. Nat Nanotechnol 2010;5:565–69; with permission.)

protons acidifies the cytoplasm, causing a reduction in both the proton gradient and enzyme activity.

Current information indicates that in addition to enolase, F^- also inhibits the membrane-bound, proton-pumping H+/adenosine triphosphatase (ATPase), which is involved in the generation of proton gradients through the efflux of protons from the cell at the expense of adenosine triphosphate. Thus, fluoride has the dual action of dissipating proton gradients and preventing their generation through its action on H+/ATPase.

The collapse of transmembrane proton gradient, in turn, reduces the ability of cells to transport solutes via mechanisms involving proton motive force. Despite these known effects on the bacterial cell, there is no general agreement that the antimicrobial effects of fluoride contribute to the anticaries effect.

Topical application is the most common form of fluoride delivery in the forms of paste, rinses, and varnishes, whereas systemic intake is available through supplemental tablets or water. The latter is more advantageous during tooth development in adolescents. Its incorporation inhibits demineralization and enhances remineralization of partially dissolved enamel or dentin crystals by combining with calcium and phosphate found in saliva. Its presence accelerates remineralization, forming the FAP surface complex on the remineralized crystal remnants inside the carious lesion.[20]

Chlorhexidine

Developed in the 1940s by Imperial Chemical Industries, United Kingdom, chlorhexidine was not marketed until 1954 as an antiseptic for skin wounds. Its

Table 4
Common commercially available fluoride products available in dentistry

Product	Manufacturer	Name	Active Content and %	Additional Benefits
Toothpaste	3M ESPE	Clinpro 5000	1.1% sodium fluoride	Tricalcium phosphate
	Colgate-Palmolive	Prevident 5000	1.1% sodium fluoride	
	Colgate-Palmolive	Colgate Total Advanced	0.75% sodium monofluorophosphate (calcium-containing paste) or 0.24% sodium fluoride	0.30% triclosan
	Sensodyne (GlaxoSmithKline)	Nupro	1.1% sodium fluoride	Novamin
	Sensodyne (GlaxoSmithKline)	ProEnamel	0.15% sodium fluoride	5% Potassium nitrate (sensitivity)
	Crest (Proctor & Gamble)	ProHealth	0.454% stannous fluoride	
	Aquafresh (GlaxoSmithKline)	Extreme Clean	0.15% sodium fluoride	
Fluoride gel	Colgate-Palmolive	Phos-Flur Gel	1.1% sodium fluoride	Phosphate gel
	Closys		0.24% sodium fluoride	
Fluoride varnish	Medicom	Duraflor	5% sodium fluoride	
	Waterpik	UltraThin	5% sodium fluoride	
	Preventech	Vella	5% sodium fluoride	Xylitol
	Medicom	Halo	5% sodium fluoride	
	Crosstex	Sparkle V	5% sodium fluoride	Xylitol
	Denticator	Zooby	5% sodium fluoride	Xylitol
	Sultan	Durashield	5% sodium fluoride	
	Sunstar Butler	Butler	5% sodium fluoride	
	DMG America	Kolorz Clear Shield	5% sodium fluoride	Xylitol
	Pascal	Fluorilaq	5% sodium fluoride	
	IBT Med	Heritage 7	5% sodium fluoride	
	GC America	MI Varnish	5% sodium fluoride	Recaldent

application soon gained popularity in surgery and medicine, including gynecology, urology, obstetrics, and as a presurgical preparation, for both the patient and the surgical team.

The application of chlorhexidine in dentistry and specifically the inhibition of bacterial plaque proliferation was studied by Loe and Schiott in 1970. These investigators showed that the use of chlorhexidine twice per day reduced the regrowth of plaque and the development of gingivitis.

The strong base and dicationic nature of chlorhexidine make it very reactive with anions, which has a direct impact on its efficacy. It targets both gram-positive and gram-negative bacteria, and has both a bacteriocidal and bacteriostatic mechanism of action (Wade & Addy 1989), and works by binding to the bacterial cell membrane.

At low concentrations, there is an increase of permeability and leakage of intracellular components (Hugo & Longworth 1964, 1965). At higher concentrations, chlorhexidine causes precipitation of the cell cytoplasm, leading to cell death (Hugo & Longworth 1966).

The extended bacteriostatic effect of chlorhexidine has been shown to last in excess of 12 hours (Schiott 1970). The attachment of the chlorhexidine molecule to the negatively charged pellicle-coated surface of the teeth is the contributing property that allows the extended efficacy (Jenkins and colleagues 1988). The attachment of 1 cation to the pellicle surface leaves the second cation to attach to the bacteria attempting to attach to the tooth. This model can be supported by the decreased inhibitory effects of chlorhexidine when using anion substances such as fluoride or sodium lauryl sulfate–based toothpaste shortly after.

Xylitol

Xylitol was discovered in the late nineteenth century in Europe as a safe sweetener alternative for people with diabetes, because it does not affect insulin levels. Its application in dentistry did not occur until the late 1970s. This sugar alcohol is found in the fibers of various fruits and vegetables, including corn husk, sugar cane, and birch wood. It is a member of a family of sugar alcohols that includes sorbitol, saccharin, and aspartame (**Table 5**).

Table 5
Summary of calcium phosphate therapies

	Brand Name	Description	Mechanism of Action
Amorphous calcium phosphate	ACP	ACP is a reactive and soluble calcium phosphate compound	ACP releases calcium and phosphate ions to convert to apatite and remineralize when it comes in contact with saliva. ACP forms on the tooth enamel within the dentinal tubules and provides a reservoir in the saliva
Casein phosphopeptide amorphous calcium phosphate	CPP-ACP or Recaldent	Recaldent is casein phosphopeptide (CPP) and ACP/CPP is an organic molecule that is able to bind calcium, phosphate ions, and stabilize ACP. CPP-ACP is a milk derivative	The Ca and PO contained in the milk-derived peptide bind to the tooth surface. ACP is released during acidic challenges
Calcium sodium phosphosilicate	CSP or NovaMin	Novamin is a calcium sodium phosphosilicate, which contains calcium, phosphorus, sodium, and silica	Novamin reacts with saliva, releasing Ca^{2+}, P^{5+}, and Na^+ into the environment. First the Na^+ buffers the acid and then the charged Ca^{2+} and P^{5+} ions saturate saliva, precipitating into demineralized areas to form a new layer of hydroxyapatite filling the demineralized lesions

Data from Hurlbutt M. Caries management with calcium phosphate. Dimens Dent Hyg 2010;8(10):40, 42, 44–46.

The use of xylitol chewing gum has been related to decreased colony counts of *S mutans*, decreased adherence of *S mutans* to the tooth structure, and enhancing the remineralization of subsurface lesions (**Table 6**).[21] Several studies have shown that the use of xylitol chewing gum showed an altered expression of the gene gftB specific to *S mutans*. The gftB gene is responsible for the production of the insoluble glucan found on the bacterial cell wall that enables the adherence to the tooth surface.[22,23]

Xylitol is also believed to have a direct effect on cell toxicity, and works similarly to the fructose metabolic pathway in bacterial cells. After the transport of xylitol into the cell, it is phosphorylated to xylitol-5-phosphate (X5P), which cannot be metabolized further. The accumulation of X5P leads to intracellular toxicity and glycolytic enzyme inhibition.

Efficacy is dose dependent, showing minimal clinical benefits when dosage decreases lower than 7 g per day, and no additional benefits higher than 10 g per day. Potential complications in the consumption of xylitol may involve minor gastrointestinal irritation.

Calcium Phosphate

Calcium phosphate, the principle mineral in tooth enamel, is a normal component in salivary secretion. It has significant contributions to the remineralization process, with the ability to neutralize acid levels and precipitate on the enamel surface, making calcium and phosphate ions readily available for uptake.

There are 5 calcium phosphate–based technologies available in the United States; HAP, amorphous calcium phosphate (ACP), casein phosphopeptide ACP (CPP-ACP), calcium sodium phosphosilicate (NovaMin) and tricalcium phosphate.[24]

ACP technology is considered unstable because calcium and phosphate salts are delivered separately, then precipitate on the tooth surface, forming a reservoir of Ca^{2+} and PO_4^{3-} ions, allowing mineral deposition to occur. Fluoride used in conjunction with ACP acts as a catalyst in the remineralization process. The application of fluoride (anion) coats the enamel surface attracting calcium (cation), changing carbonated apatite to the more acid resistant FAP (**Table 7**).

ACP, unless stabilized in some way, transforms to a thermodynamically more stable calcium phosphate phase or undergoes an autocatalytic solution-mediated crystallization process. CPP is a milk protein derivative and acts mainly

Table 6		
Comparison of sugar alcohol		
Sugar Alcohols	**Sweetness Relative to Sucrose**	**Food Energy (kcal/g)**
Arabitol	0.7	0.2
Erythritol	0.812	0.213
Glycerol	0.6	4.3
Hydrogenated starch hydrolysates	0.4–0.9	3.0
Isomalt	0.5	2.0
Lactitol	0.4	2.0
Maltitol	0.9	2.1
Mannitol	0.5	1.6
Sorbitol	0.6	2.6
Xylitol	1.0	2.4
Compare with sucrose	1.0	4.0

Table 7
Common commercially available calcium phosphate products available in dentistry

Product	Manufacturer	Name	Active Content	Additional Benefits
Paste	GC America	MI Paste	CPP-ACP	
	GC America	MI Paste Plus	CPP-ACP	Fluoride
	Sensodyne	NUPRO Prophylaxis Paste	Novamin	Fluoride
	Sensodyne	NUPRO 5000 ppm	Novamin	5000 fluoride
	3M ESPE	Clinpro 5000	Tricalcium phosphate	1.1% sodium fluoride
Varnish	GC America	MI Varnish	CCP-ACP	Fluoride
	3M ESPE	Vanish	Tricalcium phosphate	Sodium fluoride
Gum	Cadbury Adams USA, LLC	Trident Xtra Care	CCP-ACP	Xylitol

to stabilize Ca^{2+}, PO_4^{3-}, and F^- ions as water-soluble amorphous complexes to ensure the delivery of calcium and phosphate to the tooth before they precipitate or crystallize.

NovaMin was originally introduced to manage cold sensitivity. The precipitation of Ca^+, PO_4^-, Na^+, and bioactive silica glass aid in the reversal of white spot lesions, dentin demineralization, and the remineralization of root carious lesions.[25,26] The release of Na^+ buffers and helps neutralize acids produced by acidogenic bacteria, whereas the bioactive silica glass catalyzes the formation of crystalline HAP associated with bone replacement and repair.

Adjunctive Therapy

Sodium bicarbonate

Sodium bicarbonate ($NaHCO_3$) has a wide variety of applications in numerous fields because of its amphoteric properties, the ability to react with acids and bases. It can be added as a simple solution for raising the pH balance of water (increasing total alkalinity) in which high levels of chlorine (2–5 ppm) are present, as in swimming pools.[27] By this same property, $NaHCO_3$ can neutralize microbial acid by-products in dental biofilm in the oral cavity (**Box 1**).

Box 1
Additional applications for sodium bicarbonate

- Used in cooking as a leavening agent
- Neutralizing acids and bases
- Antacid to treat acid indigestion and heartburn
- First aid used in acidosis
- Used in tricyclic antidepressant overdose
- Used to cover an allergic reaction of poison ivy, oak, or sumac to relieve the itching
- Personal hygiene; tooth whitening and plaque removal
- A cleaning agent
- Biopesticide
- Cattle feed supplement

The hypertonic $NaHCO_3$ solution causes the more hypotonic microbial cell to lose water, causing a shift in the osmotic pressure gradient, consequently dehydrating and killing the cell.[28] The effects of $NaHCO_3$ are advantageous only for the short-term, with minimal efficacy on plaque pH and no effect on the viability of S mutans.[29]

The lack of long-term stability and efficacy of $NaHCO_3$ requires a more frequent use, especially after an acid attack. As pH decreases lower than 5.5, rinsing with a solution of water and $NaHCO_3$ can increase the pH back to a normal range, at which remineralization occurs.

Gān Cǎo (Glycyrrhiza uralensis) (Chinese licorice)

Glycyrrhiza uralensis, otherwise referred to as Chinese licorice, is a flowering plant native to Asia. The literal term is sweet herb or sweet grass, and it has been used in ancient Chinese medicine for more than 4000 years. It is used worldwide as a flavoring and sweetening agent in tobaccos, chewing gums, candies, beverages, and toothpaste.[30]

Eastern medicine believes it to have numerous applications and benefits, such as an antiinflammatory, as an antiviral, and as an analgesic.[30] Among the various properties, the contribution as an anticariogenic agent is most applicable for this discussion (**Table 8**).

Recent investigations, to isolate and identify the chemical components of Glycyrrhiza uralensis, have had remarkable results when tested against S mutans. Two components, glycyrrhizol A and 6,8-diisoprenyl-5,7,4'-trihydroxyisoflavone, have shown a specific affinity for S mutans and have the most effective concentration levels in laboratory cultures.[31]

Although the contributions to oral health are beneficial, excessive consumption of Glycyrrhiza is contraindicated in patients suffering from edema, kidney disorders, hypokalemia, hypertension, and congestive heart failure. People with heart conditions or high blood pressure should avoid ingesting extensive amounts of licorice, because it can further heighten blood pressure and lead to stroke. In addition, it can cause salt and water retention and low potassium levels, leading to heart problems.[30]

Triclosan

Introduced in 1972 as a cleansing agent, triclosan has been added to several products used routinely on a day-to-day basis, such as soaps, shaving creams, mouthwashes, cleaning supplies, deodorants, and toothpaste. Useful as a topical cleanser, it has also been infused into plastics, kitchen utensils, and clothing, increasing resistance to bacterial, fungal, and viral colonization.

At higher concentrations, triclosan acts as a biocide, with multiple cytoplasmic and membrane targets. At lower concentrations, it functions as a bacteriostatic agent, binding to and deactivating the enoyl-acyl carrier protein reductase enzyme in bacteria. This enzyme plays a key role in the fatty acid synthesis, essential for reproducing and building cell membranes.

Its effectiveness in preventing gingivitis, and therefore its application in toothpaste, was researched and approved by the US Food and Drug Administration (FDA) in 1997. Since that time, triclosan has come under strong criticism, not only in the dental community but in medicine as well. In 2005, Rule and colleagues[32] suggested that triclosan can lead to a potential interaction with chlorine in tap water to form chloroform, a known human carcinogen.[33,34] More recently, Cherednichenko and colleagues[34] have linked triclosan to impaired muscle contraction.

Table 8
Composition of toothpaste

Abrasives	Surfactants	Humectants
Alumina	Amine fluorides	Glycerol
Aluminum trihydrate	Dioctyl sodium sulfosuccinate	PEG 8 (polyoxyethylene
Bentonite	Sodium lauryl sulfate	glycol esters)
Calcium carbonate	Sodium N-lauryl sarcosinate	Pentatol
Calcium pyrophosphate	Sodium stearyl fumarate	PPG (polypropylene
Dicalcium phosphate	Sodium stearyl lactate	glycol ethers)
Kaolin	Sodium lauryl sulfoacetate	Sorbitol
Methacrylate		Water
Perlite (a natural volcanic glass)		Xylitol
Polyethylene		
Pumice		
Silica		
Sodium bicarbonate		
Sodium metaphosphate		
Gelling or Binding Agents	**Flavors**	**Preservatives**
Carbopols	Aniseed	Alcohols
Carboxymethyl cellulose	Clove oil	Benzoic acid
Carrageenan	Eucalyptus	Ethyl parabens
Hydroxyethyl cellulose	Fennel	Formaldehyde
Plant extracts (alginate,	Menthol	Methylparabens
guar gum, gum arabic)	Peppermint	Phenolics (methyl, ethyl,
Silica thickeners	Spearmint	propyl)
Sodium alginate	Vanilla	Polyaminopropyl
Sodium aluminum silicates	Wintergreen	biguanide
Viscarine		
Xanthan gum		
Colors	**Film Agents**	**Sweeteners**
Chlorophyll	Cyclomethicone	Acesulfame
Titanium dioxide	Dimethicone	Aspartame
	Polydimethylsiloxane	Saccharine
	Siliglycol	Sorbitol

Currently, the FDA is working to incorporate the most up-to-date data and information into the regulations that govern the use of triclosan in consumer products. The FDA communicated the findings of its review to the public in winter, 2012.

Sodium Hypochlorite

Sodium hypochlorite has been used as a disinfectant for more than 100 years and as an endodontic irrigant for more than 75 years. It possesses many properties of an ideal antimicrobial agent, including rapid bactericidal action, relative nontoxicity at use concentrations, no color, no staining, ease of access, and very low cost and is lethal to most bacteria, fungi, and viruses.[35] Lobene and colleagues[36] showed that subgingival irrigation of 0.5% sodium hypochlorite caused significantly greater and longer-lasting reduction in plaque and gingivitis than irrigation with water alone.[37,38]

Hypochlorite solutions lose strength and efficacy with time, thus fresh solutions should be prepared daily. A working solution of 4.92 mL to 250 mL of water is efficient to have an effect on oral bacteria. The lowest concentration of chlorine that has any efficacy against test bacteria in vitro is 0.01%.[39]

More recently, a stabilized chlorine dioxide oral rinse was developed. Its composition is free from alcohol and sodium lauryl sulfate but pH balanced and effective for eliminating the bacteria that initiate oral malodor.[40,41]

The Oral Care Path

Modern research has led to significant progress in the understanding of the histopathology of caries in enamel and dentin, microbial risk factors, physiology and pathology of saliva, and an understanding of the mechanisms of actions of fluorides. The development of new preventive interventions and restorative materials has had a significant impact on the restoration of decayed teeth and the retention of teeth for life.[37,42–44]

CAMBRA assesses the degree of risk for an individual and then specifically combats those risk factors that cause caries, periodontal disease, recession, and xerostomia for the prevention of tooth loss. Risk factors vary during life and change as individuals age.

The microflora of dental plaque biofilms from diseased sites is distinct from that found in health. In dental caries, there is a shift toward community dominance by acidogenic and acid-tolerant gram-positive bacteria (eg, mutans streptococci and lactobacilli) at the expense of the acid-sensitive species associated with sound enamel.[14]

The oral care path is a systematic approach, through CAMBRA principles, to diagnose and identify an individual's risk. Once all the risk factors have been identified, a series of products can be prescribed to offset the effects of those risks (**Fig. 3**).

Changes in lifestyle, diet, recreational habits, medical health, and prescription medications contribute to an imbalance of risk factors and protective factors, expressing a need for changes in the care path. Dietary modification, the most readily controlled factor, is essential as the risks are identified. Fermentable carbohydrates, acidic beverages, and high-fructose diets are the most readily available and therefore are the most common food sources. In combination with xerostomia, an increase in the need for neutralization of acid and an increased pH essential to the longevity of the tooth enamel.

The oral cavity exists as a balanced ecosystem under continual stress, internal and external. Controlled changes in the ecology of the oral environment do not necessarily combat the oral microbes directly but instead alter the equilibrium and create an environmentally inhospitable atmosphere for microbes.

Abrasion, erosion, and abfraction are forms of noncarious cervical lesions (NCCLs). Although they may be the result of several events, there is evidence that NCCLs are strongly associated with mechanical brushing with highly abrasive dentrifices. Dzakovich and Oslak[41] compared the effect of low-abrasive, medium-abrasive, and high-abrasive commercial toothpastes versus brushing with water only; all brushing with toothpastes created significant NCCLs.

Recession leading to the development of abrasive, erosive, or abfraction lesions calls for an altered care path using soft bristle brushes, a less abrasive dentrifice, and a modified brushing technique in a circular motion rather than horizontal can reduce the damage to exposed cementum structures.

When active caries and periodontitis are accompanied by inflammation, recession, and possibly erosion, antimicrobial therapy is initiated to control the major bacteria, S mutans and Lactobacillus sp. Exposed tooth surfaces and demineralized enamel need protection and often restoration.

Aging has a strong affiliation with increased risk factors attributed by health changes, genetics, and lifestyle challenges. Diet, mobility, and cognitive mental health may also change. Adjunctive therapies must be considered to reduce and control the cause of the oral disease rather than merely restore the missing tooth structures.

CAMBRA CAries Management By Risk Assessment   PATIENT CARE PATH MANAGEMENT PROGRAM

Caries, Xerostomia & Periodontal Diagnosis, Prevention & Treatment   All risk levels need good oral hygiene, diet & health (Modify Behavior)

RISK LEVEL	RISK FACTORS MEDICAL CONDITIONS	FLUORIDE & CALCIUM PROTECTION	ADJUNCTIVE THERAPY	ANTIMICROBIAL & ANTIFUNGAL THERAPY
LOW/MODERATE No Decay No Periodontitis Inflammation Recession Erosion	Health Conditions Age Diet Genetics Lifestyle	OTC Fluoride Toothpaste (0.15% NaF) Rx Fluoride Toothpaste (1.1% NaF) Fluoride Varnish (5% NaF) MI Paste /Plus (CCP-ACP/ Fluoride) MI Varnish (CCP-ACP/Fluoride)	4 Xylitol Mints (2 gum or candies) WOW Sodium Bicarbonate (2-3 times daily) pH Control Frequently	Antiseptic Antibiotics Antifungals Peroxide Sodium Hypochlorite CloSys
HIGH 1-2 Carious Lesions Periodontitis + Bone Loss Recession Erosion Inflammation	Xerostomia Sjogren's Syndrome Celiac Disease Stress or Other Eating Disorders GERD Smoking, Alcohols Excess Bisphosphonates	OTC Fluoride Toothpaste (0.15% NaF) Rx Fluoride Toothpaste (1.1% NaF) Fluoride Varnish (5% NaF) MI Paste /Plus (CCP-ACP/ Fluoride) MI Varnish (CCP-ACP/Fluoride)	4 Xylitol Mints (2 gum or candies) WOW (2-3 times daily) Sodium Bicarbonate (between meals to buffer pH) pH Control Frequently	Chlorhexidine (brush 1 minute daily at bedtime for 1 week each month) Sodium Hypochlorite (once everyday for 1 week each month) CloSys (once everyday for 1 week each month)
EXTREME 3+ Carious Lesions Periodontitis + Bone Loss Recession, Erosion and Inflammation Oral Prosthetic Rehabilitation	All the above: IV Bisphosphonates Chemotherapy Pregnancy Diabetes Alzheimer's or Dementia Sleep Apnea	OTC Fluoride Toothpaste (0.15% NaF) Rx Fluoride Toothpaste (1.1% NaF) Fluoride Varnish (5% NaF) MI Paste /Plus (CCP-ACP/ Fluoride) MI Varnish (CCP-ACP/Fluoride) Protect Bond & Surface Coat	4 Xylitol Mints (2 gum or candies) WOW (2-3 times daily) Sodium Bicarbonate (between meals to buffer pH) pH Control Frequently Herbal Lollipops (10-12 days every 2-3 months.)	Chlorhexidine (brush 1 minute 2x daily) Sodium Hypochlorite (once everyday for 1 month) CloSys (once everyday for 1 month) Antibiotics Therapy (amoxicillin & metronidazole) Mucositis (the answer, caphosol, miraisol, aloe, vitc, folic acid)

DIET FACTORS:

Alcohol	Wine
Coffee	Drugs
Sport Drinks	Pastries & Snacks
Citric & Carbonated Sodas	Fresh Citrus Fruits & Juices
Candy	Pickles or Vinegar
Indigestion & Heartburn	Energy Drinks
Gum with Sugar	

ONLINE RESOURCES

www.midentistry.com	www.Drjohns.com
www.drbicuspid.com	www.carifree.com
www.gcamerica.com	www.wowonalcare.com
www.nuvoramic.com	www.xylitoldepot.com
www.3m.com/dental/ prevention	www.amazon.com
www.CDAfoundation.org	www.cpadential.com
	www.xlear.com

Fig. 3. Caries management by risk assessment. (*Adapted from* Kutsch VK, Bowers RJ. Balance: a guide for managing dental caries for patients and practitioners. Llumina Press; 2012.)

The prosthodontic patient is greatly challenged with microbial management in the continued effort to prevent the recurrence of disease and maintenance of oral health. The team of therapists must constantly support the patient in their education and practice of oral hygiene maintenance within their physical and financial means.

SUMMARY

Current trends in dental disease management are centered on the identification or presence of disease and the mechanical elimination of the infected structures. The development of an oral care path redirects the focus on the identification of the early indicators of disease, before its existence. Once the risks have been identified and diagnosed, then, the proper therapies can be selected and prescribed.

The initial protocol of Featherstone's research centered on the wide spectrum of caries from the white demineralized lesions to severe loss of tooth structure. He emphasized the effects of established preventive measures of xylitol, chlorhexidine, fluorides of increasing strengths, including varnish applications, and diet control.

Some of the results are NCCLs, whereas some are contributed by bacteria-induced inflammation, whereas others include bacteria-saturated harmful biofilm, contributing to the effects on damaged tooth structure, lost supporting periodontium, multiple restorations, and missing teeth.

The experienced practitioner must meld clinical experience and observation with rapidly evolving, evidence-based scientific dentistry and information on the treatment and prevention of continued disease for the prosthodontic patient after the restorations have been completed. The incorporation of dental implants, once thought of as a 98% successful procedure, has not allowed for the various complications of caries and periodontal disease on teeth and implants. Thus, osseoseparation is necessary for justification of continued maintenance.

REFERENCES

1. US Census Bureau, Population division, population projections branch. National population projections I: summary files. Total population by age, sex, race, and Hispanic origin. Available at: http://www.census.gov/population/www/projections/natsum-T3.html. Accessed May 8, 2007.
2. Pjetursson BE, Brägger U, Lang NP, et al. Comparison of survival and complication rates of tooth supported fixed dental prostheses (FDPs) and implant supported FDPs and single crowns (SCs). Clin Oral Implants Res 2007;18(Suppl 3): 97–113.
3. Goodacre CJ, Bernal G, Rungcharasseng K, et al. Clinical complications with implants and implant prostheses. J Personal Disord 2003;90(2):121–32.
4. Phipps KR, Stevens VJ. Relative contribution of caries and periodontal disease in adult tooth loss for an HMO dental population. J Public Health Dent 1995;55: 250–2.
5. Niessen LC, Weyant RJ. Causes of tooth loss in a veteran population. J Public Health Dent 1989;49:19–23.
6. Chauncey HH, Glass RL, Alman JE. Dental caries. Principal cause of tooth extraction in a sample of US male adults. Caries Res 1989;23:200–5.
7. Burt BA, Ismail AI, Eklund SA. Periodontal disease, tooth loss, and oral hygiene among older Americans. Community Dent Oral Epidemiol 1985;13:93–6.
8. Suddick RP, Harris NO. Historical perspectives of oral biology: a series. Crit Rev Oral Biol Med 1990;1(2):135–51.

9. Loesche WJ. Role of *Streptococcus mutans* in human dental decay. Microbiol Rev 1986;50:353–80, 17.
10. Bowden GH. Microbiology of root surface caries in humans. J Dent Res 1990;69: 1205–10, 18.
11. Marsh PD. Microbiologic aspects of dental plaque and dental caries. Dent Clin North Am 1999;43:599–614, 19.
12. Becker MR, Paster BJ, Leys EJ, et al. Molecular analysis of bacterial species associated with childhood caries. J Clin Microbiol 2002;40:1001–9.
13. Marsh PD. Dental plaque as a biofilm and a microbial community–implications for health and disease. BMC Oral Health 2006;6:S14.
14. Marsh PD. Are dental diseases examples of ecological catastrophes? Microbiology 2003;149:279–94.
15. Sreebny LM, Schwartz SS. A reference guide to drugs and dry mouth: 2nd edition. Gerodontology 1997;14(1):33–47.
16. USA Today/Kaiser Family Foundation/Harvard School of Public Health, The Public on Prescription Drugs and Pharmaceutical Companies. 2008.
17. LeGeros RZ. Calcium phosphate in enamel, dentine and bone. In: Meyers HM, editor. Calcium phosphates in oral biology and medicine, vol. 15. Basel (Switzerland): Karger; 1991. p. 108–29.
18. Wang Z, Fox JL, Baig AA, et al. Calculation of intercrystalline solution composition during in vitro subsurface lesion formation in dental minerals. J Pharm Sci 1996; 85:117.
19. Hamilton IR. Biochemical effects of fluoride on oral bacteria. J Dent Res 1990;(69 Spec No):660–7.
20. Featherstone JD. The science and practice of caries prevention. J Am Dent Assoc 2000;131:887–99.
21. Featherstone J, Singh S, Curtis D. Caries risk Assessment and Management for the Prosthodontic Patient. Journal of Prosthodontics 2011;20:2–9.
22. Lee YE, Choi YH, Jeong SH, et al. Morphological changes in *Streptococcus mutans* after chewing gum containing xylitol for twelve months. Curr Microbiol 2009; 58:332–7.
23. Miyazawa H, Iwami Y, Mayanagi H, et al. Xylitol inhibition of anaerobic acid production by *Streptococcus mutans* at various pH levels. Oral Microbiol Immunol 2003;18:215–9.
24. Hurlbutt M. Caries management with calcium phosphate. Dimens Dent Hyg 2010; 8(10):40, 42, 44–46.
25. Andersson OH, Kangasniemi I. Calcium phosphate formation at the surface of bioactive glass in vitro. J Biomed Mater Res 1991;25:1019–30.
26. Hench LL, Polak JM. Third generation biomedical materials. Science 2002;295: 1014.
27. Outdoor fun: pool care. Arm & Hammer Baking Soda. 2003. Available at: www.armandhammer.com. Accessed 2007-09-26.
28. Lawrence CA, Block SS. Disinfection, sterilization, and preservation. Philadelphia: Lea and Febiger; 1968. p. 641.
29. Barnes CM. An evidenced-based review of sodium bicarbonate as a dentifrice agent. Compendium 1999;4(1):3–11.
30. Chen J, Chen T. Chinese medical herbology and pharmacology. Chapter 17, section 1. Art of Medicine Press; 2004.
31. He J, Chen LI, Heber D, et al. Antibacterial compounds from *Glycyrrhiza uralensis*. J Nat Prod 2006;69:121–4.

32. Rule KL, Ebbett VR, Vikesland PJ. Formation of chloroform and chlorinated organics by free-chlorine-mediated oxidation of triclosan. Environ Sci Technol 2005;39(9):3176–85. http://dx.doi.org/10.1021/es048943.
33. US Department of Health and Human Resources; US Food and Drug Administration.
34. Cherednichenko G, Zhang R, Bannister RA, et al. Triclosan impairs excitation-contraction coupling and CA2+ dynamics in striated muscle. Proc Natl Acad Sci U S A 2012;109(35):14158–63.
35. Slots J. Selection of antimicrobial agents in periodontal therapy. J Periodont Res 2002;37:389–98.
36. Lobene RR, Soparkar PM, Hein JW, et al. A study of the effects of antiseptic agents and a pulsating irrigating device on plaque and gingivitis. J Periodontol 1972;43:564–8.
37. Palmer S. Secondary decay. Dent Cosmo 1880;22:15–21.
38. Bisnoff HL. Remineralization. Dental Items of Interest 1939;61:881–7.
39. Rutala WA, Cole EC, Thomann CA, et al. Stability and bactericidal activity of chlorine solutions. Infect Control Hosp Epidemiol 1998;19:323–7.
40. Drake D, Villhauer AL. An in vitro comparative study determining bacterial activity of stabilized chlorine dioxide and other oral rinses. J Clin Dent 2011;22:1–5.
41. Dzakovich JJ, Oslak RR. In vitro reproduction of noncarious cervical lesions. J Prosthet Dent 2008;100:1–10.
42. Ismail AI, Hansson H, Sohn W. Dental caries in the second millennium. NIH Consensus Development on Dental Caries Diagnosis and Management. March 26–28, 2001.
43. Darby ET. The etiology of caries at the gum margins and the labial and buccal surfaces of the teeth. Dent Cosmo 1884;26:218–32.
44. Knapp J. Hidden dental caries. Am Dent Assoc Trans 1868;8:108–12.

A Critically Appraised Topic Review of Computer-Aided Design/Computer-Aided Machining of Removable Partial Denture Frameworks

Lisa A. Lang, DDS, MS, MBA*, Ibrahim Tulunoglu, DDS, PhD

KEYWORDS

- Computer-aided design • Computer-aided machining • CAD/CAM
- Removable partial denture • Critically appraised topic (CAT)

KEY POINTS

- Manufacturing techniques and systems have been introduced into dentistry. Computer-aided design (CAD)/computer-aided machining (CAM) systems are commercially available for virtual, three-dimensional design and fabrication of a removable partial denture (RPD) framework.
- Dental laboratory fabrication of a framework and the subsequent prosthesis remains a labor-intensive, experience-dependent task usually performed by a dental laboratory technician. Many commercial dental laboratories in North America have adopted this technology for the fabrication of RPDs.
- Evidence-based practice is based on the premise that critical review of the literature should be performed to make good practice decisions in adopting new innovative technologies.
- The current literature available provides low levels of evidence for CAD/CAM RPD fabrication. There is a preference for laboratory and clinical research before making recommendations in support of use in the clinical care of patients.

Removable partial dentures (RPDs) are used to restore patients' oral function and maintain health. There is an increase in demand for comfortable, high-quality RPDs with the increase in an aging population. In a 2000 study, 76% of the patients surveyed stated lack of fit as a common source of dissatisfaction with a prosthesis.[1] Only a

The authors have nothing to disclose.
Department of Comprehensive Care, School of Dental Medicine, Case Western Reserve University, 2124 Cornell Road, Cleveland, OH 44106, USA
* Corresponding author.
E-mail address: lisa.lang@case.edu

limited number of studies have attempted to evaluate the fit of RPD frameworks. Perhaps this is because of the difficulty in evaluating the complexity of RPD framework designs.

Standards of care have been published related to principles, concepts, and practices in prosthodontics.[2] These standards describe 8 categories for assessment: stress distribution, force control, base extension, occlusal contact, base support, rest seat form, framework fit, and retention.

In a study by Frank and colleagues,[1] fit of the framework was assessed by visual and tactile examination using a mirror and explorer. Fit was rated good if all rest seats appeared to be seated, all rigid elements touched the teeth, and the major connector did not impinge on the underlying soft tissue or had visible relief space greater than 1 mm. Silicone material was placed beneath the framework to confirm displacement of the soft tissue when impingement was observed. Although 52% of the mandibular distal extension RPDs made in community practices failed to meet more than half of the 8 standards, researchers found that 32% of the frameworks evaluated had a poor fit.

Stern and colleagues[3] evaluated rest seat adaptation. They attempted to quantify fit between castings and tooth structure by using polyether impression material samples, which represented the space between rest seat and rests collected from clinically acceptable RPDs. The polyether material was imbedded in a special medium to create samples that were measured in 4 zones: marginal ridge, the center, and the lingual and buccal contact zones.

A total of 79% of the 47 occlusal rests evaluated demonstrated at least 1 point where the distance between the RPD rest and the rest seat was 50 μm or less. Twenty-one percent of the rests did not contact at any point. Closer adaptation of the metal framework was found to exist on the marginal ridge zone of occlusal rests than the other zones for all types of RPDs. Mandibular Kennedy class I and II RPDs were significantly closer in average overall fit than mandibular Kennedy class III and IV RPDs. The difference was not identified between maxillary class I and II and maxillary class III and IV RPDs.

Twenty years later, the fit of conventionally fabricated RPD frameworks is still a problem. In a 2006 study, Dunham and colleagues[4] evaluated the fit of RPDs using a methodology similar to the 1986 study by Stern and colleagues.[3] When evaluating the fit between the framework rests and the prepared rest seats of the teeth, their findings showed that 76% of the rest seats had no contact at the deepest portion of the rest.

In the last 100 years, dental materials and dental technologies for the fabrication of prostheses have advanced remarkably. Manufacturing processing techniques and systems have been introduced into dentistry. In the 1970s and 1980s, computer-aided design (CAD)/computer-aided machining (CAM) systems were introduced for the fabrication of crowns and fixed partial dentures.

Several CAD/CAM software programs are now available commercially for virtual three-dimensional (3D) designing of dental restorations on a computer. When the design of the restoration is complete, the CAM software uses an additive rapid prototyping technology to produce a physical 3D object. This stereolithographic process is often called printing. The printed object (master pattern) can then be cast using conventional techniques, or can be produced directly in metal.

Dental laboratory work remains a labor-intensive and experience-dependent task. Many dental laboratories in the United States and Canada have adopted this technology into their RPD fabrication process. New innovative techniques such as CAD/CAM RPD systems could improve the quality of fit of RPD frameworks. The purpose of this report was to perform a systematic review of the literature to determine what level of evidence exists to support the current use of this technology.

MATERIALS AND METHODS

An electronic search was performed in PubMed using Boolean operators for articles published between 1950 and October 2012. The purpose of the search was to obtain all in vivo and in vitro articles published on the subject of CAD/CAM RPD frameworks. The following describes the key word combinations used and the number of articles produced through each search:

1. "CAD/CAM and removable partial dentures" 24 articles
2. "CAD/CAM and removable dentures" 130 articles
3. "CAD/CAM and removable prostheses" 40 articles
4. "CAD/CAM and removable frameworks" 10 articles
5. "Rapid prototyping and removable partial dentures" 8 articles
6. "Rapid prototyping and removable prostheses" 9 articles
7. "Rapid prototyping and removable frameworks" 5 articles
8. "Computerized and removable dentures" 30 articles

The titles from each search were reviewed for duplication yielding 181 publications. The electronic search was supplemented by searches for selected articles obtained from the references of the articles produced by the electronic search, and manual searches of articles published in 2012 in the *Journal of Prosthetic Dentistry, Journal of Prosthodontics*, and the *International Journal of Prosthodontics*. The titles and abstracts of all articles were reviewed for possible inclusion. **Box 1** presents the inclusion criteria. On identification for inclusion, the full text of the article was reviewed. Each article was characterized by the study design and the level of evidence it provided.[5,6]

Glover and colleagues[5] further developed the hierarchy of evidence pyramid developed by Sackett and colleagues.[6,7] In this refinement, the highest level of evidence is characterized as filtered information. The studies fall into 3 categories: systematic reviews, critically appraised topics (CATs) in which the evidence is synthesized, and critically appraised individual articles in which the publication is merely a synopsis of the literature. The types of articles in this category are listed in the hierarchy of evidence from highest to lowest.

The next level of evidence is considered unfiltered information. Randomized clinical trials (RCT), cohort studies, case-control studies/case series/reports, and background information/expert opinion are all considered unfiltered information. Within this category, RCTs are regarded as the highest level of evidence, whereas expert opinion is deemed to be the lowest level. Cohort studies, case-control studies, and case reports are listed in their respective hierarchy of evidence. In vitro studies are considered to be a lower level of evidence than in vivo studies.

Box 1
Inclusion criteria
In vitro or in vivo study
Study published in peer-reviewed journal
Study published in English
Removable partial denture framework fabricated using CAD

Rosner[8] reexamined the principles of evidence-based medicine citing the exclusion of numerous sources of research information (basic research, epidemiology, and health services research) as problematic. He therefore further refined the hierarchy pyramid to include animal research and in vitro studies. Combining the works of Glover and colleagues[5] and Rosner,[8] **Table 1** defines the hierarchy of study design scores, whereas **Table 2** defines the level of evidence score based on the Oxford Center for Evidence classification system.[9]

Using these classifications, the articles[10-18] were assigned a study design score ranging from 1 to 12 and a level of evidence score ranging from 1 to 5 (Oxford Center for Evidence[9]) independently by 2 reviewers. Where the scores assigned were different, a consensus score was then reach by the 2 examiners.

RESULTS

After excluding those articles that did not meet the inclusion criteria (English and pertaining to CAD/CAM RPDs), 9 publications remained. These articles were reviewed and analyzed for the level of evidence they provide to the dental profession. **Table 3** lists the design scores and level of evidence for each article reviewed. For both parameters, lower scores denote better design or evidence level. The articles are listed in order of publication year.

Seven of the articles[10,11,14-18] were development of concept/position papers. Two of these could be categorized as a review of the literature. Miyazaki and colleagues[16] reviewed the current use of CAD/CAM systems in dentistry. Although the primary focus of the article was on the fabrication of crowns and fixed partial dentures, the investigators discussed the increasing use of CAD/CAM technology and the future demand for its use with RPDs. Jones and colleagues[18] reviewed the current and future treatment options of RPDs. A small section of this publication discussed the use of CAD software programs in the development of RPD frameworks along with the additive CAM method of rapid prototyping. These technologies were discussed as the future of RPD fabrication; however, no clinical studies were cited as research evidence to support its use.

Table 1	
Articles were characterized by research design	
Study Design	**Design Score**
Filtered Evidence	
Systematic review/meta-analysis of RCT	1
CATs (evidence synthesized)	2
Critically appraised individual articles (article synopsis)	3
Unfiltered Evidence	
RCT	4
Prospective cohort/trial with controls (nonrandomized)	5
Retrospective cohort: treatment outcomes	6
Case-control study	7
Case series (<10); no controls or comparisons	8
Case report; cross-sectional study	9
Opinion/position paper, expert review	10
Animal research	11
In vitro studies	12

Table 2
Articles were characterized by level of evidence

Therapy	Level
Systematic review (with homogeneity) of RCTs	1a
Individual RCT (with narrow confidence interval)	1b
Systematic review (with homogeneity) of cohort studies	2a
Individual cohort study (including low-quality RCT; eg, <80% follow-up)	2b
Outcomes research, ecological studies	2c
Systematic review (with homogeneity) of case-control studies	3a
Individual case-control study	3b
Case series (and poor-quality cohort and case-control studies)	4
Expert opinion without explicit critical appraisal, or based on physiology, bench research or first principles	5

Data from Phillips B, Ball C, Sackett D, et al. Oxford centre for evidence-based medicine - levels of evidence. 2009. Available at: http://www.cebm.net/?o=1025. Accessed October, 2012.

Table 3
Summary of design score and level of evidence by article citation

Author, Year of Publication	Journal	Title	Design Score	Level of Evidence
Williams et al,[10] 2004	J Prosthet Dent	A technique for fabricating patterns for RPD frameworks using casts and electronic surveying	12	5
Eggbeer et al,[11] 2005	Proc Inst Mech Eng H	CAD and rapid prototyping fabrication of RPD frameworks	12	5
Williams et al,[12] 2006	J Prosthet Dent	Use of CAD/CAM technology to fabricate an RPD framework	9	4
Bibb et al,[13] 2006	Proc Inst Mech Eng H	Trial fitting of an RPD framework made using computer-aided and rapid prototyping techniques	9	5
Williams et al,[14] 2008	Pract Proced Aesthet Dent	CAD/CAM fabricated RPD alloy frameworks	10	5
Kibi et al,[15] 2009	J Oral Rehabil	Development of an RPD CAD system with finite element stress analysis	12	5
Miyazaki et al,[16] 2009	Dent Mater J	A review of dental CAD/CAM: current status and future perspectives from 20 y of experience	10	5
Han et al,[17] 2010	Int J Prosthodont	A preliminary report on designing a specifically developed software package	12	5
Jones et al,[18] 2010	Tex Dent J	RPDs: treatment now and for the future	10	5

Two publications[10,11] defined the techniques and discussed the concept development in great detail. In their 2004 article, Williams and colleagues[10] described the process of computerized designing to create a pattern for investment step by step. This article was followed by a 2005 article by Eggbeer and colleagues[11] in which, through the use of a desktop computer, programing software, and a haptic stylus, a virtual cast was surveyed and a framework designed. In both publications, the investigators discuss the theory behind the creation of these systems to minimize the sources of error associated with fit of conventional fabrication of RPDs. The possible sources of errors associated with CAD/CAM systems were contrasted to those of the conventional method by Eggbeer and colleagues.[11]

In the study by Eggbeer and colleagues,[11] 4 rapid prototyping (stereolithography) methods and 2 types of resins to produce patterns were compared. One pattern from each method was created. Problems associated with particular pattern manufacturing systems included fragility of the wax pattern, distortion of the pattern when handled, and difficulty spruing to the thin framework pattern. However, both resin-based systems produced acceptable patterns. These patterns were durable enough to be cast without difficulty. Frameworks were polished, fitted, and visually inspected on dental casts for fit. The fit was deemed satisfactory by the investigators. No clinical patient-based evaluation was made. Because only 1 specimen for each type of production method was produced and the evaluation of the framework fit was against a cast, this article provides a low level of evidence.

Innovators of the CAD/CAM process for removable prosthesis (RP) fabrication recognized early on that milling RP frameworks similar to fixed prosthesis frameworks would be difficult because of the complexity and delicate nature of RP framework designs. Williams and colleagues[14] wrote an expert opinion paper in 2008 outlining the CAD/CAM process for fabrication of RP frameworks. In this article, they defined the rapid manufacturing process as an alternative to milling. The investigators proposed the use of selective laser melting rapid manufacturing to produce the frameworks. Using this technology, the framework is built in layers using a manufacturing process in which a layer of powdered alloy is positioned by the computer and a fiber laser then melts the layers together in a stepwise fashion copying the layering of a virtual pattern until a complete framework is generated.

Currently, chromium cobalt, stainless steel, and titanium are the only alloys suitable for rapid prototyping technology. According to the investigators,[14] the chromium cobalt alloy is similar to dental alloys. However, these rapid manufactured metals have not been toxicology tested for use in human dental restorations. By 2008, no toxicologic studies or long-term prospective evaluations of any kind had been made on humans. Most fit evaluations have been made on dental casts with the exception of 1 clinical case report[12] in which a framework was fitted to a single patient and evaluated for fit.

Kibi and colleagues[15] performed a feasibility study using finite element analysis. The purpose of this study was to analyze a CAD system for molar tooth arrangement in unilateral distal extension bases. This system was used to design the functional tooth segment of the prostheses and was not specific to the framework design. Furthermore, the study was an evaluation of the tooth arrangement on a virtual rim and simulation of the stress distribution under the occlusal forces of the virtual teeth rather than for evaluation of the framework. This article is included in this review for completeness because it fitted the search criteria of a CAD of an RPD framework.

As interest in CAD/CAM RPDs has gained popularity, there has been increased development and improvements in existing software. Han and colleagues[17] introduced a new CAD/CAM software design specifically for RPD framework design and fabrication. Two frameworks (maxillary and mandibular) were designed, manufactured, and fitted to dental casts. Using this system, metal frameworks were created using rapid prototyping technology (selective laser melting). The type of metal used was not described. After polishing and finishing, the frameworks were evaluated by visual inspection and pressure evaluation for movement such as rocking on the dental cast. The frameworks were characterized as having a satisfactory fit on the casts.

Only 2 of the articles[12,13] evaluated the CAD frameworks clinically. In a 2006 case report by Williams and colleagues,[12] the treatment plan for a 75-year-old woman included use of CAD/CAM technology to fabricate the metal RPD framework. The haptic interfaced software package created a virtual design from the scan of the patient's master cast. A chromium cobalt direct manufactured framework was made using selective laser melting technology. The rapid prototype framework was finished and polished using conventional laboratory procedures. A prosthodontist evaluated the framework on the master cast, and then fitted the framework to the patient.

Evaluation of the framework revealed slight surface porosities in a few small areas. These imperfections were not deemed to be of any consequences as they were "not considered to likely prohibit normal function."[12] The fit was classified as excellent. The framework was judged to be comparable with those produced by conventional methods. The accuracy and quality of fit was deemed to be clinically acceptable.

Bibb and colleagues[13] also documented the fit of a CAD/CAM framework on a patient. The cast of a patient was scanned. CAD/CAM and rapid prototyping technology were used to develop a pattern that was sprued, cast, finished, and polished using conventional methods. The framework was adjusted to fit the patient. After trial fitting, the framework was judged to be clinically acceptable.

DISCUSSION

This study systematically searched for evidence to support the use of CAD/CAM RPD systems. Because there were no RCTs performed to evaluate CAD/CAM RPD technologies, this report cannot be considered a systematic review in its purest definition. Therefore, we chose to perform a CAT review and included both in vivo and in vitro studies.

Nine articles were reviewed and evaluated according to research design and level of evidence. Although 1 article[15] met the inclusion criteria, it did not address the question regarding whether there was evidence to support the use of CAD/CAM RPD design and fabrication; rather it dealt with of areas of the RPD (tooth arrangement). Excluding that article, 8 articles addressed the research question in some manner.

The research design of 4 articles[10,11,15,17] was characterized as design level 12 (in vitro), whereas 3 articles[14,16,18] were classified as level 10 (expert review or position paper; see **Table 3**). Two articles[16,18] were quasireviews of the literature and mentioned CAD/CAM technology for fabrication of RPD frameworks as the wave of the future. Four articles[10,11,14,16] were concept development or proof of concept papers. In these publications, the investigators presented the concept of using CAD/CAM technology to design and fabricate RPD frameworks. RPD frameworks were fabricated in 3 of the 4 articles either through direct rapid prototyping selective laser melting or through casting of a rapid prototyping pattern. The level of evidence for these studies was determined to be evidence level 5 (first principles) or bench research (see **Table 3**).

Two articles[12,13] were clinical case reports; study design level 9. These studies reported the fit evaluation of an RPD framework fabricated using CAD/CAM technology on a single patient. The level of evidence for these studies was characterized as level 4.

Advantages claimed by investigators and early adapters of this technology are improved fit, decreased time for fabrication, less labor required, and less sources of error (ie, miscasts, casting porosity, and so forth). There are no clinical studies to support these claims.

Williams and colleagues[12] stated cost and the initial time required to learn to design using the software as disadvantages of the system. We believe that as with most new processes, once the learning curve is reached, time and efficiency of the system will improve. The investment costs associated with CAD/CAM systems (scanner, haptic device, software) are high. The initial investment will pay off if the proclaimed advantages prove to be true. Better fit leading to fewer remakes, time efficiency leading to decreased labor time and costs could outweigh the investment costs. However, at this time, there is no evidence to support these claims.

Clearly, only low levels of evidence exists to support this technology at this time. Although this innovative technology may be the fabrication method for RPDs of the future, in light of the need for evidence-based practice, further higher levels of research evidence must be provided to support its use.

SUMMARY

The purpose of this report was to perform a systematic review of the literature to determine what level of evidence exists to support the use of CAD/CAM RPD systems to improve the quality of RPD frameworks. A PubMed search yielded 9 articles that met the inclusion criteria. In the hierarchy of research evidence, the 9 articles were deemed to be in the lower levels of the pyramid.

As with any innovative technology, clinical studies to support its use must be undertaken. Currently, no clinical outcomes research has been published to support the use of CAD/CAM RPDs.

REFERENCES

1. Frank RP, Brudvik JS, Leroux B, et al. Relationship between the standards of removable partial denture construction, clinical acceptability, and patient satisfaction. J Prosthet Dent 2000;83:521–7.
2. Principles, concepts, and practices in prosthodontics – 1994. Academy of Prosthodontics. J Prosthet Dent 1995;73:73–94.
3. Stern MA, Brudvik JS, Frank RP. Clinical evaluation of removable partial denture rest seat adaptation. J Prosthet Dent 1985;53:658–62.
4. Dunham D, Brudvik JS, Morris WJ, et al. A clinical investigation of the fit of RPD clasp assemblies. J Prosthet Dent 2006;95(4):323–6.
5. Glover J, Izzo D, Odato K, et al. EBM pyramid and EBM page generator. Trustees of Dartmouth College and Yale University; 2006.
6. Sackett DL, Strauss SE, Richardson WS. Evidence-based medicine: how to practice and teach EBM. 2nd edition. Edinburgh (United Kingdom): Churchill Livingstone; 2000.
7. Sackett DL, Rosenberg W, Gray J, et al. Evidence based medicine: what it is and what it isn't. BMJ 1996;312(7023):71–2.
8. Rosner AL. Evidence-based medicine: revisiting the pyramid of priorities. J Bodyw Mov Ther 2012;16:42–9.
9. Phillips B, Ball C, Sackett D, et al. Levels of evidence. Oxford Centre for Evidence-based Medicine; 2009.

10. Williams RJ, Bibb R, Rafik T. A technique for fabricating patterns for removable partial denture frameworks using casts and electronic surveying. J Prosthet Dent 2004;91:85–8.
11. Eggbeer D, Bibb R, Williams R. The computer-aided design and rapid prototyping fabrication of removable partial denture frameworks. Proc Inst Mech Eng H 2005;219:195–202.
12. Williams RJ, Bibb R, Eggbeer D, et al. Use of CAD/CAM technology to fabricate a removable partial denture framework. J Prosthet Dent 2006;96:96–9.
13. Bibb RJ, Eggbeer D, Williams RJ, et al. Trial fitting of a removable partial denture framework made using computer-aided design and rapid prototyping techniques. Proc Inst Mech Eng H 2006;220:793–7.
14. Williams RJ, Bibb R, Eggbeer D. CAD/CAM fabricated removable partial-denture alloy frameworks. Pract Proced Aesthet Dent 2008;20:349–51.
15. Kibi M, Ono T, Mitta T, et al. Development of an RPD CAS system with finite element stress analysis. J Oral Rehabil 2009;36:442–50.
16. Miyazaki T, Hotta Y, Kuni J, et al. A review of dental CAD/CAM: current status and future perspectives from 20 years of experience. Dent Mater J 2009;28:44–56.
17. Han J, Wang Y, Lü P. A preliminary report of designing a specifically developed software package. Int J Prosthodont 2010;23:370–5.
18. Jones JD, Turkyilmaz I, Garcia LT. Removable partial dentures – treatment now and for the future. Tex Dent J 2010;127:365–72.

Index

Note: Page numbers of article titles are in **boldface** type.

Dent Clin N Am 58 (2014) 257–264
http://dx.doi.org/10.1016/S0011-8532(13)00111-0
0011-8532/14/$ – see front matter © 2014 Elsevier Inc. All rights reserved.

dental.theclinics.com

Moving?

Make sure your subscription moves with you!

To notify us of your new address, find your **Clinics Account Number** (located on your mailing label above your name), and contact customer service at:

Email: journalscustomerservice-usa@elsevier.com

800-654-2452 (subscribers in the U.S. & Canada)
314-447-8871 (subscribers outside of the U.S. & Canada)

Fax number: 314-447-8029

**Elsevier Health Sciences Division
Subscription Customer Service
3251 Riverport Lane
Maryland Heights, MO 63043**

*To ensure uninterrupted delivery of your subscription, please notify us at least 4 weeks in advance of move.

Printed and bound by CPI Group (UK) Ltd, Croydon, CR0 4YY

03/10/2024

01040478-0009